EUTHANASIA AND THE NEWBORN

PHILOSOPHY AND MEDICINE

Editors:

H. TRISTRAM ENGELHARDT, JR.

Center for Ethics, Medicine, and Public Issues,
Baylor College of Medicine, Houston, Texas, U.S.A.

STUART F. SPICKER

School of Medicine, University of Connecticut Health Center,
Farmington, Connecticut, U.S.A.

VOLUME 24

EUTHANASIA AND THE NEWBORN.

Conflicts Regarding Saving Lives

Edited by

RICHARD C. McMILLAN

Mercer University, School of Medicine,
Macon, Georgia, U.S.A.

H. TRISTRAM ENGELHARDT, JR.

Center for Ethics, Medicine, and Public Issues,
Baylor College of Medicine,
Houston, Texas, U.S.A.

and

STUART F. SPICKER

School of Medicine,
University of Connecticut Health Center,
Farmington, Connecticut, U.S.A.

D. REIDEL PUBLISHING COMPANY

A MEMBER OF THE KLUWER ACADEMIC PUBLISHERS GROUP

DORDRECHT / BOSTON / LANCASTER / TOKYO

Library of Congress Cataloging-in-Publication Data

CIP

Euthanasia and the newborn.

(Philosophy and medicine; v. 24)
Based on a symposium entitled "Conflicts with Newborns: Saving
Lives, Scarce Resources, and Euthanasis," held May 10–12, 1984, at
the Mercer University School of Medicine, Macon, Ga.
Includes bibliographies and index.
   1.   Infants (Newborn)–Diseases–Treatment–Moral and ethical
aspects–Congresses.   2.   Euthanasia–Moral and ethical aspects–
Congresses.   3.   Infants (Newborn)–Diseases–Treatment–Government
policy–Congresses.   I.   McMillan, Richard C.   II.   Engelhardt, H.
Tristram (Hugo Tristram), 1941–   .   III.   Spicker, Stuart F.,
1937–   .   IV.   Series. [DNLM: 1.   Ethics,
Medical–congresses.   2.   Euthanasia–in infancy & childhood–
congresses.   3.   Handicapped– congresses.   W3 PH609 v.24 / W 50 E902]
RJ253.E88   1987   174'.24   86–33835
ISBN 90–277–2299–4

Published by D. Reidel Publishing Company
P.O. Box 17, 3300 AA Dordrecht, Holland

Sold and distributed in the U.S.A. and Canada
by Kluwer Academic Publishers,
101 Philip Drive, Norwell, MA 02061, U.S.A.

In all other countries, sold and distributed
by Kluwer Academic Publishers Group,
P.O. Box 322, 3300 AH Dordrecht, Holland

Printed in The Netherlands.

TABLE OF CONTENTS

EDITORIAL PREFACE

The essays in this volume, with the exception of Gary Ferngren's, derive from ancestral versions originally presented at a symposium, 'Conflicts with Newborns: Saving Lives, Scarce Resources, and Euthanasia,' held May 10–12, 1984, at the Mercer University School of Medicine, Macon, Georgia. We wish to express our gratitude to the Georgia Endowment for the Humanities for a generous grant for the symposium and to Mercer University and the Medical Center of Central Georgia for additional financial support. The views expressed in this volume do not necessarily represent those of the Georgia Endowment for the Humanities, Mercer University, or the Medical Center of Central Georgia. We have endeavored to bring together a group of individuals with contrasting viewpoints to display some of the range of approaches to a major problem in public policy: medical decisions regarding the treatment of defective newborns.

So many persons contributed to the symposium that acknowledgment of each would be impossible. Although unnamed, we express our sincere appreciation to each. Three individuals, however, must be recognized: R. Kirby Godsey, President, Mercer University; William P. Bristol, Dean, Mercer University School of Medicine; and Kenneth C. Henderson, Medical Director and Director of Medical Education, Medical Center of Central Georgia. Without their support, the symposium could not have succeeded and this volume would not have been possible. We wish also to express our gratitude to S. G. M. Engelhardt and Mary Ann Gardell, who helped transform the contributions of this symposium into the present volume. Over a period of nearly two years, manuscripts have been further developed and essays added to produce this work. The result is a volume that takes into account the development of law, public policy, and scholarship over the intervening period in an attempt to contribute to the ongoing debate.

November 1, 1986   RICHARD C. MCMILLAN
                                    H. TRISTRAM ENGELHARDT, JR.
                                          STUART F. SPICKER

vii

INTRODUCTION

Modern medicine aspires to transcending limits, which can never be set aside. Physicians often act as if they could indefinitely postpone death or make people whole despite disease, deformity, and disability. Up to a point such aspirations have virtue without hubris. They direct physicians to work to the utmost, often while exhausted, to attempt to save or cure their patients. They motivate researchers to look for ways of solving yet insoluble problems. Such aspirations have been powerfully heuristic. There are, however, costs. When one is caught up in dedication to progress or in attempts to save lives against all doubt and despair, it is difficult not to act even when intervention is refused. It is at times hard to recognize when appropriate maximum treatment is supportive or suffering-suppressing. As a result, some oncologists see cancer patients who 'prematurely' refuse treatment as quitters. The matter is even worse for physicians in neonatal intensive-care units, when parents do not want all of what the neonatologists have to offer. The neonatologists may feel that the child is being shortchanged. They know that if most parents choose against full curative interventions, there will be fewer opportunities to make progress so that future children can survive with a good quality of life in circumstances currently not possible. The advances of medical technology and its commitment to success have led to a technological imperative. Anything less than full treatment appears suspect. Many see a duty to save life at all costs. Against the backdrop of this ethos, one can understand the genesis of the Baby Doe regulations, which have attempted to force parents to provide all plausible life-saving treatment to their newborn children without consideration of their physical or mental handicaps or of costs [35].

The various Baby Doe regulations or proposed regulations [7]–[10] and the court cases [11, 39, 40] associated with them reflect major conflicts among fundamental values in our culture. First, there is the interventionist impetus of high-technology medicine just mentioned.

R. C. McMillan, H. T. Engelhardt, Jr., and S. F. Spicker (eds.),
Euthanasia and the Newborn, ix–xxx.
© 1987 by D. Reidel Publishing Company.

Those dedicated to saving lives often find foregoing curative treatment unacceptable. Second, there is a major state and societal commitment to securing the protection and nurture of newborns. This commitment is reflected in the parens patriae doctrine, the doctrine that the government is the parent of the fatherland. Finally, in potential conflict with these first two, there is the family as a sovereign moral unit. It is parents who produce children, often with well-formed objectives in mind. They want a child to help around the ranch, plow the fields, attend their alma mater, pursue a particular vocation, care for them in old age, or embrace a particular religious, political, or ideological commitment. Of course, the state may also regard children as future taxpayers, soldiers, and workers, and therefore support policies that favor birth and survival. The result is a fundamental conflict between the interests of the state, on the one hand, and of the family, on the other, with medicine taking one side or the other, depending on the dispositions of the physicians involved.

Though these tensions have a considerable lineage, they tended to be less acute before recent technological advances in neonatal care. Severely handicapped newborns often did not survive. Moreover, the costs involved for children who did were, up until the end of the last century, primarily those of special attention and perhaps moderate health care costs. With the advent of successful medical treatments, matters changed radically. Newborns can now be saved who could never have been saved in the past. But the saving often entails major costs. Moreover, the child saved may be profoundly mentally and physically handicapped. One might think here of extreme cases of children with I.Q.s below 20 and concomitant severe neuromuscular handicaps. The decision to treat or not to treat a deformed or severely handicapped newborn must also be set against the fact that in many cases one can prenatally diagnose and abort fetuses with severe defects. Insofar as prenatal diagnosis and abortion are acceptable, one is confronted with the question whether selective non-treatment of the severely handicapped is not acceptable as well. Does passage through the birth canal confer the rights of persons, or are they conferred through acceptance by a community of actual moral agents? [16]

Moral analysis of the questions occasioned by the birth of mentally and physically handicapped neonates must focus on a cluster of fundamental questions. First, there are questions of authority. Who has the authority to intervene with force to resolve areas of moral dispute? If the child cannot be in authority over itself, then who should be? The major contenders for that office are the state, the health care profession, and the parents. An answer to the question regarding authority requires addressing a second one, that of the status of newborns. Are young children best understood as the property of their parents? Do newborns have the same moral standing as adult humans or as children who have been accepted into a family? Many societies have formally or informally recognized a distinction between newborns who have not yet been accepted within a family whose death through neglect or action was allowable, and children accepted within a family who would be pro- tected against neglect and murder [18]. A third problem is also involved: the problem of deciding what is the right thing to do. This issue itself involves a set of subsidiary issues: (a) What is the best thing to do for the child? (b) When do burdens on the parents and/or society outweigh concerns for the child? (c) Are there certain actions that are to be forbidden on principle, such as active euthanasia?

Even if one can determine the level of treatment morally required for handicapped newborns, it does not follow from this that one has the moral authority to give treatment against the wishes of the parents. Coercive actions require authority in addition to rectitude. Insofar as children belong to their parents, parents may do things with their children that are morally wrong. And even if one has the authority to impose treatment, all impositions may not be prudent. Good public policy not only accomplishes with authority that which is right, but in addition takes into account the costs and benefits of the policy. One may pardon an individual worthy of punishment whom one has the authority to condemn. This point bears generally on the development of public policy. In summary, to establish that coercive governmental imposition of a policy is appropriate, one must determine (1) that the policy is morally acceptable, (2) that one has authority to impose it by force, and (3) that the imposition is prudent or worth imposing, given the range of one's moral concerns.

I. PARENTS, CHILDREN, AND THE SOVEREIGNTY OF THE FAMILY

How decisions are made regarding the selective non-treatment of new- borns with significant mental and physical handicaps depends in great measure on the extent to which the family is recognized as having special rights over children. If the family is seen as having no special authority, then parents have no more right than strangers to determine the treatment of their children. Who then is the best judge of the best interests of the child? Unless parents are seen to be in a special privileged position, there is no reason to presume that they are better judges of the best interests of their children than physicians or government bureaucrats. Unless parents have a special authority over their children or are better judges of their best interests, there may be no reason why they should have the right to decide in grey areas in favor of minimizing their costs or in terms of their idiosyncratic views of the best interests of their child.

The character of decision-making in 'grey areas' merits comments on its own. There are many circumstances in medicine where the probabilities of success are unclear, or it is unclear how to weight the character of different outcomes. If, for example, accepted medical authorities make contrary claims regarding the benefits of exclusive possibilities for treatment, and there is no clear, independent evidence to determine which group of authorities is correct, who gets to decide? Can the person (e.g., the parents) who decides in such areas of uncertainty choose that therapeutic approach least costly or least traumatic to the decision maker, since, as far as anyone can establish, either line of treatment is equally defensible?

Consider the problem of comparing different outcomes. What if one therapeutic approach will increase the child's quality of life but involves a significant risk of death? How is such a therapy to be compared with other approaches involving less risk of death, but entailing more long-term suffering and circumscription of the child's abilities? Depending on how a decision-maker ranks probabilities of longer life with probabilities of preserving more functional abilities and avoiding suffering, one choice or the other will be plausible. Unless one can appeal to a canonical disinterested observer to decide which ranking of values is to be endorsed, there can be no definitive judgment as to which choice is proper. The central philosophical problem lies in the fact that if the disinterested observer is sufficiently disinterested, it will not be able to choose between the options. In order to make the disinterested observer a criterion for choice, one has to impute to it a particular moral sense or endorsement of a particular hierarchy of values and harms. But then one is back to the question of whose moral sense and whose hierarchy of harms ought to be endorsed ([17], pp. 17–65).

The question becomes: who is in authority to make decisions when there is no authoritative view as to which decision is correct? Unfortunately, this puzzle is very frequent in medicine, for it is often unclear as to which therapeutic intervention will benefit the child. In addition, it is often the case that therapeutic choices entail trade-offs between probabilities of dying and probabilities of enhancing quality of life and avoiding suffering. The more the family is recognized as having some sovereign power, the more the onus lies on the shoulders of those who would intervene and impose treatment against parental wishes, especially in such areas of unclarity. Those who bear the burden of proof, the onus probandi, must show that they are in the right and that their intervention is worth the costs it entails. As a result, if the family is not recognized as having some degree of sovereign power, then it may find itself having to shoulder the onus of demonstrating that its treatment choices, even in such areas of unclarity, are in the best interests of the child.

The disputes raised by the Baby Doe regulations turn on very fundamental issues. If one sees authority coming from God or reason down through the government to the people, then it is plausible that parents should be put in the position of justifying their decisions. If, on the other hand, authority comes from the people to the government, then it is plausible that the choices of competent parents regarding their incompetent children must be presumed to be correct until shown otherwise. This second alternative is more credible, the more it becomes doubtful that an appeal to God is appropriate in a secular pluralist society or that an appeal to reason will successfully establish what is correct to do in these matters.

II. THE STATUS OF NEWBORNS

Newborn infants are not moral agents. Adult chimpanzees and dolphins have more serious claims to the title. Though newborn infants may be the object of substantial moral concern and play important roles in major social and moral institutions, they cannot be held responsible for their actions nor in any nonmetaphorical sense possess duties to others. They have no free will to respect, no autonomy to honor, and no views of their own best interests. As a result, other persons must decide the best interests of newborns. Insofar as infants are not moral agents, one may be brought to considering them not as persons in the strict sense but as entities to whom many of the rights of persons are imputed. If that is the case, the special moral standing that distinguishes human newborns from adult non-human primates who have a better articulated plan of life than they, must be secured through the social and moral practices within which infants are integrated.

The question then arises of the moral status of newborns who have not yet been fully accepted within such moral institutions. The way in which newborn infants were regarded in Athens for the first week after their birth, and before they were enrolled in their deme, provides an example, one explored in this volume by Darrel Amundsen. Until the child had been given rights against the community, its claims were not seen to be as strong as those of older children. There appears, in fact, to be a subtle and implicit distinction made even now between the status of newborns versus older children to whom full familial commitments have been made. This is as one would expect. The bonding to a newborn infant is less complete than that to a child that has been taken home with the full hope and expectation that it will grow to be an adult. One might note, for example, that even in Judaism there was a hesitation to give full communal commitment to a child that died before it was 30 days old.[1] The more one has lived with a child and the more one has made commitments to it, the more difficult it is to hold back from treating. In any event, many have found it plausible that less than full curative treatment need be given to all defective newborns [14, 28, 33, 37]. It should be noted that some have continued to endorse the selective provision of supportive care [22].

III. BEST INTERESTS: WHO DECIDES WHAT THEY ARE

In summary, it is morally difficult to make therapeutic choices about newborns because (1) others must decide the nature of their best interests, in that they cannot speak for themselves, and (2) those who have produced them, their parents, usually claim special sovereignty over them. Newborns are in the *de facto* possession of their parents. The first is the theme of authority as expertise: who is *an* authority? Who is the best judge of the best interests of the newborn? Here one may have conflicts between more interventionist-oriented pediatric surgeons and parents who may understand better the context in which the child will live. The second is the question of who is *in* authority to make choices between competing views of what is in the best interest of the newborn or simply to select a particular therapeutic option.[2]

In the case of those who can speak their own minds, though they may in fact be mistaken about the character of their best interests and some third party may be a better judge, they can at least claim the right to make their own choices, however misguided. They can participate in and contribute to disputes concerning the nature of their best interests. But, in the case of newborns, the newborn cannot judge, nor does it have authority over itself. The question is then not simply who is most able to judge correctly the newborn's best interests, but also who has the right to make the decision, even if that person is a flawed judge of the newborn's best interests.

IV. QUALITY OF LIFE, BEST INTERESTS, BURDENS TO OTHERS

Recent discussions about selecting the proper level of treatment for a newborn with physical and/or mental handicaps have focused on best interests in a way that has brought quality-of-life discussions into question. This is the case, for example, in a statement by the American Academy of Pediatrics:

When medical care is clearly beneficial, it should always be provided. When appropriate medical care is not available, arrangements should be made to transfer the infant to an appropriate medical facility. Considerations such as anticipated or actual limited potential of an individual and present or future lack of available community resources are irrelevant and must not determine the decisions concerning medical care. The individual's medical condition should be the sole focus of the decision. These are very strict standards [1].

At the same time, the American Medical Association maintained an approach accenting the role of quality-of-life judgments. It held that "quality of life is a factor to be considered in determining what is best for the individual" ([2], p. 10). Parents were recognized as the proper persons to decide treatment.

In desperate situations involving newborns, the advice and judgment of the physician should be readily available, but the decision whether to exert maximal efforts to sustain life should be the choice of the parents. The parents should be told the options, expected benefits, risks and limits of any proposed care; how the potential for human relationships is affected by the infant's condition; and relevant information and answers to their questions. The presumption is that the love which parents usually have for their children will be dominant in the decisions which they make in determining what is in the best interest of their children. It is to be expected the parents will act unselfishly, particularly where life itself is at stake. Unless there is convincing evidence to the contrary, parental authority should be respected ([2], p. 11).

This statement, offered under the rubric of quality of life, departs clearly from the position of the American Academy of Pediatrics and the Baby Doe regulations, in including consideration of the infants' "potential for human relationships". Reticence on the part of some to refer explicitly to quality-of-life judgments may draw from the ambiguity of the term itself. It is used to identify how life will be experienced by the person living in it, as well as how the person's life will be appreciated by others.

Many are reluctant to acknowledge that burdens to others should play a role in decisions whether or not to save a person's life. Yet it is clear that the lives of individuals cannot be saved at any cost. If there were a treatment that could regularly save the lives of a large number of children who would otherwise die and the treatment cost a significant amount of money, for example, $100,000,000, most would agree that the duty to treat would be defeated. There are limits to the burdens that must be borne to save the lives of others. This view is not only easily arguable in terms of secular morality, but it has been maintained as a central element of certain traditions of moral theology. For example, Dominicus Banez held that one was obliged to spend at most 3000 ducats to save one's own life [5]. This level of financial burden was translated into modern terms by Father Edward J. Healey in the 1940s. Healey held that even a rich man was not obliged to expend more than $2000 on saving his own life ([24], p. 162). Such understandings have been transferred to considerations of the duty to save the lives of others. For example, Father Charles A. McFadden, O. S. A., argued that one is usually obliged only to provide ordinary treatment to severely deformed newborns (that treatment that does not involve an undue burden), not extraordinary treatment (that which would involve an undue burden) ([31], p. 141). The duty to save the life of others is not absolute.

The extent to which burdens defeat a duty to treat is context-specific, as Pope Pius XII argued in a 1957 allocution.

[N]ormally one is held to use only ordinary means – according to the circumstances of persons, places, times, and culture – that is to say, means that do no involve any grave burden [aucune charge extraordinaire] for oneself or another. A more strict obligation would be too burdensome [trop lourde] for most men and would render the attainment of the higher, more important good too difficult ([34], pp. 395–96).

Since the Pope, as others in this tradition, believed in an after life, prolonging life was only of relative significance. It was in terms of man's transcendent destiny that duties were in the end to be understood.

Within this tradition, commitment to saving life at any costs would be idolatrous. Even to have understood it as a relative duty, but as one that did not take into account burdens to parents, society, and others would involve a grievous moral error of not acknowledging competing, at times more important obligations.

In addition, there is no reason to restrict defeating burdens to those that are monetarizable. If the provision of a treatment entails severe emotional or psychological burdens, these burdens can also defeat duties to treat. Here again one must note that such an approach was recognized in moral theology, which held that one need not accept a treatment involving a *horror magnus* [27]. Further, one of the maxims was that an obligation to treat existed only if there were hope of offering a benefit [30]. The tradition set major limits to the obligation to treat [6, 25]. This idea of limits was expressed in a number of formulas, such as one derived from Sanchez, *si sit spes salutis*, which indicated that one is obliged to treat only if there be hope of recovering health. By implication, this maxim incorporates considerations of quality of life.

Duties to treat are stronger, the fewer the costs involved in their provision. If one holds that there is an obligation to treat handicapped newborns, but recognizes that there are limits to that obligation, then that obligation can be defeated by sufficient burdens such that after a point the decision to treat is not one of obligation but of supererogation. After the point where treatment becomes supererogatory rather than obligatory, one may morally decide whether or not to treat in ways that discriminate against newborns with physical and mental handicaps. Such discrimination would only be immoral where there is in fact an obligation to treat. Where no such obligation exists, one might decide to go the extra mile, or the additional hundred thousand dollars, to save the life of a child, which if saved would live without any or few physical or mental handicaps. Of course, those who hold that quality of life may be taken into consideration in deciding whether one has an obligation to treat, would hold that a poor quality of outcome could also defeat the duty to provide costly medical interventions [3]. The less there is to achieve, the less the obligation to achieve it.

One can express these considerations in terms of an algorithm that displays the relations between the duty to treat on the one hand, and costs of treatment and quality and quantity of outcome on the other.

$$\text{Duty to treat} = \frac{P \times L(Q_1 + Q_2 + B_1 + B_2 + B_3)}{P \times L(C_1 + C_2 + C_3 + C_4)}$$

P = probability of success of attempt to save the newborn
L = length of newborn's life if treated
Q_1 = quality of the newborn's life as it is and will be experienced by the newborn
Q_2 = quality of the newborn's life as it is and will be appreciated by others
B_1 = benefits of the newborn's life for the parents
B_2 = benefits for future newborns who may be saved because of the experience in treating the instant case
B_3 = benefits the newborn's life is likely to confer on society generally (e.g., future economic productivity)
C_1 = costs (e.g., suffering) to the newborn from the attempt to save it (including the suffering and other costs from its continued life)
C_2 = costs to the parents from attempting to save the newborn (including the suffering and other costs from its continued life)
C_3 = costs to the health care providers (e.g., psychological exhaustion) from attempting to save the newborn (including the suffering and other costs from its continued life)
C_4 = costs to society from attempting to save the newborn (including the suffering and other costs from its continued life)
Costs and benefits must be calculated in terms of the units of life L.

In applying this algorithm, one must decide how to weigh different costs and benefits. For example, one might have arguments to justify weighting benefits to the patient more highly than costs to third parties. One must also decide where along a decreasing ratio of benefits to costs the duty to treat is defeated. At some point, it will be proper for the parents to decide that their attempt to have a child has failed, and it is best to let the infant die and, if possible, to try again to become pregnant and produce the child they had hoped to have.

V. AN OVERVIEW OF THE VOLUME AND THE ISSUES

The volume opens with an assessment of the roots of modern Western attitudes towards infanticide and the care of defective newborns. As Darrel Amundsen's overview of classical Western attitudes toward defective newborns shows, the value of human life was primarily social in nature and determined by social potential. No major pagan philosopher or jurist appears to have argued that human beings have intrinsic value. Rather, capacities in social contexts were seen to be the source of human value. Pagan society did not possess an analogue to the modern notion of the sanctity of life, in that the value of human life was seen to be acquired, not inherent. Infanticide was widely practiced in the case of defective infants, at times on eugenic grounds. Furthermore, the morality of killing defective newborns was not widely questioned, as far as

extant sources permit judgment. Since classical antiquity was characterized by a diversity of viewpoints, there were, as Amundsen emphasizes,
exceptions to this dominant view. Within certain subcultures, such as
the Jews, infanticide was condemned on all grounds. But it was not until
the rise of Christian influence that such practices were widely condemned.

There was also no notion of a right to life, as we currently understand
the term. Our modern notions of rights are not to be found in Graeco-
Roman or Judeo-Christian origins, but rather have substantial roots in
Germanic pagan notions that depended on a view of individual prerogatives over against the government and/or community. This pagan tradition saw members of the community as inviolable, in the sense of not
being open to being touched by others without their permission ([26],
pp. 24–25, [12, 13]). Here one must add that it would appear that infants
did not have the rights of others until they had been accepted by the
father and had been given suck ([20], pp. 15–16). Prior to becoming a
moral agent and a member of the community and thus having rights on
one's own terms, rights were conveyed socially.

In contrast, the predominant Mediterranean view saw 'rights' as
derived from God, society, or reason. There was little talk of people
having rights. Rather, something was right in the sense of *fas*, according
to morality, or *ius*, somewhat similar to our current notion of 'just'. A
distinction was also drawn between those things that are in accord with
customary law, *mos*, and those things that are in accord with statutory
law, *lex*. There was as well the notion of things being done according to
accepted usage, *consuetudo*. These various concepts supported ideas of
what was right or wrong to do. They did not sustain a notion of rights as
claims of individuals against society and the state. It is the old Germanic
barbarian notion of rights that developed through Anglo-Saxon law that
lies behind the Anglo-American recognition of individual rights over
against the state and society, so that persons have the right to do certain
things, even if they are wrong. This use of right is already found in the
Anglo-Saxon *riht*. Consider one of the provisions in the laws of King
Edward dating from between A.D. 900 and 925. "Now his [Edward's]
concern is that no man shall withhold from another his rights [ryhtes]"
([4]; II Edward sec. 2). This notion of the rights of individuals against
others was rearticulated in the Magna Carta, a document influenced by
Viking law [15]. One must add that such notions of right were also well
developed among the pagan Icelanders. Such concepts of rights were

independent of notions of sanctity of life and depended instead on the limits of communal and state authority.

As Gary Ferngren shows, one of the major elements in the development of the concept of the sanctity of life was the notion of the *imago dei*. Jews and Christians saw humans as made in the image and likeness of God. This understanding of the relationship between humans and the Deity not only led to the proscription of abortion and infanticide by Christians, it also underscored the importance of the body against pagan ascetics, who saw the body as evil. The *imago dei* led not to a right to life, which one could exercise or relinquish, but to a concept of the sanctity of life, which also supported the condemnation of suicide. Christian notions of the *imago dei* and the sanctity of life brought dramatic changes in public policy. This was especially the case after 392, when the Emperor Theodosius began the official persecution of pagans. But already in the time of Constantine, legal changes had been put in place to discourage infanticide. Among these was the legalization of the sale of children. One might wonder whether Christians who currently oppose abortion might not find in such a policy a promising way of encouraging pregnant women to bring their children to term.

The analysis of the ideas underlying modern Western attitudes toward defective newborns is continued by Kenneth Vaux. He underscores the ambivalence that Luther and others have had toward severely deformed newborns: such infants were at times considered monstrosities rather than humans. Exposing such entities could be treated as an act other than infanticide. Or even if regarded as human, there are circumstances when the usual duties of protection and nurture appear to be defeated. The difficulty, as Vaux' analysis suggests, is to determine how to create workable exceptions to general rules enjoining the protection and nurture of infants.

The essays by Amundsen, Ferngren, and Vaux, in illustrating the influence of Christian thought on Western custom and practice, raise a major problem for public policy, as Engelhardt shows. Insofar as contemporary society is no longer Christian but pluralist and secular in nature, there is a question of the extent to which such policy should be governed by the assumptions of the Judeo-Christian tradition. In the ancient world, children were seen as the product of parents and therefore open to exposure immediately after birth. Christianity, in contrast, saw children as gifts of God and, with a few notable exceptions, held that infanticide was impermissible. In contemporary society, as Christian influence weakens and as the government is no longer seen as the instrument of a particular church or religious view, should public policy return to the pagan viewpoint of the ancients? Engelhardt argues that such a return has been avoided in part by regarding children as wards of the state. But this practice collides with a contrary understanding, that of family sovereignty. As one becomes skeptical regarding the authority of the state, one should become skeptical as well regarding its authority to intervene in familial decisions.

Nancy King begins this volume's explicit analysis of the so-called Baby Doe regulations, which are prime examples of attempts by the state to control physician and parental decision making. As King indicates, the Health and Human Services regulations place the Federal government in a role the state has traditionally claimed, that of acting as the protector of the child's best interests when parental judgment is found in some way inappropriate. It has been argued that parents are likely to choose inappropriately when their interests and the best interests of the children seriously conflict, when they simply do not know what is best or when they are not capable of providing it. In such cases, the state has often intruded. However, assumption of the parental role by the government requires at least a demonstration that: (1) the parents, along with their physicians, cannot or will not make an acceptable decision, (2) the government can make a better decision, thereby protecting the best interests of the infant, and (3) the government has the right to do so over the protests of the parents.

Even if one held that the state ought to intrude in some cases of parental decision-making, as King argues, one might still hold it should not intrude in the way that the Baby Doe regulations provide. As King indicates, it is the consensus of the legal community that decision-making should rest with the parents, unless it can be shown that their decisions fall outside the realm of those that can be viewed as in the child's best interests, In addition, King argues that the courts, not bureaucratic agencies, provide the least intrusive means for identifying inappropriate decisions. The courts, unlike governmental agencies, tend to examine a parental decision, not to determine whether it is *the* correct decision, but rather whether it falls within a range of permissible decisions. In contrast, the various Baby Doe regulations placed the burden of proof on the shoulders of the parents.

Matters are even more complicated, since one must recognize, as Margery Shaw argues, that treatment interventions not only provide benefits but harms as well. The decision to treat an infant often entails pain and suffering to the infant, in addition to a probability of increasing life expectancy and longterm quality of life. A difficulty arises of how to balance concerns to avoid pain and suffering with concerns to increase the possibility of survival. In addition, treating an infant may impose serious pyschological and financial burdens on the parents. The review by Shaw and King of possible legal intrusions into parental decision making discloses difficulties that may lead parents to choose prenatal diagnosis and abortion. The legal, bureaucratic, and financial difficulties that parents are likely to experience with neonatal decision making, should they have a child with mental and physical disabilities, may well constitute for some a ground for an abortion, when there is evidence that the fetus is deformed.

The cumbersome character of the bureaucratic regulation of parental decision making regarding the treatment of defective newborns is further underscored by Stuart Spicker. He, too, argues that the best fora for resolving cases of true controversy are the courts. Following Margery Shaw, he contends that courts should take into consideration the harms that treatment can do to patients, not just the harms that may result from the failure to provide treatment. The Baby Doe regulations place burdens on parents and physicians that are inordinate and to the detriment of good medical decision making. The concern to avoid all quality of life decision has led to a law that is, if not unfollowable, at least very unwise.

The next section turns to the issue of constructing a defensible public policy for the care of seriously ill newborns. John Freeman poses a provocative two-part question. First, would the legalization of active euthanasia with sufficient review and control mechanisms eliminate the need for passive euthanasia? Second, might not the legalization of active euthanasia encourage physicians to embark on heroic therapy that might on balance save more lives? After all, if one cannot end a life when treatment fails and leads to an unacceptable quality of life, one may tend not to use therapies that involve both a chance of saving life with an acceptable quality of life, as well as a chance of saving life with an unacceptable quality of life. If active euthanasia is permitted, one will be encouraged to treat maximally, knowing that if the treatment fails in the sense of producing an unacceptable quality of life, one can then have that life terminated. One must also note that, if one relies on passive euthanasia for death in such circumstances, one may then impose on the person dying, not to mention those in attendance, unnecessary pain and suffering, which could have been avoided through a policy that allowed active euthanasia.

Apart from the issue of euthanasia, one is forced to examine the public policy implications of the decision to treat high-risk newborns. Very low birth-weight infants provide an excellent illustration of how recent advances in treatment raise problems for public policy. John Sinclair examines the effectiveness and efficiency on neonatal intensive care, so that both costs and outcomes can be taken into account in providing an economic evaluation of a particular health program, such as the treatment of very low birth-weight infants in neonatal intensive care units. As Sinclair argues, such an evaluation is necessary to answer whether the return from such treatment programs is worth the costs. Considering the fact that our resources are finite and that neonatal intensive care is expensive, one must ask whether there are other health care programs that might be better pursued for the benefit of society. Sinclair makes it clear that such an analysis differs from usual medical decision making in that it is not patient specific but addresses health care programs and groups of patients. In terms of program evaluation, a number of difficult moral and philosophical issues must be confronted: (1) whose preferences should count in assessing the cost-effectiveness of health care programs; (2) how does one decide between effectiveness and efficiency (i.e., between those programs that may dramatically increase survival for a particular group but at great costs, versus those that slightly increase survival for a larger group but at moderate costs, such that the latter produce more years of lives saved per dollar); (3) under what circumstances can a rationale for health care decisions be justified; and (4) can rational decisions be made in an equitable fashion? The problem is not simply determining the correct answer to the correct question. There may not be a correct answer to discover. Or in many cases it may not be clear which answer is correct, though one may assume that a correct one exists. In such circumstances of ambiguity, one confronts the equally, if not more, vexing question of who should be in authority to choose what will be done.

Richard Brandt begins his essay by arguing that public policy is morally justified if: (1) it is informed, rational, and what a normal person would wish for a society in which he expected to live out his years, and (2) it is the policy that is most beneficial for society in the long run. In addressing this issue, Brandt turns to an analysis of the President's Commission's recommendations regarding the treatment of new-borns. He critically examines three of the Commission's recommen-dations. First is the recommendation that costs to others must be ignored in treatment decisions. Brandt rejects this, arguing one should take into account not only the net benefit of the treatment for the infant, but the impact of the treatment on the family as well as society. Second is the Commission's recommendation that treatment may be withheld if it would not benefit the infant. Brandt asks how we should determine benefit for severely handicapped infants. For infants that are so defec-tive as to appear to have little potential benefit from life, Brandt concludes that this question should be answered in terms of what support services and facilities would be available to care for them. Finally, Brandt takes exception with the Commission's position regard-ing who is to make these decisions. Brandt rejects, as a matter of public policy, the primacy of parents and physicians, and opts instead for use of hospital ethics committees. Brandt's conclusion is that non-treatment may be recommended, not simply for the dying, but also for those whose prospects are far less than acceptable life, taking into considera-tion not only the 'infant's' point of view, but also the burdens that treatment will impose on the family and society. Brandt supports this conclusion through a utilitarian test for public policy.

The problem of comparing the harms and benefits promised by different levels of intervention is addressed in the fourth section of this volume. Shelp in particular addresses the fact that decisions with regard to defective newborns are decisions made in a context of tragedy. Such decisions involve parents who love their children and wish, as far as possible, to set their physical and mental handicaps aside, and to offer them a long and healthy life. Yet in many cases, such hopes are tragically foreclosed. Parents are forced to choose between outcomes, all of which involve pain, suffering, and the loss of aspirations for their children. As a result, parents with severely defective newborns must often choose between natural, if not moral, evils. Indeed, often a choice that involves death may involve the lesser of evils. Marvin Kohl de-velops this theme further in order to indicate circumstances under which active euthanasia may be justified. Death is not always a harm, as Kohl argues, because life is not always a good. This is particularly the case when the prospects for future sapience are dramatically restricted and the likelihood of suffering considerable.

Death is typically viewed as an evil, and this view, according to

Richard McMillan, unduly and seriously complicates treatment/non-treatment decisions for profoundly defective newborns. Death, rather than an evil to be resisted at all costs, is a fact of biological life. It is, rather, the conditions of death that may be evil, and we are normally selective in our judgment of those conditions. These judgments are made by human beings who are moral agents, persons. It is McMillan's contention that the usual ways in which we speak of death or life having negative or positive value for individuals cannot be carried over to the care of the profoundly defective newborn, if that infant has no potential for personhood. Contrary to much contemporary wisdom, McMillan then argues that decisions regarding the treatment of profoundly defective newborns cannot be made in a relational vacuum; such decisions simply cannot ignore the impact of the newborn on others and the impact of others on the newborn. As we can only with difficulty and only partially empathize with the profoundly defective newborn, we can neither judge best interests nor net benefit for the infant in the manner in which these criteria are commonly employed. We must employ long-term relationship considerations that, in some cases, may lead decision-makers to conclude that death is the most humane choice.

The volume concludes with an essay by two physicians who contributed importantly to the modern examination of the issue of the proper level of treatment to be given to defective newborns. Raymond Duff and Alexander Campbell distinguish three prognostic groups: a group for whom available treatment is usually successful, a group for whom available treatment will be of doubtful benefit, and a group for whom all treatment will be futile. As a result of technological advances, the second group has become more visible, and it is with regard to this group that decisions are most difficult. The authors emphasize a family oriented approach to decisions in this area. This approach places individuals, with their subjective feelings about the meaning of life, at the center of such deliberations. Duff and Campbell argue that the law should leave such decisions to the privacy of informal moral communities. They also reject ethics committees and contend that the attending physician should provide the professional guidance required. The locus of decision-making should rest with those involved with the consequences of the decision. Duff and Campbell argue that only caring persons can make caring decisions; the more remote the decision-maker, the more remote the decision. Only caring, responsible, and moral communities can determine a course of action when only tragic choices exist.

VI. LOOKING TO THE FUTURE

The choice of treatment for severely defective newborns engenders moral problems because of conflicting goals. We generally intervene and treat with vigor, for generally such a policy benefits the child. Difficulties arise when exceptions suggest that this general moral maxim at times entails costs that defeat its claims. It is because the lives of severely defective infants entail substantial costs both to them and to their parents that infanticide has been formally or informally accepted not only in the distant past, but recently as well [32, 38]. The advent of modern medical technology has solved some problems and created new ones. Many defects can now be prevented through genetic counselling, contraception, and selective abortion. Other defects can be remedied by surgical and other interventions. Yet still others are 'caused' through medicine's capacity to save lives of severely defective or premature newborns who would otherwise have died and who now survive with considerable unremediable limitations.

There are other tensions as well. Our concern to reproduce responsibly has led to tort for wrongful life and wrongful birth suits, through which parents have not only sued for having children born to them with defects they could have avoided through abortion or contraception, had they had sufficient information, but also through which children have sought recovery for having been born with defects that could have been prevented by preventing the children from coming into existence through contraception, sterilization, or abortion. Public policy appears to be on a collision course with itself, where on the one hand tort law gives incentives for the avoidance of the birth of defective newborns, while on the other hand severely restricting opportunities to forego extending the life of defective newborns once they are born ([36], pp. 393–397). This circumstance may not be as paradoxical as it at first blush seems. One is not obliged to produce defective persons, while on the other hand one may have strong obligations to respect and even support defective persons, once they do indeed come into existence. The source of the paradox may be where few are willing to acknowledge. The question may very well turn on the reasonableness as a matter of public policy of imputing at birth to humans the full rights to beneficence accorded to members of a community. It may spring from the fact that societies have generally allowed some amount of infanticide and that strict proscriptive rules are difficult, if not clearly impractical [29]. The result of the Baby

Doe regulations is that it is now more difficult to withhold or withdraw curative and life-prolonging treatment on infants than on adults, even incompetent adults [21]. It is as if we had lost sight, with regard to infants, of the general medical truth that the maximum commitment to appropriate medical treatment for a patient may often involve only supportive treatment aimed at minimizing pain and suffering, not at prolonging death or extending life.

The fact that the question of the choice of medical treatment for defective newborns has now engendered a case that has gone to the Supreme Court of the United States [39] indicates the depth of the conflict [3].

The Supreme Court ruled that the original Baby Doe regulations of March 7, 1983, July 5, 1983, and January 12, 1984, were without legislative authority, though the Court did not address the rules made pursuant to the Amendments to the Child Prevention and Treatment Act (October 9, 1984). The plurality held that "[s]ection 504 does not authorize the Secretary to give unsolicited advice either to parents, to hospitals, or to state officials who are faced with difficult treatment decisions concerning handicapped children" [*Bowen vs. American Hospital Association*, 84–1529, June 9, 1986].

These are conflicts that are part and parcel of technological success. The fact that we can now prolong death and extend life means that we must now decide when we ought to prolong death or extend life. Technology brings with it unwanted responsibilities. As Stuart Spicker indicates in this volume, there are ways in which some of the conflicts can be avoided. But these also involve the use of technology in ways that conflict with important values. One might think here again of the use of genetic counseling with contraception and sterilization or prenatal diagnosis with abortion. However, often the solutions are less overladen with deep moral disputes. For example, of the infants born with a birthweight less than 750 grams, 23% were born of mothers with cervical incompetence, and 43% with chorioamnionitis, suggesting that a significant proportion of such premature births could have been avoided ([23], p. 664). One sees here a repeating theme. The use of technology invites the further use of technology. The invitation is not one engendered by mere curiosity but by concerns to secure important human goals. The problem of using and controlling technology is central to our culture. Decisions of when to use or forego curative treatment are inescapable as our technologies expand in their capacities and their costs. This volume offers a sketch of the anatomy of the conflicts that are part of our learning to use our medical technologies that can both benefit and harm newborns.

November 1, 1986   H. TRISTRAM ENGELHARDT, JR.

Center for Ethics, Medicine, and Public Issues,
Baylor College of Medicine,
Houston, Texas, U.S.A.

NOTES

[1] Orthodox Judaism does not require one to mourn the death of a child who dies before the age of 31 days; see *Kitzur Shulhan Arukh* by Rabbi Solomon Ganzfried. The standard condensed version of the Code of Jewish religious law, entitled *Shulhan Arukh*, compiled by Joseph Karo (1488–1575), states that ". . . if an infant dies within the first 30 days of its life, or even on the 30th day of its life, and even if there has been growth of its hair and nails, you do not follow any of the observances of mourning, because it is as if there had been a miscarriage" Section 203, Paragraph 3 [adapted and translated by the late Professor Isaac Franck].

[2] Two important ideas must be distinguished: (1) the notion of an individual *in* authority over others, and (2) the notion of an individual as *an* authority concerning a particular issue. A discussion of these distinctions is provided by Richard Flathman [19].

BIBLIOGRAPHY

1. American Academy of Pediatrics: 1984, 'Principles of Treatment of Disabled Infants', *Pediatrics* **73**, 559.
2. American Medical Association: 1984, *Current Opinions of the Judicial Council of the American Medical Association – 1984*, American Medical Association, Chicago.
3. Angell, M.: 1986, 'The Baby Doe Rules', *New England Journal of Medicine* **314**, 642–644.
4. Attenborough, F. L. (trans. and ed.): 1922, *The Laws of the Earliest English Kings*, University Press, Cambridge, England.
5. Banez, D.: 1614, *Scholastica Commentaria in partem Angelici Doctoris S. Thomas*, Tom. IV, *Decisiones de Jure et Justitia*, in II: II, 1. 65, art. 1, Duaci.
6. Cronin, D. A.: 1958, *The Moral Law in Regard to the Ordinary and Extraordinary Means of Conserving Life*, Typis Pontificiae Universitatis Gregorianiae, Rome.
7. Department of Health and Human Services: 1983, 'Nondiscrimination on the Basis of Handicap, Interim Final Rule', *Federal Register* 48 (March 7), 9630–32.
8. Department of Health and Human Services: 1983, 'Nondiscrimination on the Basis of Handicaps Relating to Health Care for Handicapped Infants' Proposed Rules', *Federal Register* 48 (July 5), 30846–52.
9. Department of Health and Human Services: 1984, 'Nondiscrimination on the Basis of Handicap; Procedures and Guidelines Relating to Health Care for Handicapped Infants; Final Rule', *Federal Register* 48 (January 12), 1622–54.

10. Department of Health and Human Services: 1985, 'Child Abuse and Neglect Prevention and Treatment Program; Final Rule', *Federal Register* 50 (April 15), 14878–901.
11. Doe v. Bloomington Hospital, Indiana Ct. App. (Feb. 3, 1983), *cert. denied*, 104 S. Ct. 394 (1983).
12. Drew, K. F. (trans.): 1972, *The Burgundian Code: Book of Constitutions or Law of Gundobad*, University of Pennsylvania Press, Philadelphia.
13. Drew, K. F. (trans.): 1973, *The Lombard Laws*, University of Pennsylvania Press, Philadelphia.
14. Duff, R. S. and Campbell, A. G. M.: 1973, 'Moral and Ethical Dilemmas in the Special Care Nursery', *New England Journal of Medicine* **289**, 890–94.
15. Dufwa, T. E.: 1963, *The Viking Laws and the Magna Charta*, Exposition Press, New York.
16. Engelhardt, H. T., Jr.: 1984, 'Viability and the Use of the Fetus', in W. B. Bondeson *et al.* (eds.), *Abortion and the Status of the Fetus*, D. Reidel, Dordrecht, pp. 183–209.
17. Engelhardt, H. T., Jr.: 1986, *Foundations of Bioethics*, Oxford University Press, New York.
18. Feen, R. H.: 1983, 'Abortion and Exposure in Ancient Greece', in W. B. Bondeson *et al.* (eds.), *Abortion and the Status of the Fetus*, D. Reidel, Dordrecht, pp. 283–300.
19. Flathman, R. E.: 1982, 'Power, Authority, and Rights in the Practice of Medicine', in G. J. Agich (ed.), *Responsibility in Health Care*, D. Reidel, Dordrecht, pp. 105–125.
20. Foote, P. and Wilson, D. M.: 1970, *The Viking Achievement*, Sidgwick & Jackson, London.
21. Gostin, L.: 1985. 'A Moment in Human Development: Legal Protection, Ethical Standards and Social Policy on the Selective Non-Treatment of Handicapped Neonates', *American Journal of Law & Medicine* **2**, 31–78.
22. Gross, R. H. *et al.*: 1983, 'Early Management and Decision Making for the Treatment of Myelomeningocele', *Pediatrics* **72**, 450–58.
23. Hack, M. and Fanaroff, A. A.: 1986, 'Changes in the Delivery Room Care of the Extremely Small Infant', *New England Journal of Medicine* **314**, 660–664.
24. Healy, E.: 1942, *Moral Guidance*, Loyola University Press, Chicago.
25. Kelly, G.: 1950, 'The Duty of Using Artificial Means of Preserving Life', *Theological Studies* **11**, 203–20.
26. Lea, H. C.: *Torture*, University of Pennsylvania Press, Philadelphia.
27. Lessius, L.: 1622, *De Justitia et Jure*, Lugduni, Lib. IV, Cap. 31, dub. 8, n. 60.
28. Lorber, J.: 1971, 'Results of Treatment of Myelomeningocele', *Developmental Medicine and Child Neurology* **13**, 279–303.
29. Lund, N.: 1985, 'Infanticide, Physicians, and the Law: The "Baby Doe" Amendments to the Child Abuse Prevention and Treatment Act', *American Journal of Law & Medicine* **2**, 1–29.
30. McCartney, J. J.: 1980, 'The Development of the Doctrine of Ordinary and Extraordinary Means of Preserving Life in Catholic Moral Theology Before the Karen Quinlan Case', *Linacre Quarterly* **47**, 215–24.
31. McFadden, C. A.: 1949, *Medical Ethics*, F. A. Davis, Philadelphia.
32. Moseley, K. L.: 1986, 'The History of Infanticide in Western Society', *Issues in Law & Medicine* **1**, 345–361.
33. Pell, R.: 1972, 'The Agonizing Decision of Joanne and Roger Pell', *Good Housekeeping* (Jan.), 76–77, 131–35.

34. Pope Pius XII: 1958, 'Address to an International Congress of Anesthesiologists', *The Pope Speaks* **4** (Spring), 393–98.

35. Rhoden, N. K.: 1985, 'Treatment Dilemmas for Imperiled Newborns: Why Quality of Life Counts', *Southern California Law Review* **58** (Sept.), 1283–1347.

36. Rosenblum, V. G.: 1986, 'The Legal Response to Babies Doe: An Analytical Prognosis', *Issues in Law & Medicine* **1**, 391–404.

37. Shaw, A.: 1973, 'Dilemmas of Informed Consent in Children', *New England Journal of Medicine* **289**, 885–90.

38. Turnbull, H. T.: 1986, 'Incidence of Infanticide in America: Public and Professional Attitudes', *Issues in Law & Medicine* **1**, 363–389.

39. United States v. University Hospital, State University of New York at Stony Brook, 575 F. Supp. 607 (E.D.N.Y. 1983), *aff'd*, 729 F. 2d 144 (2d Cir. 1984).

40. Weber v. Stony Brook Hosp., 60 N.Y.2d 208, 456 N.E.2d 1186, 469 N.Y.S.2d 65 (1983).

SECTION I

WESTERN ANTECEDENTS AND DEFECTIVE NEONATES

DARREL W. AMUNDSEN

MEDICINE AND THE BIRTH OF DEFECTIVE CHILDREN: APPROACHES OF THE ANCIENT WORLD

So diverse are the varied strands of ancient Greek and Roman cultures that it is dangerous – indeed probably irresponsible – to speak of any universal ancient attitudes and practices, unless significant qualifications are placed upon any assertions other than the most specific and limited. Now in attempting accurately to describe – or, more correctly, to reconstruct – the response of people in antiquity to the defective newborn, it is necessary first to provide the broader context of values that informed – or actually formed – that response. And that broader context of values involves such issues as human worth, human dignity, value of life, and human rights, inalienable and otherwise.

John M. Rist recently published a very perspicacious monograph entitled *Human Value: A Study in Ancient Philosophical Ethics*. In his introduction Rist maintains that the view that such rights as "the right to life, to have enough to eat, to live without fear of torture or degrading punishments, the right to work or to withhold one's labour" or that any other rights "are the universal property of men as such was virtually unknown in classical antiquity". He further asserts that classical antiquity had no theory "that all men are endowed at birth (or before) with a certain value . . . though some of its philosophers took certain steps toward such a theory" ([40], p. 9).

It is especially in the literature of political philosophy that theories of human value are developed. The most famous representative of this genre is Plato's *Republic*, which must be supplemented by the *Statesman* and the *Laws* to provide a thorough picture of Plato's ideal society. There has been considerable scholarly discussion of Plato's conception of human value within the ideal state. Does the ideal state exist for its inhabitants or do the latter exist for the sake of the state? It seems as though both are true in Plato's view. Private worth, which is possession of the virtues, will inevitably lead to the seeking of the public good. While personal worth or value is always manifest in one's social utility,

R. C. McMillan, H. T. Engelhardt, Jr., and S. F. Spicker (eds.),
Euthanasia and the Newborn, 3–22.
© 1987 *by D. Reidel Publishing Company.*

and thus contributory to the common good, Plato seems to hold that personal worth is the *telos* of the ideal state (as the best environment for growth in personal virtue), rather than that the state is the *telos* of personal value. But the relationship is transparently circular, cause and effect, means and end being inextricably interwoven.

Within Plato's ideal state, failure to contribute renders one worthless. And there are levels of worth; some people are superior to others. The Guardian class, of course, has an intrinsic value that exceeds that of slaves whose only value is in their material contributions to the state. But slaves aside, even among the Guardian class there are grades of worth. Although Plato views men and women of the Guardian class as fully equal, the qualities of this class are starkly masculine, suggesting that the most virtuous (i.e., valuable) women are those who are most like men in their developed character. The children of superior adults clearly possess a potential worth that increases as they come closer to maturity. However, children's worth is not intrinsic but only potential, and they are valued in respect to their approximation to the ideal adult. They must be malleable, disposed to virtue, and physically fit.

Plato's concern for healthy children is clearly seen in his marriage regulations. The maximum number of superior adults should couple with others of equal worth. The number of inferior types coupling with others of similar value should be kept at a minimum. Since adults who are too young or too old produce less vigorous children than do those who are of ideal age for procreation, people should be prevented from having children except during their ideal years for producing robust offspring.[1] Indeed the purpose of marriage is first to produce children to ensure the continuity of the state and second to improve human stock ([34], 773D, 783D–E).

In such a society where absolute value is always seen through the grid of social value, those who are physically defective, or at least those who are chronically ill, should not be kept alive by diet, drugs, and regimen since such people will likely reproduce similarly wretched offspring and be of use neither to themselves nor to society ([35], 407D–E, 410A). Indeed, the only legitimate claim to medical care is the continued social usefulness of the one desiring care.

Aristotle's view of human value is expressed in a variety of his works, ranging from the biological to the political and ethical. He clearly postulates a hierarchy of worth within the species. Men with fully developed virtues(s) are most fully human, thus of the greatest value both to themselves and to society. There are, of course, gradations within this group. All other humans are, by comparison, defective by nature or in their present state. Those who are defective by nature are especially those whom Aristotle calls 'natural slaves', i.e., individuals who have a capacity to acknowledge reason but not to conceptualize or to engage in rational activity. They are somewhat like domesticated animals; defectives by nature. Also defective by nature, but having considerably greater range of capacity for virtue than natural slaves, are those women who themselves are not natural slaves. They are naturally defective by virtue of being women but yet, in unnatural or unusual circumstances, may demonstrate a kind of female excellence. But at the best they are defective males.

Quite distinct from natural slaves and women are children. Children may be natural slaves – a condition not immediately discernible – or female and thus limited in potential. But all male children, except for those who prove to be natural slaves, are potentially virtuous men, therefore potentially fully human. Children, however, resemble natural slaves and animals more than they do virtuous men, because they lack the developed capacity for rational thought and behavior.

For both Plato and Aristotle, then, human value is primarily social value and is determined by potentiality.[2]

Do the positions taken by Plato and Aristotle reflect the values of classical society? The answer to that question must be a highly qualified, yet hearty, affirmative; qualified, because there was a tremendous diversity of values in classical antiquity; a hearty affirmative for two reasons: (1) No pagan, whether philosopher or jurist, appears to have asked the question whether human beings have inherent value, or possess intrinsic rights, ontologically, irrespective of social value, legal status, age, sex, and so forth. (2) Connected with the first reason is a fundamental, though primitive and residual, principle that, as Thrasymachus expresses it, "justice is the will of the stronger." Rights are recognized only by their enforceability. It was against the idea that might makes right that various philosophers, including Plato and Aristotle, reacted. Power must be checked by justice, justice being essentially the definition and enforcement of rights. Rist observes that

Instead of starting with a consideration of human rights, or of basic rights, [the ancients] start with theories of power and of how power shall be tempered by justice. As their thought proceeds, they come to recognize that certain types of people, for various reasons, are in fact possessed of rights. . . . [T]he moral problem is not viewed in terms of enlarging or protecting the rights of the weak, but of controlling and rationalizing the power of the strong ([40], p. 131).

Rist's comments certainly appear valid when one considers the various legal systems of classical antiquity. Among the Greeks the exclusivistic atmosphere of the polis fostered a definition of rights focusing on citizens, more on males, who possessed the franchise, than on females, who did not. The rights of their dependents (wives, to a certain degree, and children) and human possessions (slaves) were essentially developed with a view to protecting the rights of the adult males on whom they depended or to whom they belonged. This prevailed even in the highly developed law of the Roman Empire, though its more cosmopolitan character is reflected in its extension of various, if limited, rights to a broader spectrum of society than had typically been the center of Greek attention. Yet the emphasis remains the rights of the adult male citizen primarily, with a variety of rights defined for women, rights essentially resulting from the limitations of their fathers' or husbands' power and authority, and even for slaves, in slight limitations being placed on the absolute power of owners.

In part, some of the changes that we see during the early centuries of the Empire were the result of what some have hailed as a growing humanitarianism, a by-product of a sentiment, although not of egalitarianism, at least of the brotherhood of man proclaimed especially by the Stoicism of this period. This found its way into the medical ethics of probably a minority of physicians in an ethic of respect for life that condemned both abortion and active (although not passive) euthanasia, and a broader sentiment of generosity and altruism, a philanthropy predicated upon the unexpressed and ill-defined feeling that somehow people have a value to which our compassion is owed.

Even this pagan humanitarianism, however, was not grounded on a principle of inherent value of life. A stand against abortion and active euthanasia by the probably Pythagorean author of the so-called Hippocratic Oath and such physicians as Scribonius Largus and Soranus, both of whom lived in the early Empire, was based less upon an idea of inherent value or sanctity of life than on an abhorrence of a physician's using his art in actively terminating life (fetal or otherwise); and especially in the case of abortion, an enduring, if not always articulated principle that value is more potential than ontological.

The strongly-held idea that human value is acquired rather than inherent was nearly pervasive in classical antiquity, even among those pagans who condemned abortion. It was so central to ancient conceptions of value that a fully-developed principle of sanctity of human life was never achieved in pagan society. This is particularly easily demonstrated by considering the status of the newborn and their treatment. Once more I quote John Rist:

It was almost universally held in antiquity that a child has no intrinsic right to life in virtue of being born. What mattered was being adopted into a family or some other institution of society. Both Plato and Aristotle, as well as the Stoics, Epicurus, and presumably Plotinus, accept the morality of the exposure of infants . . . on eugenic or sometimes on purely economic grounds. . . . We see here further clear evidence of the ancient view that somehow value is acquired, either by the development of intelligence or by the acceptance into society. There is no reason to think that the philosophers made substantial advances on the assumptions of the general public in this regard ([40], pp. 141–142).

Rist is absolutely correct in this assertion. Some clarification, however, is necessary. To say that the attitude in antiquity that "a child has no intrinsic right to life in virtue of being born" was "almost universal", is somewhat misleading. Since there indeed were some pagans who did condemn exposure[3] of healthy children for any reason, is Rist referring to these by his qualifying 'almost'? That would imply that such individuals condemned exposure of healthy infants on the grounds that there is an "intrinsic right to life in virtue of being born." Or is Rist suggesting that there were some – that few permitted by his 'almost' – who unequivocally condemned all infanticide, including exposure of healthy infants and the disposal of the defective? If there actually were any pagans in the second of these categories, they most certainly had not formulated an ethic of intrinsic human value, any more than had those who were in the first category. His 'almost' cannot include any – even the most humanitarian – pagans, not even those who were adamant in condemning abortion.

Although Rists' first qualifier, the adverb 'almost', can be misleading, his second qualifying phrase is more helpful, i.e., that various philosophers accepted the morality of exposure of infants "on eugenic or sometimes on purely economic grounds". If we take the term 'eugenic' in a broad sense, we can apply it to the disposal of defective infants as distinct from the exposure of healthy infants for economic (or other non-eugenic) reasons. These two categories must be kept distinct if we are to understand the response of pagans in classical antiquity to defective infants.

First of all it can be categorically asserted that there were no laws in classical antiquity, Greek or Roman, that prohibited the killing, by exposure or otherwise, of the defective newborn. Further, it is unlikely that there actually were any laws that classified exposure (as distinct from other forms of killing) of the healthy newborn as parricide or homicide, or prohibited the practice on other grounds, except, perhaps, in some limited regions or under unusual circumstances before the Christianization of the Roman Empire. If any such law or laws existed, there appears to have been little or no effort to enforce them.[4]

As already mentioned, there were some pagans who opposed the exposure of healthy infants. Aristotle implies in the *Politics* ([3], 1335b) that there was in Greece some sentiment against exposure of healthy infants or traditions hostile to the practice, when he recommends that, if there are already too many children, abortion – before sensation (πϱὶν αἴσθησιν)[5] – be practiced in those regions where "the regular customs hinder any of those born being exposed:" (ἐὰν ἡ τάξις τῶν ἐθῶν κωλύῃ μηδὲν ἀποτίθεσθαι τῶν γιγνομένων). The second-century B.C. historian, Polybius, critizes the practice of child exposure, which he saw as one of the causes of the serious depopulation of Greece that occurred in the second century B.C., attributing the act to people's "pretentious extravagance, avarice and sloth" ([38], 36.17). The Stoic philosopher Epictetus, who lived in the late first and early second centuries A.D., criticizes Epicurus for approving the exposure of children, saying that even a sheep or a wolf does not abandon its own offspring. His argument is that we ought not to be more foolish than sheep or more fierce than wolves, but rather yield to our natural impulse to love our own offspring ([17], 1.23). It is significant that he uses στέϱγειν here, the obvious word for having 'natural affection' as distinct from other Greek words that are translated by the English word 'love'.

Many of the examples of condemnation of child exposure found in classical authors are in descriptions of the practices of other cultures. The novelist Heliodorus (third century A.D.), in *An Ethiopian Romance*, has an Ethiopian gymnosophist say that he found and reared an exposed girl, "because for me it is not permissible to disregard an imperiled soul once it has taken on human form. This is a precept of our gymnosophists" ([24], p. 61). These attitudes were divergent enough from typical classical values that some authors were sufficiently intrigued to tickle their readers by relating such strange customs of exotic peoples. Others who decried various practices of their own societies describe the contrasting purity of other cultures. Tacitus, a contemporary of Epictetus, does both. He finds it remarkable that among the Germans it was regarded as shameful to kill any 'late-born' child, that is, an unwanted child ([45], 19). He uses nearly an identical sentence when he attributes the same peculiarity to the Jews, a people whose customs he usually finds strange and obnoxious ([46], 5.5).

That Jews of Tacitus' time regarded the killing of infants as a reprehensible act, violating sacred law, is evident from the writings of Philo Judaeus ([22], pp. 115–116) and Josephus ([26], 2.24). Relying on the writings of Hecataeus of Abdera (sixth/fifth centuries B.C.), Diodorus Siculus remarks that Moses required the Jews "to rear their children" (τεκνοτρόφειν [14], 40.3), and says virtually the same thing about the Egyptians, i.e., that are they required "to raise all their children" (τὰ γεννώμενα πάντα τρέφουσιν [14], 1.80). Oribasius (personal physician to Julian 'the Apostate') maintains that Aristotle also attributed this same practice to the Egyptians (τὸ τρέφειν πάντα τὰ γινόμενα [33], vol. 4, pp. 99–100). And the geographer Strabo (first centuries B.C./A.D.) asserts that the Egyptians most zealously observe the custom of raising every child who is born (τὸ πάντα τρέφειν τὰ γεννώμενα παιδία) [44], 172.5).

The expressed or implied motivations behind these condemnations of exposure differ. Epictetus obviously regards it as a violation of natural law. Polybius regards those who engaged in it as selfish and immoral. Tacitus says that the Germans held this practice (as well as any limitation of the number of their children) as *flagitium* (a disgraceful or shameful deed) and says of the Jews that they saw it as *nefas* (contrary to divine law, impious), a word much more charged with moral principle than that descriptive of German sentiment. Josephus maintains that it was forbidden by the Law, and Philo condemns it as murder, a perversion of natural law. Diodorus Siculus implies that the Jews were motivated to condemn the practice by a desire to increase their population, the motive specified by the same author for the Egyptians' forbidding the act. And Heliodorus' imaginary Ethiopian gymnosophist regarded it as morally wrong at least for his exclusive group of gymnosophists.

Now these instances of condemnations of child exposure, or of infanticide in the broader sense of the word, whether by some few Greeks or Romans, or by exotic peoples, both Jews and pagans, can be taken to include the condemnation of the killing of the defective newborn and not to be limited to the exposure of healthy infants. There is no qualifying phrase introduced by 'except'. The statements are generally quite specific and seem to imply that all which is born is raised, the word translated 'raised' meaning 'nourished' and the word translated 'born' either the word commonly used for giving birth or else the word for becoming or coming into existence. These phrases certainly would, on the surface, seem all-inclusive. Aristotle, you recall, recommends early abortion as a means of population control in the event that "regular customs hinder any of those born being exposed" ([3], 1335b). Such a statement seems inclusive, even in the English translation. But it most certainly is not, for it follows directly on this: "As to exposing or rearing the children born, let there be a law that no deformed child shall be reared" (περὶ δὲ ἀποθέσεως καὶ τροφῆς τῶν γιγνομένων ἔστω νόμος μηδὲν πεπηρωμένον τρέφειν).

Aristotle, in writing the *Politics*, is describing 'the best state'. As we have just seen, in such a state he thinks there should be a law that no deformed child should be reared. While the practice of exposing or killing deformed infants was, as we shall see, common enough in classical antiquity, suggesting a law which would make it mandatory was not by any means typical. Quintus Curtius, writing in the first century A.D., thought it was worthy of note to inform his readers that at the time of Alexander the Great it was supposedly the custom in part of India not to permit parents to determine whether their children should be reared, but the decision was in the hands of "those to whom the charge of the physical examination of children had been committed. If these have noted any who are conspicuous for defects or are crippled in some part of their limbs, they give orders to put them to death" ([13], 9.1.25). This sounds very similar to the well-known custom ascribed to the Spartans in Plutarch's *Life of Lycurgus:*

Offspring was not reared at the will of the father, but was taken and carried by him to a place . . . where the elders . . . officially examined the infant, and if it was well-built and sturdy, they ordered the father to rear it . . . but if it was ill-born and deformed, they sent it to . . . a chasm-like place at the foot of Mount Taÿgetus, in the conviction that the life of that which nature had not well-equipped at the very beginning for health and strength, was of no advantage, either to itself or to the state. ([37], 16).

The explanation given for this practice is a concern for eugenics. We can assume the same in the case of Aristotle's ideal state and the supposed custom in India. Another feature that they have in common is that the parents have no say in the matter. Both of these aspects are present in a passage from Plato's *Republic*: ". . . the offspring of the inferior, and any of those of the other sort who are born defective, they will properly dispose of in secret, so that no one will know what has become of them" ([35], 460C). This passage has been the focus of much controversy, with some scholars maintaining that this has nothing to do with exposure.[6] Irrespective of that debate, we need to step back for a moment and look at the vocabulary in these four passages used to describe the infants in question.

The child is described as ἀνάπηρον (mained, crippled) by Plato. Aristotle uses a related word, πεπηρωμένον, meaning essentially the same thing. The text of Quintus Curtius is somewhat corrupt, but the basic meaning is defective or crippled. Plutarch uses two terms, the first of which, ἀγεννές, is quite unusual, having the meaning unborn or uncreated, *perhaps* grossly deformed, the second, ἄμορφον, meaning misshapen or disfigured. Aside from the fact that the vocabulary is frustratingly imprecise, we should note that there appears to be nothing superstitious in the procedures or decision-making described. The conditions are assumed to be natural defects, of no numinous or ominous character. The situation changes when we look at the Roman scene.

The first-century B.C. historian Dionysius of Halicarnassus attributes to Romulus, the legendary founder of Rome, the following law. Explaining how Romulus had made the city large and populous, Dionysius maintains that

he obliged the inhabitants to bring up all their male children and the first born of the females, and forbade them to destroy any children under three years of age unless they were maimed or monstrous from their very birth. These he did not forbid their parents to expose, provided they first showed them to their five nearest neighbors and these also approved ([15], 2.15).

Irrespective of the very questionable historicity of this 'law', an important element is introduced. There are two different categories of defective infants here: ἀνάπηρον˙ the same word that Plato used, translated maimed, and τέρας, a noun meaning a sign or wonder, a marvel, portent or anything that serves as an omen, as, for instance, here a strange creature or monster. What is probably meant is a grossly deformed infant, perhaps the type implied by Plutarch's word ἀγεννές. The significant difference is that Plutarch's adjective is devoid of superstitious meaning, while the word τέρας is supernatural to the core. While the infant in Plutarch's account is probably no more or less grotesque than that in Dionysius', the response that each elicits is different, the response at least of the two authors as revealed in their choice of vocabulary.

Much more commonly in Roman than in Greek society was the occurrence of *prodigia* (= τέρατα, plural of τέρας), unnatural and inexplicable events, such as the birth of a lamb with five legs, a human hermaphrodite, and the like. While some *prodigia* on record are so bizarre that their historicity must be discounted, many, perhaps most, are well within the realm of possibility, especially after exaggeration is subtracted from the account. A *prodigium* had enormous significance; it was itself a message from the supernatural powers, more often than not a warning, eliciting a communal fear and guilt in Roman society, particularly during the Republican period. The message had to be discerned by *haruspices* (soothsayers), the unnatural thing destroyed, and a *piaculum*, that is, an expiatory rite, performed. Consider the following event which occurred in 207 B.C., as recorded by the first-century B.C. historian, Livy:

Relieved of their religious scruples, men were troubled again by the report that at Frusino there had been born a child as large as a four-year-old, and not so much a wonder for size as because . . . it was uncertain whether male or female. In fact the soothsayers summoned from Etruria said it was a terrible and loathsome portent; it must be removed from Roman territory, far from contact with earth, and drowned in the sea. They put it alive into a chest, carried it out to sea and threw it overboard. The pontiffs likewise decreed that thrice nine maidens should sing a hymn as they marched through the city ([28], 37.27).

Such events abound in the extant literature.[7] The motivations for the killing of such newborn are different from the primarily eugenic concerns of the other authors whom we have considered thus far. The response to *prodigia* is rooted in some very deep-seated fear, guilt, and shame that are only slightly evident in the response to the birth of sickly, maimed or moderately deformed infants. Maimed, deformed, monstrous, constitute a continuum that can accommodate both superstitious and eugenic concerns. A law requiring the killing of deformed infants would include so-called monstrous births as well, motivated perhaps by both eugenic and superstitious responses. Such seems to underlie a law in the ancient Twelve Tables, a code thought to have been compiled in Rome in the fifth century B.C., to which Cicero alludes. This law required that a *puer ad deformitatem* be killed quickly ([10], 3.8). While modern translators render this 'terribly deformed', that seems stronger than the Latin, which appears to accommodate the entire continuum described above.

The continuum broadens when we consider a passage in a treatise *On Anger* 1.15 written by the first-century A.D. Stoic philosopher, Seneca:

Mad dogs we knock on the head; the fierce and savage ox we slay; sickly sheep we put to the knife to keep them from infecting the flock; unnatural progeny we destroy; we drown even children who at birth are weakly and abnormal. Yet it is not anger, but reason that separates the harmful from the sound ([41], vol. 1, pp. 144–145).

Here we see *portentosi*, that is, unnatural or monstrous births; *debiles*, that is, sickly or weak infants; and *monstrosi*, that is, deformed or abnormal newborn. We should note that Seneca is neither recommending nor condemning this practice. He simply gives it as an example, along with several others, of violence or ostensibly destructive activity, in which his society engaged as a matter of course, that did not involve anger or hatred but was motivated by a concern for individual or social good. The two sentences immediately preceding the section quoted say, "Does a man hate the members of his own body when he uses a knife upon them? There is no anger there, but the pitying desire to heal."

It should be clear that in Roman culture the killing of defective newborn was common, even apparently required in the case of those infants so grossly deformed or unusual as to appear to be *portentia* or monstrous births. For Greece, however, we have seen only the anomalous conditions in Sparta and the 'ideal' practices suggested by Aristotle and Plato. These really tell us little about conditions in Greek society during the classical period. There is, however, a passage in Plato's *Theaetetus* that is very revealing. The man whose name supplies the title for this dialogue has suggested that knowledge is nothing more than perception. Socrates wishes to subject this 'brain-child' to examination to see whether it is worth rearing. Socrates had earlier warned him that that was precisely what he was going to do once Theaetetus gives birth to his idea:

I suspect that you, as you yourself believe, are in pain because you are pregnant with something within you. Apply, then, to me, remembering that I am the son of a midwife and have myself a midwife's gifts, and do your best to answer the questions I ask as I ask them. And if, when I have examined any of the things you say, it should prove that I think it is a mere image and not real, and therefore quietly take it from you and throw it away, do not be angry as women are when they are deprived of their first offspring. For many, my dear friend, before this have got into such a state of mind towards me that they are actually ready to bite me, if I take some foolish notion away from them, and they do not believe that I do this in kindness . . . ([36], 151B–C).

After Theaetetus elaborates his theory, Socrates says, "Shall we say that this is, so to speak, your newborn child and the result of my midwifery? Or what shall we say?" Theaetetus replies, "We must say that, Socrates." Socrates then continues:

Well, we have at least managed to bring this forth, whatever it turns out to be; and now that it is born, we must in very truth perform the rite of running around with it in a circle – the circle of our argument – and see whether it may not turn out to be after all not worth rearing, but only a wind-egg, an imposture. But, perhaps, you think that any offspring of yours ought to be cared for and not put away; or will you bear to see it examined and not get angry if it is taken away from you, though it is your first-born? ([36], 160E–161A).

First of all, it is self-evident that the whole comparison would be sheer nonsense unless a custom prevailed of disposing of defective newborn, even defective first-born, at least at Athens at that time. Second, we may note that some mothers typically were angry when their first-born were taken from them. Apparently they were better able to cope with losing a defective infant if they already had at least one healthy child. Third, it is evident that the examination of a new-born infant was part of a midwife's responsibilities. There is relatively little attention given in ancient medical literature to the duties of midwives. However, Soranus, a physician who lived in Rome in the first and second centuries A.D., wrote a gynecological treatise – the best that has survived from antiquity – that was designed for midwives. A passage in this treatise is entitled 'How to Recognize the Newborn That is Worth Rearing'. It reads:

Now the midwife, having received the newborn, should first put it upon the earth, having examined beforehand whether the infant is male or female, and should make an announcement by signs as is the custom of women. She should also consider whether it is worth rearing or not. And the infant which is suited by nature for rearing will be distinguished by the fact that its mother has spent the period of pregnancy in good health, for conditions which require medical care, especially those of the body, also harm the fetus and enfeeble the foundations of its life. Second, by the fact that it has been born at the due time, best at the end of nine months, and if it so happens, later; but also after only seven months. Furthermore by the fact that when a woman puts it on the earth it immediately cries with proper vigor; for one that lives for some length of time without crying, or cries but weakly, is suspected of behaving so on account of some unfavorable condition. Also by the fact that it is perfect in all its parts, members and senses; that its ducts, namely of the ears, nose, pharynx, urethra, anus are free from obstruction; that the natural functions of every [member] are neither sluggish nor weak; that the joints bend and stretch; that it has due size and shape and is properly sensitive in every respect. This we may recognize from pressing the fingers against the surface of the body, for it is natural to suffer pain from everything that pricks or squeezes. And by conditions contrary to those mentioned, the infant not worth rearing is recognized ([43], pp. 79–80).

While this passage from Soranus gives concrete evidence for what was undoubtedly a common practice both in Greek and Roman cultures, it is not, strictly speaking, a medical pronouncement upon the decision-making processes involving the care of the defective newborn. It is written on the assumption that a defective infant is *eo ipso* not worth rearing. The question is simply how to determine most easily and efficiently which infants are worth rearing. Even this was a question seldom addressed by ancient medical authors. It was a midwife's concern – which is why we encounter this guidance in a gynecological treatise written for midwives. Not that medical authors, as well as natural philosophers, were uninterested in the questions why some infants were born defective and how to try to prevent this. Various intriguing suggestions were advanced and theories developed which are not germane to this study.

Two conclusions can now be drawn. One is that the *care* of defective newborns simply was not a medical concern in classical antiquity.[8] The second is that the morality of the killing of sickly or deformed newborns appears not to have been questioned, at least not in extant sources, either by non-medical or by medical authors. Interestingly enough, Soranus, who was atypical of the ancient medical authors in condemning abortion, not only raises no objection to the rejecting of defective newborns but also, as we have seen, quite dispassionately provides the criteria to be used by midwives in determining which newborns are worth rearing.

I have earlier asserted that the idea that human value is acquired rather than inherent was so central to ancient conceptions of value that a fully-developed principle of sanctity of human life, such that includes even the defective newborn, was never achieved in pagan antiquity. For apparently no pagan raised the question whether human beings have inherent value, or possess intrinsic rights, ontologically, irrespective of social value, legal status, age, sex, and so forth. The first espousal of an idea of inherent human value in Western civilization depended on a belief that every human being was formed in the image of God. We shall return shortly to this principle of *imago Dei* as a basis for inherent human value.

It is unlikely, however, that the earliest Christians formulated a concise definition of human value based upon the concept of *imago Dei*. The condemnation of acts which would later be viewed as violations of a person's rights as one formed in God's image were, in the earliest

Christian literature, part of a broad moral indignation against those aspects of Greco-Roman culture which stand in the starkest contrast to the most basic principles of the Gospel of love, mercy and compassion, salvation from sin to holiness and purity. All aspects of pagan brutality and immorality were condemned, all of which seemed to early Christian apologists to be common and related features of society that they viewed as corrupted to its very core by the disease of sin. Apologists condemned in the same breath gladiatorial shows, grossly cruel executions conducted as spectator sports, abortion, infanticide, and a broad and imaginative variety of sexual deviations. Some apologists saw abortion as a sexual crime in that it was done to destroy the results of a sexual act that was lust when engaged in for other than the purpose of procreation. Infanticide had the same motive, as did exposure, except that the latter created a potential for another sexual sin, i.e., incest, since exposed children often ended up in brothels.[9]

So common, indeed universal, among Christians in the early centuries of Christianity was the condemnation of abortion and infanticide, to include exposure,[10] that I shall only mention a few features. Some apologists point out that the practice of infanticide among the pagans is not surprising, in light of a tradition of the sacrifice of infants in various cults – a practice in which some cults still engaged, although it was strictly forbidden by law; a practice, incidentally, of which early Christians were themselves slanderously accused. Further, these apologists claim, the pagan myths are full of tales of infanticide that set a precedent of approbation. Further, some early Church Fathers contrast active infanticide with exposure, asserting that exposing a baby to cold, hunger, and carnivorous animals is more cruel than simply strangling it. But, they tell us, many pagans, thinking that it is impious to kill the infant with one's own hands, kill it by the less messy means of a slow death out of their sight.

None of the early Christian condemnations of infanticide make any reference to the condition of the baby, whether it is healthy or defective, or consider a possible eugenic motivation for the active or passive killing of a newborn. But while I asserted that the relatively rare instances of pagan condemnations of exposure would not have included the killing of the defective, I shall maintain even more categorically that early Christian condemnation of exposure and other forms of infanticide would have included any and every form of infanticide, active or passive, of the newborn, whether they be healthy, sickly, or deformed.

There are three reasons that immediately come to mind for this attitude. One, which I shall mention only in passing, is the significantly different attitude of Christianity to children generally. In classical society, even in its more humanitarian movements, children were essentially viewed as potential adults, their value residing in what they would become. We moderns, in a child-oriented society, generally do not appreciate just how revolutionary was Jesus' teaching that unless you become as little children, you cannot enter the kingdom of God. Second, the social thrust of early Christianity was demonstrably and spectacularly oriented to helping the helpless, caring for the destitute, succoring the deprived.

The third reason requires a little more space than the first two. I made reference earlier to the concept of people being created in God's image as ultimately providing the basis for a Christian theology of human value. I shall leave aside such questions as the relationship of image and likeness of God and the extent to which these concepts are entangled by patristic authors with the Platonic conception that likeness to God is the *telos* of human endeavor. The earliest Christian apologist who seems to imply the concept of *imago Dei* as a basis for the condemnation of abortion and infanticide is Clement of Alexandria (second century, [40], pp. 162–163). Even if the *imago Dei* may be defaced by human will, obstinacy, and sin, such could not be the case with the fetus and the newborn infant. Such an assertion obviously would include the sickly and deformed newborn as possessing the *imago Dei*. But what of the extreme end of the continuum of which I spoke earlier, the monstrous or grossly deformed?

Augustine, in the *City of God* 16.8, comments on the tremendous diversity among people, enormous racial differences, and whole tribes of people who seem to us to be monstrous. He then says,

If whole peoples have been monsters, we must explain the phenomenon as we explain the individual monsters who are born among us. God is the Creator of all; He knows best where and when and what is, or was, best for Him to create, since He deliberately fashioned the beauty of the whole out of both the similarity and dissimilarity of. its parts. . . . I know men who were born with more than five fingers or toes, which is one of the slightest variations from the normal, but it would be a shame for anyone to be so silly as to suppose that, because he did not know why God did this, the Creator could make a mistake in regard to the number of fingers on a man's hand. Even in cases of greater variations, God knows what He is doing, and no one may rightly blame His work. . . . It would be impossible to list all the human offspring who have been very different from the parents from whom they were certainly born. Still, all these monsters undeniably owe their origin to Adam ([4], vol. 7, pp. 502–503).

Later in the same work (22.12), Augustine says that pagans mock the idea of the resurrection of the dead, referring to various physical defects as well as "all the human monstrosities that are born", and then ask, "What kind of resurrection will there be in cases like these?" [(4], vol. 8, p.459). Augustine, in his *Enchiridion* 87, specifically addresses the question of the resurrection of the grossly deformed or human 'monstrosities'.

. . . concerning monsters which are born and live, however quickly they die, neither is resurrection to be denied them, nor is it to be believed that they will rise again as they are, but rather with an amended and perfected body. God forbid that that double-membered man recently born in the East – about whom most trustworthy brethen, who saw him, have reported, and Jerome the priest, of holy memory, left written mention – God forbid, I say, that we should think that at the resurrection there will be one such double man, and not rather two men, as would have been the case had twins been born. And so all other births which, as having some excess or some defect or because of some conspicuous deformity, are called monsters, will be brought again at the resurrection to the true form of human nature, so that one soul will have one body, and no bodies will cohere together, even those that were born in this condition, but each, apart, for himself, will have as his own those members whose sum makes the complete human body ([4], vol. 4, pp. 442–443).

The *imago Dei*, with its attendant value, rights, and responsibilities, attached in early Christian thought to the newborn, whether healthy or sickly, maimed, deformed, monstrous, indeed to that whole continuum of the defective, in vivid contrast to the attitudes and practices of pagan antiquity. The Christian concept of *imago Dei* provided both the basis and the structure for the idea of inalienable rights and of intrinsic human value that has prevailed in Western society nearly until the present.

Western Washington University
Bellingham, Washington, U.S.A.

ACKNOWLEDGEMENT

This publication was suported in part by NIH Grant LM04108 from the National Library of Medicine. I wish to thank Dr. Gary B. Ferngren for his criticism of an earlier draft of this paper.

NOTES

[1] Plato variously recommends that women not bear children before age 20 ([35], 460E) or age 16 ([34], 785B). Aristotle recommends 18 as the minimum age ([3], 1335a). Their concern is with eugenics.

[2] For a discussion of Plato's and Aristotle's views on human value, see [21] and [40].

[3] The prevalence of exposure in classical antiquity has been debated by modern scholars. For some specialized studies see [5, 7, 9, 16, 19, 39, 48]. Engels' assessment appears correct: "After careful analysis of the literacy evidence, earlier studies concerning the exposure of children (and any resultant infanticide) have established that the practice was of negligible importance in Greek and Roman society" ([16], p. 112). It has been popularly assumed that the exposure of female newborns was extremely common. Engels convincingly argues that the high level of female infanticide assumed for classical antiquity by some scholars would have produced demographic consequences of a catastrophic nature. It is, of course, important to bear in mind that exposure is an ambiguous word and that very likely exposure, unless excessive, may well have affected the population relatively little since probably the majority of exposed infants were reared. Sometimes exposure is infanticide; sometimes it is simply abandonment.

[4] J. W. Jones writes of Ancient Greece generally that "neither Greek public opinion nor Greek law frowned on the practice [of exposure], if the exposure was not delayed beyond a few days after birth" ([25], p. 288). Thebes, during the early centuries of the Christian era, may possibly be an exception, if Aelian (*Varia Historia* 2.7) can be trusted (for which see [19], p. 289). Speaking only of Athens, Harrison says that while "there seems general agreement that there was probably no explicit enactment conferring the right to expose", nevertheless there is "no reason to doubt that the father had this absolute discretion and that the right of exposure was more than a purely formal one" ([23], p. 71 and Note 1). Putting this in other terms, he says that an Athenian father's right to expose his child is "perhaps better expressed as the absence of a duty to introduce it into the family" ([23] p. 73) or "the right to expose should perhaps be thought of as the absence of a duty to rear" ([23], p. 74 Note 2). The assertion made by the late second or early third century A.D. physician-philosopher Sextus Empiricus, in his *Outlines of Pyrrhonism* 3.211, that "Solon gave the Athenians the law . . . by which he allowed each man to slay his own child" [42] can be confidently rejected ([23], p. 71, Note 2). It can be categorically asserted that the Athenian father never "enjoyed a power remotely resembling the Roman father's *ius vitae ac necis*" ([23], p. 74), that is "power of life and death" over his children. That power is, of course, the well-known Roman father's *patria potestas*. The question of the legality of exposure in Roman law is entangled in the complexity of the changing *patria potestas* during the imperial period as well as the development of laws governing the parental reclaiming of exposed children reared by others, either as free or slaves, and the sale of free newborn as slaves. The Roman father's authority to put his children to death appears not to have been rescinded until the reign of the first Christian emperor, Constantine, who in 318 promulgated a law concerning parricide, i.e., the killing of parents and children (*Codex Justinianus* 9.17.1, [12], vol. 2, p. 379). In 374, Valentinian enacted a statute concerning homicide making the killing of an infant a capital offense (*Codex Justinianus* 9.16.7, [12], vol. 2, p. 379). In the same year he issued another statute which seems unambiguously to forbid exposure of infants. It begins, *Unusquisque subolem suam nutriat. Quod si exponendam putaverit, animadversioni quae constituta est subiacebit* ("Everyone should support his own offspring, and anyone who thinks that he can expose his child shall be subject to the penalty prescribed by law."*Codex Justinianus* 8.51.2 [12], vol. 2, p. 361). While this seems clear enough, is the penalty referred to here that of Constantine's law of 318 concerning parricide, or is there an even earlier law to which this legislation of 374 has reference? This question is raised in great part by a statement made by the great Roman jurist Paul in his *Sententiae* (third century): *Necare videtur non tantum*

is qui partum praefocat, sed et is qui abicit et qui alimonia denegat et is qui publicis locis misericordiae causa exponit, quam ipse non habet. ("Not only he who strangles a child is held to kill it, but also he who abandons it, or denies it food, as well as he who exposes it in a public place for the purpose of arousing the pity which he himself does not feel." The better manuscripts read *praefocat* = strangle; some read *perfocat* = smother. *Digest* 25.3.4, [12], vol. 1, p. 366). Paul is here obviously defining *necare*. The exact significance of the passage for the right of the Roman father to kill his children – or to expose them – cannot be dogmatically asserted. For a discussion, see [39]. On *patria potestas*, see [8], Section 38.

[5] On which see [32].

[6] See, for example [31].

[7] For an interesting discussion, see the chapter entitled *Prodigium and Morality* in [6], pp. 93ff.

[8] For an interesting discussion of the minor role of pediatrics in ancient medicine, see [18].

[9] See, e.g., Justine Martyr, *The First Apology* 27 ([27], pp. 63–64), Tertullian, *Apology* 9 [47], Clement of Alexandria, *Christ the Educator* 21 ([11], p. 217), and Lactantius, *The Divine Institute* 6.20 ([1], vol. 7, p. 187).

[10] See, e.g., Minucious Felix, *Octavius* 30 [30], *Constitutions of the Holy Apostles* 8.3 ([1], vol. 7, p. 466), Justin Martyr, *The First Apology* 27 ([27], pp. 63–64), Lactantius *The Divine Institutes* 5.9 ([1], vol. 7, p. 144–145), Tertullian, *Apology* 9 [47] and *Ad Nationes* 1.15 ([1], vol. 3, pp. 133–134), *The Didache* 2 ([2], vol. 1, pp. 310–313), *The Epistle of Barnabas* 19.5 ([2], vol. 1, pp. 402–403), and *The Epistle to Diognetus* 5.6 ([2], vol. 2, pp. 360–361). For a discussion, see Giordani, [20], pp. 243–252.

BIBLIOGRAPHY

1. *The Ante-Nicene Fathers*: various dates, A. Roberts and J. Donaldson (eds.), Eerdmans, Grand Rapids, Michigan.
2. *The Apostolic Fathers*: 1912–13, K. Lake (trans.), Harvard University Press, Cambridge, Massachusetts.
3. Aristotle: 1932, *Politics*, H. Rackham (trans.), Harvard University Press, Cambridge, Massachusetts.
4. Augustine: various dates, *Writings of Saint Augustine*, various trans., The Catholic University of America Press, Washington, D.C.
5. Bennett, H.: 1923, 'The Exposure of Infants in Ancient Rome', *Classical Journal* 18, 341–351.
6. den Boer, W.: 1979, *Private Morality in Greece and Rome: Some Historical Aspects*, E. J. Brill, Leiden, Netherlands.
7. Bolkestein, H: 1922, 'The Exposure of Children at Athens and the ἐγχυτρίστριαι', *Classical Philology* 17, 222–239.
8. Buckland, W. W.: 1952, *A Text-Book of Roman Law from Augustus to Justinian*, 2nd. ed., Cambridge University Press, Cambridge, Massachusetts.
9. Cameron, A.: 1932, 'The Exposure of Children and Greek Ethics', *Classical Review* 46, 105–114.
10. Cicero: 1928, *Laws*, C. W. Keyes (trans.), Harvard University Press, Cambridge, Massachusetts.

11. Clement of Alexandria: 1954, *Christ the Educator*, S. P. Wood (trans.), The Catholic University of America Press, Washington, D.C.
12. *Corpus Juris Civilis*: various dates, P. Krueger *et al.* (eds.), Weidmann, Dublin and Zurich.
13. Curtius: 1946, *History of Alexander*, J. C. Rolfe (trans.), Harvard University Press, Cambridge, Massachusetts.
14. Diodorus of Sicily: 1933–1957, *Library of History*, C. H. Oldfather *et al.* (trans.), Harvard University Press, Cambridge, Massachusetts.
15. Dionysius of Halicarnassus: 1937–1950, *Roman Antiquities*, E. Cary (trans.), Harvard University Press, Cambridge, Massachusetts.
16. Engels, D.: 1980, 'The Problem of Female Infanticide in the Greco-Roman World', *Classical Philology* **75**, 112–120.
17. Epictetus: 1925–1928, *Discourses*, W. A. Oldfather (trans.), Harvard University Press, Cambridge, Massachusetts.
18. Etienne, R.: 1976–1977, 'Ancient Medical Conscience and the Life of Children', *Journal of Psychohistory* **4**, 127–161.
19. Feen, R. H.: 1983, 'Abortion and Exposure in Ancient Greece: Assessing the Status of the Fetus and "Newborn" from Classical Sources', in W. B. Bondeson *et al.* (eds.), *Abortion and the Status of the Fetus*, D. Reidel, Dordrecht, Holland, pp. 283–299.
20. Giordani, I. 1977, *The Social Message of the Early Fathers*, A. Zizzamia (trans.), St. Paul Editions, Boston, Massachusetts.
21. Golding, M. P. and Golding N. H.: 1975, 'Population Policy in Plato and Aristotle: Some Value Issues', *Arethusa* **8**, 345–358.
22. Goodenough, E. R.: 1968, *The Jurisprudence of the Jewish Courts in Egypt: Legal Administration by the Jews under the Early Roman Empire as Described by Philo Judaeus*, Philo Press, Amsterdam, Holland.
23. Harrison, A. R. W.: 1968, *The Law of Athens: The Family and Property*, Clarendon, Oxford, United Kingdom.
24. Heliodorus: 1957, *An Ethiopian Romance*, M. Hadas (trans.), University of Michigan Press, Ann Arbor, Michigan.
25. Jones, J. W.: 1956, *The Law and Legal Theory of the Greeks*, Clarendon, Oxford, United Kingdom.
26. Josephus: 1926, *Against Apion*, H. Thackeray (trans.), Harvard University Press, Cambridge, Massachusetts.
27. Justin Martyr: 1948, *Writings of Saint Justin Martyr*, T. B. Falls (trans.), The Catholic University of America Press, Washington, D.C.
28. Livy: 1919–1951, *Histories*, B. O. Foster *et al.* (trans.), Harvard University Press, Cambridge, Massachusetts.
29. Lloyd, G. E. R.: 1983, *Science, Folklore and Ideology: Studies in the Life Sciences in Ancient Greece*, Cambridge University Press, Cambridge, Massachusetts.
30. Minucius Felix: 1931, *Octavius*, G. H. Rendell (trans.), Harvard University Press, Cambridge, Massachusetts.
31. Mulhern, J. J.: 1975, 'Population and Plato's Republic', *Arethusa* **8**, 265–281.
32. Oppenheimer, J. M.: 1975, 'When Sense and Life Begin: Background for a Remark in Aristotle's Politics (1335b24)', *Arethusa* **8**, 331–343.
33. Oribasius: 1928–1933, *Oribasii Collectiones Medicae*, I. Reader (ed.), Hakkert, Amsterdam, Holland.

34. Plato: 1926, *The Laws*, R. G. Bury (trans.), Harvard University Press, Cambridge, Massachusetts.
35. Plato: 1930–1935, *Republic*, P. Shorey (trans.), Harvard University Press, Cambridge, Massachusetts.
36. Plato: 1921, *Theaetetus*, H. N. Fowler (trans.), Harvard University Press, Cambridge, Massachusetts.
37. Plutarch: 1914–1926, *The Parallel Lives*, B. Perrin (trans.), Harvard University Press, Cambridge, Massachusetts.
38. Polybius: 1922–1927, *The Histories*, W. R. Paton (trans.), Harvard University Press, Cambridge, Massachusetts.
39. Radin, M.: 1925, 'Exposure of Infants in Roman Law and Practice', *Classical Journal* **20**, 337–342.
40. Rist, J. M.: 1982, *Human Value: A Study in Ancient Philosophical Ethics*, E. J. Brill, Leiden, Netherlands.
41. Seneca: 1928–1935, *Moral Essays*, J. W. Basore (trans.), Harvard University Press, Cambridge, Massachusetts.
42. Sextus Empiricus: 1933, *Outlines of Pyrrhonism*. R. G. Bury (trans.), Harvard University Press, Cambridge, Massachusetts.
43. Soranus: 1956, *Gynecology*, O. Temkin (trans.), The Johns Hopkins University Press, Baltimore, Maryland.
44. Strabo: 1917–1932, *Geography*, H. J. Jones (trans.), Harvard University Press, Cambridge, Massachusetts.
45. Tacitus: 1914, *Germany*, H. Hutton (trans.), Harvard University Press, Cambridge, Massachusetts.
46. Tacitus: 1925–1931, *The Histories*, C. H. Moore (trans.), Harvard University Press, Cambridge, Massachusetts.
47. Tertullian: 1931, *Apology*, T. R. Glover (trans.), Harvard University Press, Cambridge, Massachusetts.
48. Van Hook, L.: 1920, 'The Exposure of Infants at Athens', *Transactions of the American Philological Society* **51**, 134–145.

GARY B. FERNGREN

THE *IMAGO DEI* AND THE SANCTITY OF LIFE: THE ORIGINS OF AN IDEA

"If you don't know where you are going," said the late Archbishop of Canterbury, William Temple, "it is sometimes helpful to know where you've come from." Ours is an age in which human values, in the pluralistic context of Western culture, are in a constant state of flux and redefinition. Basic medical ethics of the Western world is deeply indebted to Graeco-Roman medicine (e.g., as in the Hippocratic Oath), as well as to the moral and ethical systems that grew out of Judaism and early Christianity. Although historical investigations do not provide ready solutions to current problems, they can prove beneficial in increasing our sensitivity to the historical and moral framework of the dilemmas of modern medicine, particularly to the concern for human values brought to the forefront of public interest by the awesome possibilities of medical technology. The concept of the sanctity or sacredness of human life is such a concern. The religious origin of the concept is indicated by the derivation of the words 'sanctity' and 'sacredness' (from the Latin *sanctus*, 'holy,' and *sacer*, 'consecrated') that have often been applied to human life in the Western tradition. They imply the divinely-sanctioned inviolability of human life, a concept which is firmly imbedded in the Judaeo-Christian heritage, and which has until recent decades been the underlying basis for the belief that every human being is born with certain inalienable rights, the chief of which is the right to live. This belief is grounded in the Jewish doctrine, which was taken over by Christianity, that man (I use the term generically) was created in the image of God (*imago Dei*).

PRE-CHRISTIAN JUDAISM

The concept of the *imago Dei* must be understood in the context of Jewish teaching about God as revealed in the Old Testament.[1] The religion of Israel was unique in the ancient world, particularly if we

R. C. McMillan, H. T. Engelhardt, Jr., and S. F. Spicker (eds.),
Euthanasia and the Newborn, 23–45.
© *1987 by D. Reidel Publishing Company.*

23

contrast it with the religious beliefs of Israel's ancient near-eastern
neighbors. The latter were polytheistic and their religion was centered
on the worship of natural forces, especially those associated with fertility. The earth, sky, and heavenly bodies were divinities. Although the
gods were often personifications of nature, they were depicted in human
or animal form. Many were national or regional gods, limited in locale
and power. By contrast, the religion of Israel conceived of only one
God. Monotheism was the chief characteristic of Israel's belief. Moreover, this God (Yahweh) was regarded as being outside and above
nature, which was created by him. He was transcendent rather than
immanent. He was also a universal God, the God of all peoples. His
power extended over all creation and all nations. Yahweh was often
spoken of in human terms and the Old Testament is rich in anthropo-
morphisms. Yet Israelites thought of them merely as a metaphorical
way of speaking, not as literal descriptions of deity. Yahweh could not
be visibly represented in any form (see Deut. 4:15–19) and Israelites were
prohibited from making idols, which were characteristic of polytheism.
This is one of the distinctive features of the Hebrew religion. Images could
only prove confusing. They revealed nothing of Yahweh's nature, since
he was conceived as a spirit who had no body, and thus their use would
have led to misrepresentation of his character and to idolatry. Precisely
because Israel's religion was rooted in monotheism, ethics and religion
were inseparable, for both were derived from Yahweh. Polytheism
presented no absolute moral standards. The gods were beings like man,
but on a superhuman scale, and not superior to him in moral or spiritual
attributes. The worship of the gods was often mechanical and formal,
based on the idea of a bargain or contract between the worshipper and
his god for their mutual advantage. There was no necessary connection
between morality and religion in the belief-systems of the ancient Near
East. Babylonians, Sumerians, and Egyptians did not ask their gods to
make them good, but to bestow on them, their community, and their
family material blessings. By contrast, the worship of Yahweh demanded holiness of conduct. Yahweh is presented not only as an
all-powerful and sovereign God, but a God of holiness (*qadosh*) whose
power is always exercised in a moral context. Yahweh delights in
goodness and truth but hates evil (Jer. 9:24). The ethical nature of
Israel's laws was rooted in the holiness of Yahweh. The law of Israel,
the Torah, was based on Yahweh's covenant with Israel. When the
Hebrews were delivered from bondage in Egypt Yahweh made a cove-

nant with Israel, which made her his special people. As a condition of maintaining the covenant, Israel was expected to reflect in her community life the character of Yahweh as revealed in the Torah. There is never in the Old Testament an appeal to abstract justice. Yahweh acts in justice; therefore he expects the conduct of his people to be marked by justice. Only by obeying his voice and keeping his commandments can they maintain the continued favor of Yahweh and become the righteous people that he wishes them to be.

In Hebrew thought the nature of Yahweh is represented not by pictorial images but by man himself. Man alone can be called the image of Yahweh because in his very nature and being he reflects his Creator. The *locus classicus* of the Hebrew conception of the *imago Dei* is Genesis 1:26–27:

> Then God said, 'Let us make man in our image, after our likeness; and let them have dominion over the fish of the sea, and over the birds of the air, and over the cattle, and over all the earth, and over every creeping thing that creeps upon the earth.' So God created man in his own image, in the image of God he created him; male and female he created them.[2]

Man is created from the dust of the earth; like the animals he too is a creature. But the manner of his creation and his spiritual nature (clearly implied in the account) set him apart from the animal kingdom. Created last, he is the highest of Yahweh's works and stands at the summit of his created order. The formulaic 'according to its kind' is omitted, as is the command to the earth or water to bring forth animal life. Yahweh resolves, 'Let us make man' (the plural may represent a plentitude of power), and man springs into being immediately at his direct command. Since Irenaeus theologians have attempted to distinguish between 'image' (*ṣelem*) and 'likeness' (*demûth*), but most recent commentators believe that the terms are synonymous. There has, however, been the widest disagreement over the precise meaning of these terms.[3] It is unlikely that a physical resemblance is indicated, for in spite of anthropomorphic imagery the Hebrews declared that Yahweh had no similitude and they were forbidden to make any image of him representing male or female (see Deut. 4:15–16). The *imago Dei* is often taken to refer primarily to man's dominion over Yahweh's creation. His dignity lies in his role as Yahweh's representative, a rational creature possessing erect posture and the faculty of speech, who rules over the animal kingdom as well as the earth generally. This role is set forth in Psalm 8 where man is said to reflect the glory of Yahweh in his rule over Yahweh's creation: "Yet thou hast made him little less than God, and dost crown him with glory and honor" (v. 5). In this capacity man is God's vice-regent on earth; he is exalted above all creation. Implied in his distinction from and superiority to the animal kingdom is his endowment with rationality, self-consciousness, volition (on man's attributes that reflect Yahweh's image see Ecclus. 17:1–11). Hence we may speak of the human personality *in toto* mirroring his image. But there is implied in the image as well the idea that man is a spiritual being capable of communion with Yahweh and morally responsible for his own actions. Man was made to have unbroken fellowship with Yahweh and as an ethical being he was given the capacity for both moral reflection and choice. In Genesis 5:3 we are told that Adam transmitted the divine image to his son Seth and the implication was drawn that by means of procreation it is passed on to successive generations. As a result of Adam's sin, however, death (both physical and spiritual) and disease were imposed as a penalty on all men. This is indicated in the story of the temptation and Fall in Genesis 3. The effect of sin on the image is alluded to in the apocryphal Wisdom of Solomon: "For God created man for incorruption, and made him in the image of his own eternity, but through the devil's envy death entered the world" (2:23–24). There is no indication in the Old Testament, however, that the image of God was believed to be lost. It was diminished because of the Fall, but not totally effaced.

That belief that the image of God in man had implications for the protection of human life is indicated in Genesis 9:6 where Yahweh tells Noah, "Whoever sheds the blood of man, by man shall his blood be shed; for God made man in his own image." According to the Hebrew concept of the human personality man was viewed as a unity rather than in dualistic terms. There were two elements in man's nature, the 'soul' (*nephesh*) and the 'flesh' (*bāśār*). The soul was the principle of life that animated the flesh, but there was no dichotomy between them. The soul was not made to exist apart from the flesh. When Yahweh formed Adam out of the dust of the ground and gave him breath he became a living soul (*nephesh*). "Man does not 'have' a soul," writes James Barr, "he is a soul" ([14], p. 932). Hence to destroy the human body was to destroy the human personality and as such it was an affront to the dignity of God, for man bore the image (and therefore the dignity) of Yahweh. Thus in Hebrew thought human life possessed intrinsic value by virtue of its divine endowment, in contrast to classical (Graeco-Roman) thought, which defined personhood judicially in terms of citizenship, i.e., membership in a family, kinship organization, and state.[4] In that sense life was regarded as sacred. This belief was to become central to Jewish concepts of personhood. According to Samuel Belkin,

the Mishnah declares that God created but a single man in order to teach mankind that whoever destroys a single individual God imputes it on him as if he had destroyed the entire world, and whoever saves the life of a single individual God imputes it on him as if he had saved the entire world ([3], p. 97).

The high value that is attached to human life extended to potential life still in the womb. The fetus was regarded as the creation of Yahweh, who formed it for his own purpose, as in Psalm 139:

For thou didst form my inward parts, thou didst knit me together in my mother's womb. I praise thee, for thou art fearful and wonderful. Wonderful are thy works! Thou knowest me right well; my frame was not hidden from thee, when I was being made in secret, intricately wrought in the depths of the earth. Thy eyes beheld my unformed substance; in thy book were written, every one of them, the days that were formed for me, when as yet there was none of them (vv. 13–16).

Yahweh is depicted as telling Jeremiah, "Before I formed you in the womb I knew you, and before you were born I consecrated you; I appointed you prophet to the nations" (Jer. 1:5; cp. Is. 49:1). Yahweh is even represented as responsible for creating human beings with physical defects. Thus he tells Moses, "Who has made man's mouth? Who makes him dumb, or deaf, or seeing, or blind? Is it not I, the Lord?" (Ex. 4:11). Perhaps it is this understanding of man (even defective man) as reflecting Yahweh's image that imparts a general humaneness to the Mosaic Law as compared with other law-codes of the ancient Near East (e.g., the Code of Hammurabi). There are many provisions of the Torah that protect the rights of the blind and deaf (see, e.g., Lev. 19:14), the weak, the poor, widows and orphans, and even foreigners and slaves, who lie outside the covenant community.

In light of the passages cited, which indicate that Yahweh creates life and sustains it in the womb, it is surprising to find that abortion was not explicitly forbidden by either the Torah or rabbinic Judaism. According to the Torah,

When men strive together, and hurt a woman with child, so that there is a miscarriage, and yet no harm follows, the one who hurt her shall be fined, according as the woman's husband shall lay upon him; and he shall pay as the judges determine. If any harm follows, then you shall give life for life, eye for eye, tooth for tooth, hand for hand, foot for foot, burn for burn, wound for wound, stripe for stripe (Ex. 21:22–25).

This passage indicates that the accidental destruction of the fetus was not a capital offense. Only monetary compensation was exacted for the miscarriage of the fetus, whereas in the case of the death of the mother the *lex talionis* required a life for a life according to the principle that "he who kills a man shall be put to death" (Lev. 24:17). The implication is that the fetus was not considered a soul (*nephesh*), while the mother was. According to the Jewish view, which was clearly enunciated later in the Mishnah, human life began at birth. To be more precise, when the greater part of the fetus had emerged from the womb it was considered a human being. Until that time the fetus could be dismembered to save the life of the mother. But once the head of the fetus had emerged it could not be sacrificed, even if the life of the mother was endangered (Mishna, Oholot, 7:6). The newborn child was regarded as a human being with the same rights as any fully-grown person. At birth every Israelite was regarded as reflecting the image of Yahweh and his life was considered sacred. Hence infanticide was absolutely prohibited. Infant sacrifice ("passing through the fire"), which was a feature of the religious practices of Israel's neighbors, was explicitly forbidden by the Torah (Lev. 18:21 and 20:2) and punished by stoning to death. Nevertheless, it was sometimes practiced during times of national apostasy (see 2 Kings 17:17 and Ps. 106:34–39), though condemned by the prophets. Exposure of infants was a sufficiently common practice to be known to the Israelites (see Ez. 16:5), but given the intrinsic right to life of the newborn it will have been regarded as homicide. Philo (ca 30 B.C. – A.D. 45), although reflecting Hellenistic influences, states the Jewish view of infanticide:

No doubt, the view that the child, while still adhering to the womb below the belly, is part of its future mother is current both among natural philosophers whose life study is concerned with the theoretical side of knowledge and so among physicians of the highest repute. . . . But when the child has been brought to the birth it is separate from the organism with which it was identified and being isolated and self-contained becomes a living animal, lacking nothing of the complements needed to make a human being. And, therefore, infanticide undoubtedly is murder, since the displeasure of the law is not concerned with ages but with a breach to the human race ([3], p. 100).

Emasculation was, like child-sacrifice, a common feature of the polytheistic religions of Israel's neighbors. The practice was condemned in Israel and eunuchs were excluded from participation in the religious life of the nation. According to the Torah, "He whose testicles are crushed or whose male member is cut off shall not enter the assembly of the Lord" (Deut.

23:1). Apparently mutilation, whether accidental or deliberate, was regarded as defacing the image of Yahweh in man ([7], p. 413). Lacking virility, a eunuch was less than a man since he had forfeited an essential part of his human nature, his sexual distinction. No other bodily defect (e.g., blindness or lameness) resulted in exclusion from the congregation of Israel; undoubtedly discouragement of the ancient near-eastern practice of religious castration was a factor in its prohibition.

In the period between the Old and New Testaments the concept of the *imago Dei* underwent development as a result of the growing belief in Judaism of the resurrection of the body. The idea of personal immortality was vague and undeveloped in early Hebrew thought. The dead were believed to go to Sheol, a place of obscurity where they were thought to lead a shadowy existence. In the later Old Testament period belief in the resurrection of the dead begins to appear (see Dan. 12:2). The concept of the immortality of the soul is a Greek idea that is foreign to both Hebrew and Christian thought. In the New as well as the Old Testament man is seen as a unity of body and soul in a mutual relationship. Both will be raised in the judgment, a belief that classical thought found repugnant. Greek thought since the third century B.C. asserted a dualism of body and soul and sought to make the soul independent of the body. This tendency, found in several Hellenistic philosophical sects (e.g., Cynicism and Stoicism), emphasized that the individual should concern himself with the care of his soul, while cultivating an attitude of indifference to or disparagement of the body. This kind of asceticism (which was imported into Christianity in late antiquity) was initially foreign to both Jewish and early Christian thinking. "The Hebrew idea of personality," writes Wheeler Robinson, "is that of an animated body, not (like the Greek) that of an incarcerated soul" ([25], p. 27). The belief that the entire personality (body and soul) shares in the resurrection is expressed in Maccabean times by a Jewish mother in the course of encouraging her sons, who were suffering torture at the hands of the Seleucid King Antiochus IV (ca 167 B.C.):

I do not know how you came into being in my womb. It was not I who gave you life and breath, nor I who set in order the elements within each of you. Therefore the Creator of the world, who shaped the beginning of man and devised the origin of all things, will in his mercy give life and breath back to you again, since you now forget yourselves for the sake of his laws (2 Mac. 7:22–23).

We find here a new aspect of the *imago Dei*. Mankind is seen as sharing in another of Yahweh's attributes, his immortality. Hence one of her sons can offer his hands and tongue to be cut off with the words, "I got these from Heaven, and because of his laws I disdain them, and from him I hope to get them back again" (2 Mac. 7:11). The theme of the resurrection of the body is taken up and developed in the New Testament.

EARLY CHRISTIANITY

The idea of the *imago Dei* undergoes a transformation in the New Testament.[5] The Old Testament concept is found without change in such passages as James 3:9 and 1 Corinthians 11:7, but the emphasis of the New Testament is soteriological and eschatalogical, i.e., it is concerned with the salvation and ultimate destiny of fallen man. The whole tenor of the New Testament represents man as suffering from the consequences of the Fall and the entrance of sin into the world. He continues to bear God's image, but it is an image that is marred and defaced. The fellowship with his Creator is broken, God's revelation of himself is spurned, and man in his character and conduct behaves in a manner that is antithetical to that for which he was made (see Rom. 1:18–2:11). Man experiences God's wrath and, alienated from his Maker, deserves eternal separation from him; unable to help himself, he needs a Saviour. Yet in spite of his sin man remains a creature of infinite value; in spite of man's unfaithfulness, God remains faithful to his covenant promises. He sends his son, Jesus Christ, into the world to be born of a woman, to partake of human flesh in order to give his life for the redemption of mankind. This is the Christian idea of the Incarnation, which is the central theme of the New Testament. It is in Christ that the image of God, obscured and blurred by sin, is restored. In three passages in the New Testament Jesus is referred to as the image of God. In 2 Corinthians 4:4 he is called "the likeness of God." In Colossians 1:15–16 he is "the image of the invisible God, the first-born of all creation; for in him all things were created, in heaven and on earth, visible and invisible, whether thrones or dominions or principalities or authorities – all things were created through him and for him." In both these passages the Greek word *eikōn* is translated 'image,' the same word that is used in the Septuagint to translate the Hebrew *selem*. In Hebrews 1:3 a different word, *charaktēr* ('an engraved stamp, impression, or image') is used, but the idea is similar: "He reflects the glory of God and bears the very stamp of his nature, upholding the universe by his word of power." Christ, then, is not viewed merely as a representation of God, but the perfect representation, the God-man in whom dwells all the fullness of the Godhead bodily. It is only through Christ that man can regain the image of God. Jesus is represented by Paul as the second Adam, who by means of his atoning sacrifice brings about the redemption of a fallen race (see I Cor. 15:42–50): "Just as we have borne the image of the man of dust, we shall also bear the image of the man of heaven" (v. 49). Christ is pictured as the prototype of a redeemed humanity. He is the 'first-born' among many brethren who are predestinated to be conformed to his image (Rom. 8:29). The Christian by repentance and faith is spiritually renewed and is changed by degrees into the likeness of Christ (2 Cor. 3:18). The old nature is to be put off with its sinful habits and the new nature put on (Col. 3:5–17), "which is being renewed in knowledge after the image of its creator" (v. 10) and results in a transformed life that is characterized by righteousness and holiness. There is an eschatalogical element in the process of the Christian's being conformed to the image of Christ. This is found in the hope of the final resurrection of the whole man, body and soul, which will become like Christ (1 John 3:2; Phil. 3:20–21; Col. 3:4). Geoffrey Bromiley summarizes these New Testament themes when he writes,

The original purpose of God, that man be created in His own image and after His likeness, will thus be brought to perfect and glorious fulfillment in the new creation, when the redeemed people of God bear the image of their Lord and Head, who bore the image of sinful man for them, and who is Himself the express image of God ([4], p. 805).

The doctrine of the Incarnation is the major contribution of the New Testament to the concept of the *imago Dei*: "And the Word (*logos*) became flesh (*sarx*) and dwelt among us" (John 1:14a). The Christian understanding of the *imago Dei*, viewed in the light of the Incarnation, was to have two important consequences for practical ethics that became increasingly apparent as Christianity began to penetrate the world of the Roman Empire. Together they represent a radical departure from the social ethics of classical paganism. The first of these consequences was the impetus that the doctrine gave to Christian charity and philanthropy. It is not an overstatement to say that the classical world had no religious or ethical impulse for charity. Philanthropy among the Greeks and Romans did not generally take the form of private charity, nor did it manifest itself in a personal concern for those in need, such as widows, orphans, or the sick.[6] Benevolence instead took the form of civic philanthropy on behalf of the community at large rather than of individuals. The motive was clearly understood to be *philotimia* ('love of honor') or *philodoxia* ('love of glory'). In spite of the growing emphasis in the teaching of the Hellenistic philosophical sects on cosmopolitanism and the brotherhood of man, private charity motivated by sympathy for those in need was discouraged. Stoicism taught a generalized 'love of mankind' (*philanthropia*), but insisted that benevolence and liberality must be based on a rational rather than an emotional response. By contrast, personal concern for the poor and needy was an important theme in the Old Testament which gave rise to the insistence in later Judaism (e.g., in the Apocrypha and the Talmud) that almsgiving is a duty and even the highest virtue. This emphasis was taken over by Christianity and is alluded to often in the pages of the New Testament, where charity is represented as an outgrowth of *agape* ('self-giving love'), which is rooted in the nature of God (1 John 4:8). It was God's great love for mankind that brought about the Incarnation (John 3:16). It was Christ's self-sacrificing love that led to his death on the cross as a ransom for man's redemption. And this same kind of love (*agape*) was expected to characterize those who professed his name. In Colossians 3, where Paul urges Christians to put on a new nature that reflects a life transformed in the image of Christ, he writes: "And above all these put on love (*agape*), which binds everything together in perfect harmony" (v. 14). Just as God loved man, so man was expected to respond to divine love by extending love to his brother, who bore the image of God (John 13:34–35). Love of God and devotion to Christ provided the motivation for love of others that had its practical outworking in charity (Matt. 25:34–40). Compassion was regarded as a manifestation of Christian love (Col. 3:12 and 1 John 3:17) and an essential element of the Christian's obligation to all men. This is succinctly expressed in the *Clementine Homilies*, which were written sometime before 380:

Ye are the image of the invisible God. Whence let not those who would be pious say that idols are images of God, and therefore that it is right to worship them. For the image of God is man. He who wishes to be pious towards God does good to man, because the body of man bears the image of God. But all do not as yet bear his likeness, but the pure mind of the good soul does. However, as we know that man was made after the image and after the likeness of God, we tell you to be pious towards him, that the favour may be accounted as done to God, whose image he is. Therefore it behoves you to give honour to the image of God, which is man – in this wise: food to the hungry, drink to the thirsty, clothing to the naked, care to the sick, shelter to the stranger, and visiting him who is in prison, to help him as you can. And not to speak at length, whatever good things any one wishes for himself, so let him afford to another in need, and then a good reward can be reckoned to him as being pious towards the image of God. And by like reason, if he will not undertake to do these things, he shall be punished as neglecting the image (6 in [24], vol. 8. p. 285).[7]

We find in this sentiment the initial basis for the whole Western tradition of philanthropy and private charity. The classical concept of *philanthropia* was not merely insufficient to provide a motivation for private charity, it actively discouraged it.[8] Christianity, on the other hand, insisted that the love of God required the spontaneous manifestation of love toward one's brothers and that one cannot claim to love God without loving his brother (1 John 4:20–21). 'Pure religion' was defined in part as visiting "orphans and widows in their affliction" (James 1:27). From its very beginning the Christian church collected funds for distribution to the poor and the sick (especially to widows and orphans) and appointed deacons to supervise their care (see Acts 6:1–6 and Justin Martyr, *Apologia* 1. 67). Numerous injunctions can be cited from the early Fathers to visit the sick and care for the poor. Ignatius regarded it as one of the marks of the heretics that "they do not care for the widow, the orphan, or the distressed" (*Epistle to the Smyrnaeans* 6). Several accounts tell of Christians who risked their lives in time of plague to care for the ill even during periods of persecution (see, e.g., Eusebius, *Ecclesiastical History* 7. 22, for a well-known instance in Alexandria in the mid-third century). After the legalization of Christianity by Constantine in 313, hospitals (*xenodochia*) began to be established by Christians in the last quarter of the fourth century. They were recognized by pagans in antiquity as distinctly Christian foundations and they furnish perhaps the most notable manifestation of Christian teaching regarding the duty of helping those in need. The rescue and care of orphans and foundlings was regarded by early Christians as a particularly Christian duty, since it involved in many cases saving the lives of children who had been exposed by their parents.[9] Hence children were often exposed at the doors of churches, where it was expected that they would be cared for. Because the exposure of newborn infants was a widespread feature of pagan society, the number of foundlings was large and Christian orphanages were established for their care. But personal adoption of foundlings remained common among Christian families, as the inscriptional evidence (particularly of epitaphs) from late antiquity attests.

The second consequence of the Christian doctrine of the *imago Dei* for practical ethics was that it provided the basis for the belief that every human life has absolute intrinsic value as a bearer of God's image and an eternal soul for whom Christ died. It has been much debated whether the classical world possessed a religious or philosophical basis for the concept of human dignity (*dignitas humana*) that applied to all mankind. Two recent studies have concluded that this idea cannot be found in classical Greek and Roman authors.[10] The classical world believed in the dignity of man, but it was in the dignity of the virtuous man, the man who possessed *arete* ('excellence, virtue'). This understanding was based on the belief that only a balanced and controlled personality that exhibited the recognized virtues could be deemed virtuous. The Roman concept of *humanitas* was used to describe the humane virtues that were expected to be possessed by educated people, but they were virtues that were thought to characterize only a small group that belonged to the upper class of Roman society. Human dignity, then, was not regarded as intrinsic. Nor was there any concept of inherent human rights. Rights were defined judicially and they depended on membership in a society (a family, kinship group, or state) that granted them. Those who lay outside (foreigners, slaves, foundlings) had no claim to any inherent rights, though in fact they might be granted certain privileges, as were foreigners and slaves on occasion. Inequality was deemed a natural feature of life in the classical world and it did not cause surprise or regret ([10], pp. 273–288). Many examples can be given of the lack of recognition that basic human rights belonged to those who lay outside the protection of society, but three will suffice. With only a few exceptions the Greek state recognized no obligation to care for orphans, who were left to look after themselves as best they could by begging or menial jobs.[11] Slaves continued throughout classical antiquity to be tortured when giving evidence in trials on the assumption that only by means of torture could they be expected to speak the truth. Finally, a recent study has discovered little sympathy in early Greek literature for the deformed or oppressed, an attitude that can be demonstrated to have characterized popular (and official) opinion in virtually every period of classical antiquity.[12] Attitudes to the deformed reflected the belief that health and physical wholeness were essential to human dignity, so much so that life without them was not thought to be worth living.[13] Citizenship, kinship, status, merit, or virtue formed the bases of claims to the possession of human rights or human worth. Those who lacked them (e.g., orphans, slaves, foundlings, the deformed, prisoners) had no claim to the rights that they alone guaranteed or even to a recognition of their human worth.

One might expect that the philosophical sects that arose in the Hellenistic age (and Stoicism in particular) would have provided by their teachings the basis for the belief that all men are endowed with value and therefore possess basic rights. Roman Stoicism was marked in the first two centuries of the Christian era by a cosmopolitanism and humanitarianism that affirmed the brotherhood of all men and the necessity of kindness, beneficence, and humane treatment of every person, civilized or barbarian, slave or free, all of whom were regarded as possessing a divine spark. As promising as this belief appears, it never developed into an explicit claim that all individuals possessed human rights, perhaps because the pantheistic theology of Stoicism prevented the uniqueness of the individual from being fully recognized ([23], pp. 145–152). There were, moreover, characteristics of Stoic doctrine that were not hospitable to the development of the idea of an intrinsic human worth that applied to all men. The Stoics cultivated an apathy to suffering because they believed that pain, sickness, and suffering were indifferent things (*adiaphora*). Hence one finds a kind of hardness in Stoic teaching that has no place for the gentle virtues. As Lecky observes, with particular reference to Stoicism, "friendship rather than love, hospitality rather than charity, magnanimity rather than tenderness, clemency rather than sympathy, are the characteristics of ancient goodness" ([19], vol. 1, pp. 190–191). Although Stoicism aimed at a very high level of moral excellence its practical influence was disappointing. Its suppression of the emotions and elevated morality aimed too high for the ordinary individual, who could not hope to rise to the standard proclaimed by Stoicism. As a result it had little influence on the morality of the masses. It is true that the influence of Stoicism on Roman law was extensive in ameliorating, for example, the treatment of slaves. But the Stoics' indifference to human suffering prevented them from actively seeking the protection of the weak. Anyone who reads very widely in classical literature notices how little human life was valued in antiquity. There was a notable strain of cruelty in Roman society that is perhaps most apparent in the gladiatorial games, which enjoyed enormous popularity among all classes of society (including both men and women) with their spectacles of blood. The games had a debasing and brutalizing effect on the Romans by rendering them insensitive to human suffering as a result of their regularly observing the most gruesome atrocities in the arena. Surprisingly enough, few philosophers raised moral objections to the games. They presumably shared the view of their contemporaries that cruel and unspeakable crimes (such as those presumed to have been committed by men compelled to fight in the arena) deserved punishment in kind. No argument that all men are brothers mitigated that belief. One finds in Stoicism (as in classical thought generally) a profound pessimism about human nature that led to quietism. The Stoics were reluctant to attempt radical change in society or the amelioration of human institutions, believing that they were for the most part incapable of improvement.

In this regard the attitude of the early Christians differed *toto caelo* from that of the Stoics. The Christian belief in the *imago Dei* led them to a stern and uncompromising condemnation of pagan morality in all its aspects. Its tolerance of the elimination of unwanted human life and of the cruelty shown to those whom society had condemned or abandoned was viewed as an indication that Roman society was incurably wicked. Abortion, infanticide, the gladiatorial games, and suicide were attacked in the strongest possible terms. Early Christians showed special concern for the protection of unborn and newborn life. Abortion, though occasionally condemned in classical antiquity, was widely practiced and the fetus (being regarded as part of its mother) enjoyed no legal protection or absolute value. As early as the first century we find abortion condemned in Christian writings for violating God's handiwork. In the Didache the aborted fetus is called a 'moulded image' (*plasma*), i.e., of God (2. 2.). In the Apocalypse of Peter (second century) abortion is said to corrupt 'the work of God who created them' (i.e., children). This theme is reiterated in the numerous examples of condemnation of abortion that are found in the church fathers.[14] The difference in Christian and pagan attitudes towards abortion reflected a difference in how the fetus was perceived. "To the Pagans," writes Lecky, "even when condemning abortion and infanticide, these crimes appeared comparatively trivial, because the victims seemed very insignificant and their sufferings very slight" ([19] vol. 2, p. 22). To Christians, however, the fetus was not only a potential human being but an eternal soul, which, if it died unbaptized, was thought to be consigned forever to limbo or hell. Abortion was regarded by some as worse than murder. Tertullian (ca 160/70 – ca 215/20) explicitly calls abortion homicide:

For us, indeed, as homicide is forbidden, it is not lawful to destroy what is conceived in the womb while the blood is still being formed into a man. To prevent being born is to accelerate homicide, nor does it make a difference whether you snatch away a soul which is born or destroy one being born. He who is man-to-be is man, as all fruit is now in the seed (*Apologeticum ad nationes* 1. 15 in [21], p. 12).

The exposure of newborn children was also condemned in early Christian writings. Whether or not it was forbidden by law under the Empire (this is disputed), it was not punished and it was almost universally practiced and viewed with general indifference. The practice was widely attacked by Christians (see, e.g., Minucius Felix, *Octavius* 30. 2 and 31. 4; and Lactantius 6. 20), who viewed it as a crime hardly less heinous than infanticide, which was apparently punishable in Roman law.

Gladiatorial combat also fell under the condemnation of Christians. The killing of a gladiator in the arena was regarded as murder and the early church refused baptism to practicing gladiators. Christians who participated in the games were excommunicated, while Christians who attended them were denied communion. The games were restricted by imperial legislation beginning with Constantine in 325 A.D. In 404 a monk named Telemachus, who had come to Rome from Asia Minor for that purpose, ran into the amphitheatre and tried to separate the gladiators. He was stoned to death by the angry spectators, but the Emperor Honorius was sufficiently impressed by his heroic attempt to end the cruelty that he abolished gladiatorial combat. The belief that human life was sacred and therefore to be protected led to the idea that the taking of any human life by a Christian was murder. Thus in the first three centuries Christians were forbidden to serve in the military, to act as executioners, or to bring capital charges. While these prohibitions were modified after Christianity became a legal (and later the official) religion of the Empire, the principle behind them continued to influence Christian opinion for centuries afterward. Finally, Christianity emphatically condemned suicide, which had been idealised in classical antiquity as a noble means of death. Christians were encouraged to endure suffering with the help of God's grace rather than to seek to put an end to their lives, and suicide was regarded as self-murder. The only serious debate over the propriety of suicide involved cases in which a woman's chastity was in danger. Augustine discussed the matter at length (*City of*

God 1. 22–27) and his condemnation of suicide (on the ground that it is homicide and precludes the possibility of repentance) proved definitive in settling the question in the early church.

The Christian condemnation of abortion, child-exposure, gladiatorial combat, and suicide, in the long run bore fruit. As the moral climate of the late Roman Empire gradually changed with the spread of Christianity, these practices came to be regarded with increasing disapproval. There were several reasons for the success of Christianity in creating a transformation of moral values in the ancient world that led to a greater sensitivity to human worth in general and to the protection of the weak in particular. In the first place Christianity provided a religious rather than a merely philosophical basis for ethical values. Stoicism had failed to communicate its moral values to the Roman populace at large, while Roman religion had no moral content. Christianity had a wide appeal to a popular audience that Stoicism could never attain even if it had tried. It took over from Judaism the concept that God demanded moral righteousness from his followers and that a failure to obey his will constituted sin. Christianity, unlike Stoicism, did not appeal to virtue; it aimed rather at the eradication of sin and its promise of bliss or suffering in the world to come furnished a powerful motivation for the pursuit of righteousness that appealed to the masses who were left untouched by philosophical argument. By grounding respect for life in the doctrine of the *imago Dei* it rendered the mistreatment of a human being a sin against God. This is expressed in the *Recognitions* of Clement:

What, then, is that honour of God which consists in running from one stone or wooden figure to another, in venerating empty and lifeless figures as deities, and despising men in whom the image of God is of a truth? Yea, rather be assured, that whoever commits murder or adultery, or anything that causes suffering or injury to men, in all these the image of God is violated. For to injure men is a great impiety towards God. Whenever, therefore, you do to another what you would not have another do to you, you defile the image of God with undeserved distresses (5. 23 in [24], vol. 8, pp. 148–149).

It was the transcendent value of human beings that required that they be treated with compassion and respect. Since every man was created in God's image no human life (whether that of a fetus, a newborn, or a deformed individual) lay outside the absolute right to protection. Moreover, Christianity taught that man's moral well-being was as important as his physical protection, that the care of his soul was as necessary as the cure of his body. By moral and spiritual improvement he could be brought closer to the image of God in which he was created. Because the mistreatment of one's fellow man was a sin against God, the early church could and frequently did impose severe sanctions against those who violated its moral teachings. Exclusion from communion, the imposition of severe penance, and excommunication (with its implication of eternal damnation) did much to inculcate the belief that abortion, exposure, and gladiatorial combat were sins of the most heinous sort. Nor did Christianity share the quietism of Stoicism (and of the ancient world generally). Christianity, with its strong strain of moralism, was uncompromising in its desire to eliminate those moral evils that it believed contaminated society. As long as Christians were in a minority they could only protest them. But when, after the conversion of Constantine, they enjoyed influence, they began to press for legislation to eradicate practices that were incompatible with the high value that they attached to human life. The legislation that was introduced in the fourth and fifth centuries concerning the protection of women, children, and slaves, and the prohibition of cruel punishments, was inadequate and inconsistent, and produced less than the intended results. It was partially successful, however, in lessening some undesirable features (such as exposure and infanticide) that had characterized pagan society for centuries.[15]

Finally, the Christian doctrine of the *imago Dei* saved Christianity from being taken captive by the denigration of the body that grew out of the belief that there is a dichotomy between the body and the soul. Dualism was widely held in late antiquity; it is found in Neo-Platonism and Neo-Pythagoreanism, as well as earlier in Stoicism. Disparagement of the body was a *Leitmotiv* of much classical philosophy and it had a strong appeal for Christians. It manifested itself particularly in the rigid asceticism that is found in early monasticism. "Pagans and Christians," writes E. R. Dodds, "(though not all pagans or all Christians) vied with each other in heaping abuse on the body; it was 'clay and gore', 'a filthy bag of excrement and urine'; man is plunged in it as in a bath of dirty water" ([9], p. 29). Against this dualism, which in late antiquity threatened to overwhelm the earlier Christian view of the basic unity of the human personality, the doctrine of the *imago Dei* was used to support a more positive teaching regarding the body. We see this in a pseudepigraphic work attributed to Justin Martyr:

But following our order, we must not speak with respect to those who think meanly of the flesh, and say that it is not worthy of the resurrection nor of the heavenly economy, because, first, its substance is earth; and besides, because it is full of all wickedness, so that it forces the soul to sin along with it. But these persons seem to be ignorant of the whole work of God, both of the genesis and formation of man at the first, and why the things in the world were made. For does not the word say, "Let Us make man in our image, and after our likeness?" What kind of man? Manifestly He means fleshly man. For the word says, "And God took dust of the earth, and made man." It is evident, therefore, that man made in the image of God was of flesh. Is it not, then, absurd to say, that the flesh made by God in His own image is contemptible, and worth nothing? But that the flesh is with God a precious possession is manifest, first from its being formed by Him if at least the image is valuable to the former and artist; and besides its value can be gathered from the creation of the rest of the world. For that, on account of which the rest is made, is the most precious of all to the maker (*On the Resurrection* 7, in [24], vol. 1, p. 297).

The belief that the body as well as the soul is of worth was often obscured in early Christianity, not only in the ascetic movements, but also in the Docetic christologies (which taught that Christ did not occupy a real material body and human nature, but only an apparent body) and in such prominent heresies as Gnosticism and Manichaeism, which held that matter is inherently evil. But as long as the Incarnation was regarded as the central tenet of Christianity and the ultimate redemption and resurrection of the body remained a hope, it was difficult for dualism to prevail in Christian thinking. "It has always been realised in the main tradition of Christianity," writes Herbert Butterfield, "that if the Word was made flesh, matter can never be regarded as evil in itself" ([5], p. 121). The consequences for Western thought were enormous.

LATER DEVELOPMENTS

Of the later developments of the concept of the *imago Dei* we need speak only briefly. Many early church fathers made a distinction between the 'image' (*imago*) and the 'likeness' (*similitudo*) of God. According to Irenaeus (fl. ca 175 – ca 195) and Tertullian the former denotes the bodily form of man and the latter his spiritual nature. Clement of Alexandria (ca 155 – ca 220) and Origen (ca 185 – ca 254) believed that the 'image' referred to man's essential human characteristics, while the 'likeness' denoted those characteristics that were not essential. The latter view was taken over and developed by the Scholastics, who defined the 'image' as that which belonged to man by nature (i.e., his inherent personal and moral endowments), and the 'likeness' as a 'superadded gift' (*donum superadditum*) of righteousness bestowed on man by God at creation and lost in the Fall, which nevertheless left his natural virtues unimpaired and his will free. The Protestant reformers denied the distinction between the *imago* and *similitudo*, Luther seeing the image of God in man's righteousness, which was lost in the Fall, and Calvin finding it in the sum of man's qualities, both natural and spiritual. Although there was a good deal of patristic and mediaeval discussion of the concept, much of it subtle and speculative, the theological refinements led to no modification of the idea of the sanctity of life, which grew out of it.

In the twentieth century the idea of the *imago Dei* has received extensive treatment by theologians. Two in particular, the Swiss Reformed theologian Karl Barth and the German Lutheran theologian Helmut Thielicke, have discussed the concept as it relates to the formulation of medical ethics. Barth sees human life as possessing great value as a creation of God and on the basis of this view he rejects both abortion (with qualifications) and euthanasia, as well as the artificial prolongation of life.[16] According to Thielicke, the basis of human dignity does not lie in an immanent quality of man, but rather in his creation by God and in the fact that Christ died for him. He speaks (as does Barth) of man's "alien dignity" (*dignitas aliena*), "a dignity which is imparted to him and which therefore partakes of the majesty of Him who bestows it" ([28], p. 172). He quotes with approval Thomas Carlyle's statement: "Gentlemen, you place man a little higher than the tadpole. I hold with the ancient Psalmist (Ps. 8): 'Thou hast made him a little lower than the angels'" ([28], p. 185). Thielicke means by this that the nature of man cannot be understood merely in terms of his evolutionary beginnings, but must take into account his status and ultimate destiny: he is a divine creation (a little less than God) who stands under God's protection and is thus inviolable. With this as his informing principle, Thielicke discusses a number of cruxes in modern medical ethics.[17]

The doctrine of the *imago Dei* provided the basis for the understanding of man in the West until the nineteenth century, when Darwin's theory of evolution dealt it a nearly fatal blow. Man came increasingly to be viewed not as God's special creation but as an integral part of the animal world, who was different from lower forms of animal life only because he had been more successful in the struggle for existence and more adaptable within the process of natural selection. Man was not unique, but an accident of nature who differed in degree, not in kind, from the primates. Nearly as revolutionary in its implications for moral and religious ideas was the influence of the new psychology in the early twentieth century. Behaviorism, which sought to study man as a purely physiological organism, was less influential than the psychoanalytic school of Sigmund Freud, which viewed man as an egoistic being motivated by the basic urges of sex, self-preservation, and power. Freud's concept of the unconscious, into which suppressed desires are driven, only to manifest themselves in neurotic behavior, gave rise to the view that man is a product of subconscious and irrational forces. As the ideas of Darwin and Freud became the common property of educated people, the older view of man inevitably declined. Like other aspects of Judaeo-Christian ethics, however, the sanctity-of-life ethic continued to be widely held for a generation or two after the breakup of the theological tradition on which it was based. But the process of secularism (quite apart from medical and scientific advance) has done much in recent years to recast the judgment that all human life is sacred. Moreover, the increasing privatization of belief and the divorce of religious sanctions from public policy and institutions have notably lessened the influence of its theological rationale. One may doubt that the idea of the sanctity of life in its traditional form can continue to exist divorced from the theological concept of the *imago Dei*. It is likely that it will maintain its influence in a pluralistic age like our own only so long as the Judaeo-Christian tradition that gave it birth continues to be a living force that is capable of relating in a meaningful way its belief in the transcendent value of all human life to contemporary (and increasingly difficult) issues in bio-medical ethics.

Oregon State University
Corvallis, Oregon, U.S.A.

ACKNOWLEDGEMENT

This publication was supported in part by NIH Biomedical Research Support Grant RR07079. I thank Dr. Darrel W. Amundsen for his helpful suggestions.

NOTES

[1] For the purpose of this paper I omit discussion of questions of authorship and divergencies of theologies in the Old Testament.
[2] All biblical quotations (including the Apocrypha) are taken from the Revised Standard Version.

[3] On these terms and the concept of the *imago Dei* in the Old Testament generally, see [20]; [30], pp. 144–150; [31], pp. 159–165; [17], pp. 22–39; [15], pp. 166–173; and [16], vol. 2, s.v., εἰκών, pp. 390–392.

[4] See [23], pp. 129–131.

[5] On the idea of the *imago Dei* in the New Testament see [16], vol. 2, s.v., εἰκών, pp. 395–397; [22], pp. 684–685; and [6], pp. 162–164.

[6] See the discussion in [13], pp. 77–88.

[7] Cp. the very similar passage (to which this is clearly related) in the *Recognitions* of Clement 5.23 (in [24], vol. 8, pp. 148–149).

[8] On the lack of a concept of neighborly love that extended to all men, see [8], pp. 62–72; and [11].

[9] In Judaism God was regarded as the father of orphans (see Ps. 68:5) who were regarded as under his protection (see Mal. 3:5 and Deut. 27:19). Perhaps this attitude influenced the early Christian feeling of obligation to care for orphans.

[10] See [23]; and [8], pp. 137–150.

[11] On the classical attitude towards orphans see [8], pp. 37–61. Den Boer observes that "warmth or tenderness are noticeably absent from the sources of the classical period that deal with the fate of orphans" ([8], p. 56).

[12] See [8], p. 128 n. 70, where den Boer refers to a study by W. Burkert. Physical deformity was regarded as a shameful thing. Thus King Croesus of Lydia did not consider his son who was deaf and dumb to be a real son (Herodotus 1. 38. 2) and the Persians were ashamed to be ruled by a governor whose ears had been cut off (Herodotus 3. 73. 1): see [10], p. 279.

[13] See [12], esp. pp. 5–9. Kudlien [18] points out that there developed a concept of relative health in Greece in the fifth century B.C. that accepted less than perfect health as necessary to a good life.

[14] For a discussion of passages from early Christian writers that pertain to abortion see [21], pp. 7–18.

[15] For a summary of the Constantinian legislation see 'Constantinus I,' in [26], vol. 1, pp. 636–637.

[16] See Barth's extensive discussion in [2]. Of particular interest are his treatment of 'Respect for Life' (pp. 324–397) and 'The Protection of Life' (pp. 397–470), which deal with a number of bio-ethical issues.

[17] See [29], pp. 146–186. For an extended discussion by Thielicke of the idea of the *imago Dei* and its implications see [28], pp. 147–170.

BIBLIOGRAPHY

1. Amundsen, D. W. and Ferngren, G. B.: 1982, 'Philanthropy in Medicine: Some Historical Perspectives', in E. E. Shelp (ed.), *Beneficence and Health Care*, D. Reidel, Dordrecht, Holland, pp. 1–31.
2. Barth, K., 1961: *Church Dogmatics III/4: The Doctrine of Creation*, G. W. Bromiley and T. F. Torrance (eds.), T. & T. Clark, Edinburgh.
3. Belkin, S.: 1960, *In His Image: The Jewish Philosophy of Man as Expressed in Rabbinic Tradition*, Abelard-Schuman, London/New York/Toronto.
4. Bromiley, G. W.: 1982, 'Image of God', in G. W. Bromiley (ed.), *The International*

Standard Bible Encyclopedia (rev. ed.), vol. 2, Eerdmans, Grand Rapids, Michigan, pp. 803–805.

5. Butterfield, H.: 1949, *Christianity and History*, Charles Scribner's Sons, New York.

6. Davidson, W. L.: 1915, 'Image of God', in James Hastings (ed.), *Encyclopedia of Religion and Ethics*, vol. 7, Charles Scribner's Sons, New York, pp. 160–164.

7. Delitzsch, F.: 1951 (rpt.), *Biblical Commentary on the Old Testament*, vol. 3: *The Pentateuch*, Eerdmans, Grand Rapids, Michigan.

8. den Boer, W.: 1979, *Private Morality in Greece and Rome: Some Historical Aspects*, E. J. Brill, Leiden.

9. Dodds, E. R.: 1968, *Pagan and Christian in an Age of Anxiety*, Cambridge University Press, Cambridge.

10. Dover, K. J.: 1974, *Greek Popular Morality in the Time of Plato and Aristotle*, Basil Blackwell, Oxford.

11. Downey, G.: 1965, 'Who is My Neighbor? The Greek and Roman Answer', *Anglican Theological Review* **47**, 2–15.

12. Ferngren, G. B. and Amundsen, D. W.: 1984, 'Virtue and Health/Medicine in Pre-Christian Antiquity', in E. E. Shelp (ed.), *Virtue and Medicine*, D. Reidel, Dordrecht, Holland, pp. 3–22.

13. Hands, A. R.: 1968, *Charities and Social Aid in Greece and Rome*, Cornell University Press, Ithaca.

14. Hastings, J., Grant, F. C., and Rowley, H. H.: 1963, *Dictionary of the Bible* (rev. ed.), Charles Scribner's Sons, New York.

15. Jacob, E.: 1958, *Theology of the Old Testament*, Arthur W. Heathcote and Philip J. Allcock (trans.), Harper & Row, New York.

16. Kittel, G. and Friedrich, G. (eds.): 1964–1967, *Theological Dictionary of the New Testament*, 10 vols., G. W. Bromiley (trans.), Eerdmans, Grand Rapids, Michigan.

17. Knight, G.: 1959, *A Christian Theology of the Old Testament*, John Knox Press, Richmond, Virginia.

18. Kudlien, F.: 1974, 'The Old Greek Concept of "Relative" Health', *Journal of the History of the Behavioral Sciences* **9**, 53–59.

19. Lecky, W. E.: 1869, 1902, *History of European Morals: From Augustus to Charlemagne*, 2 vols., Longmans Green, London.

20. Miller, J. M.: 1972, 'In the "Image" and "Likeness" of God', *Journal of Biblical Literature* **91**, 289–304.

21. Noonan, J. T., Jr.: 1970, 'An Almost Absolute Value in History', in John T. Noonan, Jr. (ed.), *The Morality of Abortion: Legal and Historical Perspectives*, Harvard University Press, Cambridge, Massachusetts.

22. Porteous, N. W.: 1962, 'Image of God', in G. A. Buttrick (ed.), *The Interpreter's Dictionary of the Bible*, vol. 2, Abingdon, Nashville, pp. 682–685.

23. Rist, J. M.: 1982, *Human Value: A Study in Ancient Philosophical Ethics*, E. J. Brill, Leiden.

24. Roberts, A. and Donaldson, J. (eds.): 1885–1896 (rpt. 1956), *The Ante-Nicene Fathers*, 10 vols., Eerdmans, Grand Rapids, Michigan.

25. Robinson, H. W.: 1926, *The Christian Doctrine of Man*, T. & T. Clark, Edinburgh.

26. Smith, W. and Wace, H.: 1877–1887, *A Dictionary of Christian Biography*, 4 vols., Little, Brown, & Co., Boston.

27. Temkin, O., Frankena, W. K., and Kadish, S. H.: 1976, *Respect for Life in Medicine, Philosophy, and the Law*, Johns Hopkins University Press, Baltimore.

28. Thielicke, H., 1966: *Theological Ethics*, vol. 1, William H. Lazareth (ed.), Fortress Press, Philadelphia.

29. Vaux, K. (ed.): 1970, *Who Shall Live?* Fortress Press, Philadelphia.

30. von Rad, Gerhard: 1962, *Old Testament Theology*, vol. 1, D. M. G. Stalker (trans.), Harper & Row, New York and Evanston.

31. Wolff, H. W.: 1974, *Anthropology of the Old Testament*, Margaret Kohl (trans.), Fortress Press, Philadelphia.

GARY B. FERNGREN

THE STATUS OF DEFECTIVE NEWBORNS FROM LATE ANTIQUITY TO THE REFORMATION

FORMATIVE INFLUENCES

The triumph of Christianity in the fourth century led to profound changes in the manners and morals of the Roman world. Although it remained an illicit religion for the first three centuries of the Christian era, Christianity grew steadily in spite of vigorous persecution. In 313 Constantine, the first Christian emperor, issued the Edict of Milan, which ended Roman persecution of Christianity and granted Christians freedom of worship. Except for Julian the Apostate, who reigned briefly (361–63), all subsequent Roman emperors were Christians. Just as earlier emperors had given state support to Roman paganism, the Christian emperors favored Christianity in both policy and legislation. They tolerated paganism, which remained for most of the fourth century the official Roman religion. It declined rapidly, however, and in 382 the emperor Gratian withdrew public support of pagan worship. Finally, in 392 the emperor Theodosius ordered the closure of pagan temples, banned all public pagan worship, and made Christianity the state religion. Thus more than a millennium of continuous religious tradition came to an official end in Rome. Paganism continued to exist in private belief and worship, but Christianity was increasingly widely adopted. As pagan religious traditions were swept away, so too were pagan attitudes to moral questions. For some three centuries Christians had vigorously attacked the pagan acceptance of abortion, exposure, and infanticide. In the fourth century they were in a position to issue legislation that reflected Christian morals. In 318 Constantine made it a punishable offence (parricide) for a father to kill his child. In 329 he legalized the sale of children and in 331 decreed that those who had raised exposed children need not give them up to their parents. The latter two laws seem to have been intended to give to poor children who might be exposed a greater chance of being kept alive. Not until 374 was infanti-

R. C. McMillan, H. T. Engelhardt, Jr., and S. F. Spicker (eds.),
Euthanasia and the Newborn, 47–64.
© 1987 *by D. Reidel Publishing Company.*

cide punishable by law and every parent required to nourish his own
offspring. The wording of this constitution is ambiguous, but it seems to
have forbidden ordinary exposure. The prohibition of parents from
attempting to reclaim children whom they had exposed was repeated by
a constitution of 412. Justinian (529–65) extended the protection of
newborns by prohibiting their subjection to any form of servitude by
those who rescued them. Children who had been exposed were granted
absolute freedom from both their natural parents and their adoptive
parents. Abortion, though repeatedly condemned by Christian moralists, seems not to have been forbidden by law even under Christian
emperors.

Roman legislation regarding the protection of newborns was perhaps
less extensive after the legalization of Christianity than one might expect
and it is not likely in itself to have seriously diminished the practices that
it prohibited. Far more significant, and ultimately more influential, were
the decisions taken by early church councils, both local and ecumenical.
The period between 300 and 600 witnessed the earliest conciliar legislation regarding abortion and infanticide.[1] The first council to speak
specifically to the practice of infanticide was the local council held at
Elvira in Spain in about 305. Two canons dealt with infanticide (the
definition seems to have included abortion as well). Canon 63 excluded
a baptized woman who had committed adultery and destroyed her child
even from death-bed communion. According to Canon 68 a female
catechumen who had committed the same double sin could be baptized
only at the end of her life. The severe discipline of the Council (excommunication in the former case, which meant exclusion from heaven, and
lifelong penance in the latter) indicates the seriousness of the sin in the
eyes of the church. The Council of Ancyra, which met in Asia Minor in
314, while admitting that the ancient punishment for adultery and
infanticide was penance for life, nevertheless limited penance to ten
years. The Council of Lerida, held in Spain in 524, further reduced the
period of penance to seven years. The canons of the Council of Ancyra
were frequently cited in later discussions of abortion and exposure and
its penitential discipline of ten years was widely adopted in both East
and West.

The growth of the penitential system provided a powerful means of
influencing moral behavior. Behind this form of ecclesiastical discipline
lay the belief that anyone excommunicated from the visible church lost
his salvation (*extra ecclesiam nulla salus*). By virtue of the power of the

keys the church had the right to deprive communicants, either temporarily or absolutely, from fellowship, as well as to restore them, following penance, to the fold of the church. It was believed that the discipline of the church was ratified in heaven. Hence the growth of church canons, in an environment increasingly influenced by theological considerations, had much greater influence on those who sought salvation than did the law of the state. The harsh penalties imposed by successive church councils, while by no means eradicating infanticide and abortion, did much to portray them as sins of the most heinous sort, which required (in the case of baptized Christians) either lengthy penance or excommunication.

Whereas the Romans drew a marked distinction between abortion and infanticide, regarding the fetus as a *spes animantis* rather than an *infans*,[2] Christians in the early centuries of the Christian era tended to speak of them together as parricide.[3] In classical antiquity parricide was the name given to the killing of a close relative and it was regarded as the most shocking, because it was the most unnatural, of crimes. Christians applied this odious charge to the destruction of both the unborn fetus and the newborn child, and even to the use of contraception, because it prevented the existence of life.[4] Hence, in contradistinction to the Roman pagans, Christians looked at conception, gestation, birth, and nurture as a continuous process, and interference with that process at any point as obstruction of the development of human life. It was deemed as morally repugnant for parents to prevent the development of their own offspring as it was to kill their own parent. While abortion, exposure, and infanticide are each explicitly condemned in early Christian writings, they are often lumped together for practical purposes in the canons of early councils. For this reason it is sometimes difficult to determine precisely which is being discussed.

THE STATUS OF THE FETUS

In the fourth century a new feature was interjected into the Christian discussion of the value of the fetus. Theologians began to speak of the distinction between the unformed and formed fetus. The distinction was based on the Septuagint translation of Exodus 21:22–23, which requires that a life be given for a life only if the embryo is formed (a qualification that is lacking in the original Hebrew text). The earliest indication that this distinction was discussed in connection with penitential discipline comes from Basil the Great (330–379), who defines abortion as homicide and says that the 'subtle distinction' between a completely formed and an unformed fetus must be rejected (Epistle 188, Canon 2). The canons of Basil were later to exercise great influence, particularly in the Eastern church, on the subject of abortion. According to Lactantius (ca 240 – ca 320) the fetus is formed and ensouled after forty days. In a similar vein Cyril of Alexandria (d. ca 444) believed that the fetus was not human until after forty days (*De Ador. in Spir. et Ver. 8*). Both writers were probably influenced by the Aristotelian theory of the animation of the fetus. Aristotle held that the embryo at conception possesses only a nutritive soul. It later receives a sensitive soul (*De Gen. Anim.* 2.3). The formation of the fetus and the infusion of the rational soul occur in the male forty days after and in the female ninety days after conception (*Historia Animalium* 7.3).

While theologians debated for several centuries whether animation occurs at the time of the formation of the fetus, the distinction between the unformed and formed fetus came to underlie much of the discussion of abortion during the Middle Ages. It also influenced penitential discipline imposed for the sin of abortion. Augustine, commenting on the Septuagint version of Exodus 21:22–23, distinguishes between the penalty in the Mosaic law for killing an unformed fetus and that for killing a formed fetus (he used a Latin translation of the Septuagint). The embryo, he observes, was *informatus* before it was endowed with a soul and its destruction was punishable with only a fine. Once the embryo is endowed with a soul it is *formatus* and an animate being. Hence its destruction was homicide and was punished by death (*Quaestiones in Exodum* 80). Jerome, too, recognized the distinction. The killing of a fetus, he writes in a letter to Algasius, is not considered homicide until the elements that are formed in the uterus take on the appearance and limbs of a human being (Epistle 121. 4). Augustine's views were particularly influential in the subsequent discussion of the matter. Pope Gregory III (731–741) followed Basil in limiting the penance for abortion to ten years; but unlike Basil he distinguished between the formed and unformed fetus and in the latter case required only a single year's penance. The passage from Augustine, together with Jerome's opinion, was included by Gratian in his *Decretum*, which he composed in *ca* 1140 to harmonize discordant opinions of earlier canonical authorities. It thereby exercised great influence in the later Middle Ages. On the other hand, the Sixth Ecumenical Council, which met at

Constantinople in 680–81, made abortion a capital crime and recognised no distinction between earlier and later stages of embryonic formation, a practice that was consistent with earlier conciliar legislation.

We see by the sixth century the existence of two separate but parallel traditions regarding abortion in the West ([6], pp. 63–64). One (that of the penitential canons) viewed abortion only of the formed fetus as homicide. The other (that of conciliar legislation) condemned all abortions, together with infanticide, as murder. These two traditions continued throughout the Middle Ages. There is no indication that the early Christian writers on the subject of abortion intended, by making a distinction between the formed and unformed fetus, to indicate that the unformed fetus was of little value. Christian moralists had always insisted that all life, as God's creation, was sacred from the moment of conception, and that potential life was to be valued. Neither Jerome nor Augustine sanctioned the abortion of an unformed fetus; both in fact condemned it.[5] The question at issue was how the church should deal with those who were guilty of that sin. There seemed to be scriptural support for making a distinction in the required penance, and the Septuagint translation of Exodus 21:22–23 was interpreted in the light of traditional scientific theories of embryonic development. With the rediscovery of Aristotle's works in the late Middle Ages, Aristotle's distinction between the formation of the male and female fetus was adopted by scholastic theologians in discussions of the animation of the fetus. But in general one can say that by the sixth century most of the theological rationale for the church's position had been hammered out. The abortion of a formed fetus constituted homicide; that of an unformed fetus was regarded as a grave sin, but not as homicide. There was little further development during the next thousand years.

THE STATUS OF NEWBORNS

The question of ensoulment, which occasioned so much discussion among Christian theologians in late antiquity and the Middle Ages, has some bearing on the question of the status of newborns. As we have seen, early Christian writers condemned the prevention or destruction of human life at any point, whether by means of contraception, abortion, exposure, or infanticide. Both Augustine and Jerome admitted that they could not determine precisely when human life begins. Augustine, in fact, doubted that the matter was capable of solution (*De anima eius origine* 4. 4). Yet their inability to reach a satisfactory answer did not prevent them from vigorously opposing abortion, even of the unformed fetus. According to Augustine, God causes the birth of each child; it is he who forms each body and gives it life and nourishment. Just as the fetus in its earliest stages is to be protected, so newborn children are to be preserved, irrespective of the circumstances of their conception or their physical or mental condition. Augustine makes frequent reference to defective children in his treatise *Contra Iulianum*. He does so in the context of his defense of original sin (which Julianus denied) and the necessity of baptism to remove it. The child born of a prostitute, he says, is sometimes adopted by God as his own son (6. 43). Even children born of adultery are God's creation (3. 16). So too are those newborns who have deformities. Augustine believes that birth-defects are due to original sin. "Indeed, if nothing deserving punishment passes from parents to infants, who could bear to see the image of God, which is, you say, adorned with the gift of innocence, sometimes born feeble-minded, since this touches the soul itself?" (3. 4) "If there were no such sin, then infants, bound by no evil, would suffer nothing evil in body or in soul under the great power of the just God" (3. 5). God distributes physical or mental defects among men just as he distributes different personalities, according to his hidden judgement. No one can escape suffering in this life (4. 16). Deformities can be transmitted from parents to children, for God in creating persons does not act contrary to the laws that he has established in human generation (5. 14). In spite of the fact that many infants are born with defects, it is the true and good God who forms all bodies, even monsters, who are called 'errors of nature' (5. 53). Elsewhere he says that defective newborns have a place in God's design. Even though a child is born feeble-minded because of an accidental defect, he is nevertheless created a man by the work of God (*Operis imperfecti contra Iulianum* 3. 160–61). Just as Augustine is inclined to believe that aborted fetuses take part in the resurrection of the dead, so he believes that monsters (i.e., defective persons) will be raised up as well, with perfect bodies that will replace their defective bodies (*Enchiridion* 84–87).

Augustine's assertion that monsters are creatures of God who were made for a purpose, with the implication that they therefore enjoy the right to live, constitutes perhaps the earliest defence of the intrinsic personhood of defective newborns in the Western tradition. Like Augustine's concern for the unformed fetus, it grew out of the early Christian doctrine that man is created in God's image. The theological rationale is found in Judaism as well, but the implications were not as fully developed. While the rights of defective children in particular were seldom specifically mentioned by the early Christians, concern for their welfare may be surmised from two factors. The first is the strong Christian denunciation of the practice of exposure. It was always the Roman custom not to permit deformed children to live. In their blanket condemnation of exposure the Christians implicitly affirmed the right of even the defective to live. The second is the impulse to relieve human suffering, which was so prominent a part of early Christianity. One finds frequent injunctions in early Christian literature to relieve the sick and the poor, widows and orphans, and all those in need. Among those who are sometimes singled out for mention are foundlings. Many early Christian hospitals had a section (called the *Brephotropheion*) specifically set apart for foundlings. It is unlikely that defective children were not cared for. Such a distinction would violate the numerous Christian statements that called for the compassionate treatment of all, whether male or female, young or old, free or slave, healthy or ill.

If the doctrine of the *imago Dei* provided the underlying theological rationale for the belief that human life was sacred from the moment of conception, another Christian doctrine played perhaps an even more important role in limiting the exposure of newborn children, including those with defects. This was the belief that children who died without baptism were doomed to eternal perdition. From the late second century the baptism of infants was a common practice in the church. With the spread of the Latin doctrine of original sin in the fourth and fifth centuries baptism came to be regarded as necessary to wash away from newborn infants the inherited sin of Adam. In the East the Greek Fathers, lacking a formulated doctrine of original sin, placed less importance on the absolute necessity of baptizing newborn children. They regarded unbaptized children as spending eternity in limbo, where they were without physical suffering. But in the West infants who died without baptism were widely, perhaps almost universally, regarded as lost for eternity. Augustine, who espoused the doctrine, did much to popularize it in the West. The doctrine was baldly stated in the sixth century by Fulgentius in his short treatise *De Fide* (which was as late as the Renaissance ascribed to Augustine):

It is to be believed beyond doubt, that not only men who are come to the use of reason, but infants, whether they die in their mother's womb, or after they are born, without baptism, in the name of the Father, Son and Holy Ghost, are punished with everlasting punishment in eternal fire, because though they have no actual sin of their own, yet they carry along with them the condemnation of original sin from their first conception and birth (*De Fide* 27: [28], pp. 416–17).

This doctrine acted as a major deterrent both to abortion and exposure. Ordinary Christians (and not merely theologians) considered the destruction of human life in its prenatal or natal stages the damnation of an immortal soul. Abortion was regarded as a worse sin even than murder, since the fetus died unbaptized and hence without salvation. So too exposure of a newborn infant meant that the child would not be baptized. Unless infants were in danger of death their baptism was postponed until one of the holy days set aside for baptism (Epiphany, Easter, or Pentecost), when the rite was performed in a church by a member of the clergy. Thus baptism of a child (which was an elaborate rite) virtually committed the parents to raising it. This fact undoubtedly placed parents of deformed infants in a terrible quandary; yet so severe, according to the teaching of the church, were the consequences of refusing baptism that it is likely that they prevented many pious parents from exposing their defective children. The theological consequences of exposure were made clear by the canons of the church. The Council of Mentz in 852 decreed a harsher penance for a mother who had killed her unbaptized child than for one who had killed it after baptism ([28], pp. 411–12).

There existed, however, an alternative, which appears to have been practised with some frequency in the Middle Ages: the donation (*oblatio*) of infants to be raised by the church ([4], pp. 17–33). Almost from the beginning Christianity had placed orphans, along with widows, under its special protection. The rescue and nurture of deserted infants was a much-encouraged act of Christian charity. Hence infants were often left in the precincts of a church or monastery. The practice became sufficiently common that several local councils dealt with the disposition of foundlings (*alumni*). A canon of the Council of Vaison (442) was perhaps representative . In the case of a child who had been exposed the priest was to announce that the parents might reclaim it by acknowledging it within ten days; thereafter it would belong to the family that gave it shelter. Similar canons were enacted by the councils of Arles (452) and Agde (506). In the ninth century the Council of Rouen issued an invitation to women to place illegitimate infants whom they did not wish to raise at the door of the church where they would be cared for. The practice of entrusting newborns to the care of the church was referred to as well in various legal codes of the early Middle Ages. Provision is made for these foundlings in the Code of Justinian (Novel 153), in the Visigothic Law in Spain, in the Lombard Lex Romana in Italy, as well as in a Frankish capitulary of about 744.[6] One might view the oblation of unwanted or defective children in church buildings in the Middle Ages merely as a continuation of the practice of exposure that was ubiquitous in classical antiquity. But there was a significant difference. The infant would not die or be sold into prostitution, fates that were often experienced by children exposed in pagan antiquity. The child was assured of baptism and being raised by the church. Monastic records indicate that defective children were often abandoned to the care of the church ([4], p. 21). Exposure (but not oblation) was still a sin in the eyes of the church, for which lengthy penance could be fixed. An Irish canon of the seventh century decreed seven years. Nevertheless, it continued for centuries and the church gradually extended its facilities to care for foundlings. Foundlings had been cared for in *Brephotropheia*, which were a part of many Christian hospitals that came into existence in the fourth century or later, and before that were frequently raised by individual Christians. But it was not till the early Middle Ages that separate foundling hospitals were established. Mention is made of these institutions at Treves in the sixth century and at Angers in the seventh, but the earliest of which we have certain knowledge was founded in Milan in 789. It is of interest that this hospital was founded out of a concern for the eternal destiny of infants who would otherwise die unbaptized and so go to hell. In some cases the foundlings were brought up as slaves (or later as serfs) of the church.

Brephotropheia apparently existed in large numbers in the Byzantine Empire, where they seem to have enjoyed exemption from taxation ([7], pp. 248–49). We are not told whether defective children were accepted, but there is frequent reference in accounts of Byzantine philanthropy to the care of the disabled and deformed. Alexius I Comnenus (1081–1118) was one of a number of Byzantine emperors who were known for their philanthropy. He founded an orphanage with a school to provide an education for orphans. He also built a new

section near the acropolis of Constantinople, a 'second city' that con-
tained dwellings for the poor and special homes for mutilated men. His
daughter, Anna Comnena, writes:

Here you could see them coming along singly, either blind, or lame, or with some other
defect. You would have called it Solomon's porch on seeing it full of men maimed either in
their limbs or in their whole bodies. This ring of houses is two-storied and semi-detached,
for some of these maimed men and women live up above 'twixt earth and sky, while others
creep along below on the ground floor. As for its size, anyone who wants to visit them
would begin in the morning and only complete the round in the evening. Such is this city
and such are its inhabitants (Alexias 15. 7; [7], p. 128).

With this kind of attention given to disabled adults it is likely that special
care was given as well to defective infants who were taken into found-
ling-homes.

Although most of the evidence is indirect, there is reason to believe
that after the legalization of Christianity a new attitude was introduced
regarding the treatment of defective children. The church insisted, by its
teaching and penitential discipline, that defective newborns be allowed
to live and be raised. It is likely that some were raised, if not always by
their parents, at least by philanthropic institutions established by the
church, to whom they were entrusted. Behind this change in attitude,
and in great part responsible for it in the West, was the belief in the
perdition of unbaptized infants. In the East, where this doctrine was
lacking, the Byzantine emphasis on philanthropy provided the impulse
for concern for the disabled of every age.

THE LATE MIDDLE AGES AND THE RENAISSANCE

The belief that baptism was necessary to secure the salvation of newborn infants continued to be popularly held in the High Middle Ages in
spite of a good deal of debate on the matter among theologians.[7]
Thomas Aquinas, who regarded original sin (which is removed by
baptism) as a sin of nature rather than of the person, and therefore not
to be punished in the same way, expressed the opinion that an unbaptized infant who died before birth might in some way be saved. The idea
of limbo as a place for infants who died without baptism, where they
suffered the pain of loss but not of sense, only gradually gained widespread acceptance in the West. The opinion of Augustine, who held that
unbaptized infants suffer the pain of sense in hell, remained a commonly-
held view even after the Council of Trent (which did not treat the

question). In the sixteenth century both the views of Augustine and Aquinas continued to have proponents. Among laypersons, however, the traditional Augustinian view furnished the motive to save the newborn infant for baptism at all costs. The church encouraged the use of caesarean section to save the life of the infant, which might otherwise be lost in difficult labor by being dismembered, a common practice that dated from antiquity. Nevertheless, midwives were sometimes reluctant to carry out a caesarean section, preferring instead to allow the child to die in a protracted birth. Various expedients were devised (without the authority of the church) for irregular baptism in cases where midwives expected to lose the child. They included sprinkling baptismal water on the uterus and baptizing stillborn children. As late as the seventeenth century the French obstetrician François Mauriceau devised an intra-uterine syringe with a long bent extension that made it possible for midwives to baptize endangered infants *in utero*.

It has sometimes been held that exposure and infanticide (like abortion) were relatively uncommon in the Middle Ages, owing to their condemnation by the church. Recent studies have suggested that they were more common than was once thought.[8] They appear to have become more frequent in the late Middle Ages than they were earlier, as evidenced by the number of foundling homes established, particularly in Italy ([27], pp. 99–100). Perhaps the serious economic and social dislocations of late mediaeval society caused by war, the plague, and the decline of manorialism, account at least in part for this phenomenon. Infanticide by 'overlaying' (suffocation) was frequently mentioned in the late Middle Ages. It was punished by ecclesiastical rather than secular courts and in England a relatively light penance of three years (one of which had to be on bread and water) became standard. The courts often failed to determine whether the death of the child was accidental or intended ([13], pp. 369–70). In the late fifteenth and sixteenth centuries some states took over from the church the prosecution of suspected cases of infanticide. Two groups of women were most often prosecuted: unwed mothers and old women who were suspected of witchcraft. The most frequent charge against witches, in fact, was that of infanticide.

Witches were blamed not only for the death of infants, but also for the birth of deformed children. In 1573 the great French surgeon Ambroise Paré (1510–90) wrote an interesting treatise on monsters and prodigies, in which he listed the causes of monstrosity. "There are," he writes, "reckoned up many causes of monsters; the first whereof is the glory of God, that his immense power may be manifested to those which are ignorant of it." A second cause is "that God may punish men's wickednesse, or show signs of punishment at hand." He then lists several natural causes. These include "an abundance of seed and overflowing matter"; a deficiency of seed, which results in the absence of members or shortness; "the force of imagination" of the mother, which can influence the fetus; "straightnesse of the womb"; the position of the mother in sitting or lying during pregnancy; and hereditary conditions (e.g., lameness) which parents pass on to their offspring. Finally, writes Paré, "monsters are occasioned by the craft and subtlety of the Devill" ([25], pp. 926–63).

There is little originality in the list. As Paré himself observes, classical writers attributed monstrosity to several of these causes. Augustine, for example, in his *Contra Iulianum*, recognized the possibility that the mother's imagination during conception as well as hereditary deformities might produce defective offspring. A glance at the list reveals that the first, second, and last of the causes mentioned by Paré are theological (monsters reveal the glory of God, they result from God's punishment, they are produced by the devil), while the rest are natural. Paré (like Augustine) recognized both ultimate and proximate causation in the birth of defective infants. He himself was a devout Christian, who is reputed to have said often of successful surgery. "I treated him, God cured him." Most theologians and many laymen will have attributed monstrosity to one of the three theological explanations given by Paré (quite apart from the physical cause). The belief that the devil and his agents ("conjurors, charmers, and witches," as Paré describes them) were responsible for defective children was particularly widespread. In the Middle Ages the devil was popularly believed to seduce young girls, who as a result bore monsters that were sometimes smuggled into the homes of other families. Midwives might fall under suspicion of witchcraft if they delivered a deformed child. Since the time of the Babylonians, who studied fetal and adult abnormalities as a means of foretelling the future, monstrous births had been commonly regarded as prodigies that portended some great event, most often an evil one. Martin Luther regarded monstrous births as supernatural portents. In 1523 Luther and Melanchthon published a work entitled *Der Papstesel* ('The Pope's Donkey'), in which they interpreted the symbolism of an ass-like monster, which popular legend said had been seen floating down the Tiber River in Rome. Luther and Melanchthon described the monstrous animal as a sign from God that foretold the coming doom of the papacy. Luther later published a second treatise in which he attempted to show that a monstrous calf, which had been discovered at Freiburg, was a work of Satan that had symbolic meaning ([29], pp. 306–307). He believed that human monstrosities were produced by Satan, not by God, and that they had no soul or had Satan himself as their soul and therefore should be drowned.[9] On one occasion when Luther was in Dessau he heard of a twelve-year-old child who had been a monster since birth and seriously suggested that the child be thrown into the river Mulde ([22], p. 123). His attitude probably represents the outlook of the German peasantry from which he came more than a considered theological opinion. His views in this matter are likely as well to have been influenced by the 'witch-craze' of the sixteenth and seventeenth centuries, which produced widespread alarm in European society regarding demonic influences.[10]

THE PROTESTANT REFORMATION

The views of the Protestant reformers regarding status of human life in its earliest stages (both pre- and postnatal) differed in some respects from traditional Catholic teaching. Luther and Calvin condemned both contraception and abortion; Calvin called the latter 'an inexpiable crime.' He did not follow the Septuagint in distinguishing between the formed and unformed fetus and thought it 'not lacking in great absurdity' to believe that the killing of a fetus at any stage was not a capital crime ([10], p. 157). The reformers broke with traditional Catholic teaching in rejecting the Augustinian belief that unbaptized infants were eternally damned. Luther taught the necessity of baptizing infants for the remission of original sin, but he believed in the possibility that infants who were stillborn or unbaptized might be saved. While God ordinarily works through means (i.e., the sacraments), Luther wrote, he can and sometimes does save those who do not receive baptism ([21], pp. 49–50). He did not countenance the baptism of unborn infants, counselling women to pray instead for endangered fetal life ([21] p. 49) and he was reluctant to pronounce on the question of whether an unborn (and presumably endangered) child who had only a limb projecting from the womb should be baptized ([20], p. 74). In 1542, to comfort mothers who had lost children at birth, Luther wrote a small tract, *Ein Trost den Weibern* ('A Comfort to Women'), in which he stated that stillborn and unbaptized infants could be buried with the rites of the church in the hope that they would take part in the

resurrection. Calvin and the Reformed churches rejected the doctrine
that baptism was necessary to salvation (see Calvin's *Institutes* 4. 16. 26).
Calvin believed that all those who were born deserved eternal punishment because of original sin (*Institutes* 4. 15. 10), but cautiously suggested that those who were baptized into the covenant community might
be presumed to be saved (4. 16. 9). Individual salvation was, however,
determined not by baptism but by God's inscrutable decree of election.
In general Reformed Protestants showed little interest in the theological
discussion of the status of the fetus or newborn infant. In great part this
was due to their rejection of a sacramentalist understanding of baptism
and not being faced with the problems that accompanied it; and in part
to the Calvinistic emphasis on the providence of God and the wisdom
and justice of his decrees.

The Protestant Reformation introduced a renewed emphasis on marriage, the home, and the family. This emphasis grew largely out of the
reformers' opposition to the Catholic claim that celibacy was superior to
matrimony. Luther makes frequent reference in his writings to the
importance of the home in the nurturing of children, as well as to the
duties of parents to their children and children to their parents. In
children, he writes, "you may behold the providence of God, who
created them out of nothing. In a half year He gave them body and life
and all their members and also intends to support them" ([21], p. 138).
Parents must provide for them not only physical support but spiritual
nurture as well.

Therefore it is highly necessary that every married person regard the soul of his child with
greater care and concern than the flesh which has come from him, that he consider the
child nothing less than a precious, eternal treasure, entrusted to his protection by God so
that the devil, the world, and the flesh may not steal and destroy it ([21], p. 141).

Calvin's emphasis on God's providence led him to acknowledge that it
was in God's hand to give or withhold children. He regarded children as
a gift of God and a sign of his blessing. Hence Onan's sin of coitus
interruptus (Genesis 38:8–10) was 'doubly monstrous': "It is to ex-
tinguish the hope of the race and to kill before he is born the son who
was hoped for" ([23], p. 353, n. 31). While Calvin does not specifically
discuss the reasons for the birth of defective children, one surmises that
he regarded such births as providential.

Scripture, to express more plainly that nothing at all in the world is undertaken without his
determination, shows that things seemingly most fortuitous are subject to him. . . . Even

though the rich are mingled with the poor in the world, while to each his condition is divinely assigned, God, who lights all men, is not blind. And so he urges the poor to patience; because those who are not content with their own lot try to shake off the burden laid upon them by God (*Institutes* 1. 16. 6).

A few pages earlier he writes:

Carnal reason ascribes all such happenings, whether prosperous or adverse, to fortune. But anyone who has been taught by Christ's lips that all the hairs of his head are numbered will look farther afield for a cause, and will consider that all events are governed by God's secret plan (*Institutes* 1. 16. 2).

CONCLUSION

The concept of the sanctity of life in Christian thinking has from the beginning been based on theological premises, the chief of which is that human beings are created in the image of God. In the formative patristic discussions human life was defined as sacred and deserving of protection from the moment of conception. As a result, in the period under survey, Christian writers condemned contraception, abortion, exposure, and infanticide, though there was always some disagreement in drawing out the implications of the underlying premises for specific issues. If the question of the treatment of defective newborns was seldom specifically raised, it was because the matter was largely subsumed under the question of whether infants should be exposed. The church had always condemned the practice of exposure, though it was unable fully to exterminate it. "Are defective infants human beings (*homines*) who are deserving of life?" That question, if addressed to theologically-literate persons of our period, would have been answered by most in the affirmative. A variety of reasons would be given, all theological. Apparent exceptions sometimes arose. The birth of seriously defective infants might be attributed to Satan or to witches. Lacking a soul, such infants might be thought to deserve death. Monstrous births have in all ages produced terror and revulsion and it is not surprising that it must often have been difficult to discern the image of God in them. But for the most part the Western tradition from the fourth century to the Protestant Reformation accepted the belief, explicit in Christian teaching, that all newborn life ought to be protected and nourished.

Oregon State University
Corvallis, Oregon.

ACKNOWLEDGEMENT

This publication was supported in part by a research fellowship from the Oregon Committee for the Humanities. I thank Darrel W. Amundsen for his helpful criticism.

NOTES

[1] See [6], pp. 46–64.

[2] It was widely held in classical antiquity that the soul entered the body at birth. According to Tertullian, "this view is entertained by the Stoics, along with Aenesidemus, and occasionally by Plato himself, when he tells us that the soul, being quite a separate formation, originating elsewhere and externally to the womb, is inhaled when the newborn infant first draws breath" (*De Anima* 25).

[3] See [23], p. 91.

[4] For a condemnation of all three practices, see Augustine, *De nuptiis et concupiscentia* 1. 15. 17. The passage (later known as the *Aliquando*) is translated in [24], p. 16.

[5] In two passages Augustine discusses the possibility that aborted fetuses will have a part in the resurrection of the dead. In the *City of God* (22. 13), while cautious, he sees no strong reason to exclude them. In the *Enchiridion* (85), on the other hand, he thinks it likely that the formed fetus will be resurrected, while the unformed fetus will perish like semen.

[6] Several of these *Leges Barbarorum* contain provisions that prohibit both abortion and infanticide. According to Lex VII of the Lex Visigothorum those who kill their own children, whether *in utero* or at birth, will be sentenced either to public execution or the loss of both eyes. See [2], pp. 568–69.

[7] See the interesting mediaeval English poem on the subject of infant damnation, in which a midwife is upbraided by a priest for the loss of a soul and prevented from the future practice of her profession for allowing a newborn child to die without proper baptism ([8], pp. 47–49).

[8] See [11], [13], [15], and [27].

[9] For several citations to Luther's works see [1], p. 96, n. 82.

[10] On the European witch-craze see [26], pp. 90–192. On Luther's belief in witches see [16], pp. 416–423.

BIBLIOGRAPHY

1. Althaus, P.: 1972, *The Ethics of Martin Luther*, Robert C. Schultz (trans.), Fortress Press, Philadelphia.
2. Amundsen, D. W.: 1971, 'Visigothic Medical Legislation', *Bulletin of the History of Medicine* **45**, 553–569.
3. Augustine, St.: 1957, *Against Julian*, Matthew A. Schumacher (trans.), Catholic University of America Press, Washington, D.C.
4. Boswell. J. E.: 1984, '*Expositio* and *oblatio:* The Abandonment of Children and the Ancient and Mediaeval Family', *American Historical Review* **89**, 10–33.
5. Calvin J.: 1960, *Institutes of the Christian Religion*, John T. McNeill (ed.) and Ford

Lewis Battles (trans.), 2 vols., Westminster Press, Philadelphia.

6. Conner, J.: 1977, *Abortion: The Development of the Roman Catholic Perspective*, Loyola University Press, Chicago.

7. Constantelos, D. J.: 1968, *Byzantine Philanthropy and Social Welfare*, Rutgers University Press, New Brunswick, N.J.

8. Coulton, G. G.: 1918 (1968), *Social Life in Britain from the Conquest to the Reformation*, Barnes and Noble, New York.

9. Dyer, G. Y.: 1967, 'Limbo', in *The New Catholic Encyclopedia*, vol. 8, McGraw-Hill, New York, pp. 762–765.

10. Grisez, G. G.: 1970, *Abortion: The Myths, The Realities, and the Arguments*, Corpus Books, New York.

11. Helmholz, R. H.: 1974, 'Infanticide in the Province of Canterbury During the Fifteenth Century', *History of Childhood Quarterly* 2, 379–390.

12. Jonkers, E. J.: 1947, 'La législation de Justinien et la protection de l'enfant à naître', *Vigiliae Christianae* 1, 240–243.

13. Kellum, B. A.: 1973, 'Infanticide in England in the Late Middle Ages', *History of Childhood Quarterly* 1, 367–388.

14. Kelly, J. N. D.: 1960, *Early Christian Doctrines* (rev. ed.), Harper and Row, New York.

15. Langer, W. L.: 1973, 'Infanticide: A Historical Survey', *History of Childhood Quarterly* 1, 353–365.

16. Lea, H. C.: 1939, *Materials towards a History of Witchcraft*, Arthur C. Howland (ed.), vol. 1, University of Pennsylvania Press, Philadelphia.

17. Lecky, W. E.: 1865 (1955), *History of the Rise and Influence of the Spirit of Rationalism in Europe*, George Braziller, New York.

18. Lecky, W. E.: 1869 (1902), *History of European Morals: From Augustus to Charlemagne*, 2 vols, Longmans Green, London.

19. Ludlow, J. M.: 1875, 'Exposing of Infants', in W. Smith and S. Cheetham (eds.), *A Dictionary of Christian Antiquities*, vol. 1, John Murray, London, pp. 653–654.

20. Luther, M.: 1959, *Luther's Works*, vol. 36: *Word and Sacrament II*, Adbel Ross Wentz (ed.), Muhlenberg Press, Philadelphia.

21. Luther, M.: 1959, *What Luther Says: An Anthology*, compiled by Ewald M. Plass, vol. 1, Concordia, St. Louis.

22. Magnus, H.: 1908, *Superstition in Medicine*, Julius L. Salinger (trans.), Funk and Wagnalls, New York.

23. Noonan, J. T., Jr.: 1965, *Contraception: A History of its Treatment by Catholic Theologians and Canonists*, Harvard University Press, Cambridge.

24. Noonan, J. T., Jr.: 1970, 'An Almost Absolute Value in History', in John T. Noonan, Jr. (ed.), *The Morality of Abortion: Legal and Historical Perspectives*, Harvard University Press, Cambridge, pp. 1–59.

25. Paré, A.: 1634, *The Workes of that Famous Chiurgion Ambrose Parey*, Th. Johnson, T. H. Cotes, and R. Young (trans.), London.

26. Trevor-Roper, H. R.: 1956, *The European Witch-Craze of the Sixteenth and Seventeenth Centuries and Other Essays*, Harper and Row, New York.

27. Trexler, R. C.: 1973, 'Infanticide in Florence: New Sources and First Results', *History of Childhood Quarterly* 1, 98–116.

28. Westermarck, E.: 1906, *The Origin and Development of the Moral Ideas*, vol. 1, Macmillan, London.
29. White, A. D.: 1896, 1901, *A History of the Warfare of Science with Theology*, vol. 2, D. Appleton, New York.
30. Williams, G. H.: 1970, 'Religious Residues and Presuppositions in the American Debate on Abortion', *Theological Studies* **31**, 10–75.
31. Wood, H. G.: 1910, 'Baptism (Later Christian)', in James Hastings (ed.), *Encyclopedia of Religion and Ethics*, vol. 2, Charles Scribner's Sons, New York, pp. 390–406.

KENNETH L. VAUX

DANVILLE'S SIAMESE TWINS: RELIGIO-MORAL PERSPECTIVES ON THE CARE OF DEFECTIVE NEWBORNS

As a boy, Illinois' Poet Laureate Carl Sandburg would visit the circus when it came to Galesburg. He describes having seen a man with elastic skin who could pull it out from his face and neck. The circus spieler promised more such 'curi-aw-si-ties' and 'mon-straw-si-ties' inside the tent. "Years later it came over me that at first sight of the freaks I was sad because I was bashful"[1] ([21], p. 192).

Bob and Pam had awaited anxiously the birth of their first child ([25], p. 1–2). They had trained in natural childbirth and were ready for the joys of Lamaze intimacy with the new baby. Their anticipation was heightened when Pam's obstetrician detected two heartbeats and told her they should expect twins. Then, like Chang and Eng in Siam in 1811, the twins presented conjoined. Even though the parents were medically trained (she a nurse, he a physician), like the poet, they were awestruck and horrified. A decision was made to let nature take its course.

The babies, joined at the mid-section with common abdominal organs and genital systems, were left untreated for congestion and pneumonia. Respiratory assist, nutrition, and hydration were not initiated. An order appeared in the chart: "Do not feed infants, in accordance with parents' wishes." Then the experience broke into public view and became an issue we all have had to confront. A conscience-plagued nurse, an anonymous tipster, an intervention by the Illinois Department of Children and Family Services, temporary custody, custody hearings, State's Attorney charges, parents' plea of innocence, surgical separation of twins, return of custody, marital separation of the parents all followed – and yet today the drama continues. Meanwhile, the children moved toward life or death. Jeff has grown and learned to walk with a brace. After three years of life with a colostomy, ileostomy, one leg, and constant monitoring in an institution, Scott died. Though the tent is missing, the morbid circus curiosity, that strange blending of sympathy, revulsion, and fascination goes on. Like the poet, we witness with sad

R. C. McMillan, H. T. Engelhardt, Jr., and S. F. Spicker (eds.),
Euthanasia and the Newborn, 65–80.
© 1987 by D. Reidel Publishing Company.

hearts the spectacle of helpless infants and anguished parents. Even though the poignant ordeal continues, we must offer ethical reflection and formulate a moral response.

THE MORAL RESPONSE: HISTORY

Across the ages societal response to such events has been shaped by the ancient emotive responses of awe and fear. These in turn created the active dispositions of reverence and revulsion. Rudolf Otto described this mingled attraction and terror as the primal religious impulse [18]. This psychic response gave rise in primitive cultures to the sense that any exceptional birth was a supernatural event. It was a blessing or a curse, an omen, an ominous birth, a portent of the future (L. Monstrare)[2] or, retrospectively, a judgment for past wrongs. If the world is a divine milieu and all events are fraught with significance, this ancient response can be seen as the mechanism used to lift life crises to that level of meaning.

At times, the births of exceptional and abnormal creatures, mongols, conjoined twins – even separated twins – were seen as divination. The Gods, Asvin and Asva, inseparable twins of the Indian Vedas, were god-doctors who worked miracles for all who suffered. Conversely, among the North Pomo and Kato Indian tribes of California, twins were killed, sometimes with the mother, to avert ominous fortune, sibling strife and incest. Like Cain and Abel or Jacob and Esau, they represented both glory and disorder, creativity and chaos. They were seen to proceed from the hand of God or the nature demons of the underworld. Virgil chanted of twins born in the mystery of night:

There are two monsters whose name is Dire; produced together with the Tartar Magera in but a single birth, by the deep night; She with a Serpent's coils did cloak her babes and arm them well with vetose wings ([27], p. 5).

Not only do we find that psychic wrath and guilt lead to abandonment and even torture of the deformed, there was also a natural evolutionary value that shaped behavior, a biological determinant. As with animal societies, most primitive societies exposed deformed offspring. Hunting societies often practiced infanticide. Pastoral societies practiced selective infanticide, e.g., the killing of girl children in Pre-Islamic Arab cultures ([19], p. 51). The instincts at work in infanticidal impulses were, therefore, survival, altruism in the sense of kin selection, and volitional response to the noumenal power felt in experience.

This disposition began to be transformed in the Ancient Near East. As civilization dawned in Mesopotamia, Egypt, and elsewhere, we began to have both social structures and religious sanctions protecting life, even deformed life, guiding medical practice along lines of sustaining life and avoiding harm. Agrarian imperatives to have many offspring and the theological sense of murder as blasphemy commingled to form a conscientious sense of the sacredness of child-life. The harsh penalty for abortion (impaling and not burying the woman) in the 15th century B.C. Assyrian law probably typifies Ancient Near Eastern (semitic) ethics. ([1] p. 882). This perspective condemns the naturalistic desire to transmit life well (whole and healthy) to children even at the cost of abortion and selective infanticide, which was the ethic expressed most powerfully by the Greeks and Romans.

The religious morality regarding prenatal and infant life formed in the Near-Eastern Ethos is conveyed to our modern tradition by Judaism and primitive Christianity. It is based on two themes: (1) the doctrine of sanctity of life, which animates the activity of safeguarding the transmission of life to new beings and (2) the doctrine of passing on life well, which accents purity, wholeness or wellness in the offspring. These responses correspond to the dialectics of respect and rejection in our animal heritage and dialectics of reverence and revulsion in the protohuman (primitive and pastoral) response. When we observe the prohibition of infanticide in Medieval Islam (based on the prophet's sympathy proceeding from his own experience as an orphan) or the practice of 18th and 19th century Catholic societies to more readily accept the arrival of abnormal children, or the right to life commitments of 20th century Christian fundamentalism, we witness the cultural virtue of spontaneous, reverent acceptance of the grace of new life.

At the same time we know that midwives in Catholic and Protestant societies of recent centuries took deformed babies aside and neglected to slap in their respiratory reflex. We know that until this century parents commonly suffocated their sleeping children when household economy or limited coping capacity demanded. We have seen a series of devout, concerned parents from the Danville twins to Baby Jane Doe who say 'no' to heroic rescue endeavors with their own severely injured newborns. They are most often animated by the simple instinct to do better with another try.

Athenian law, one of the first great charters of social obligation, also condoned a custom allowing exposure (neglect allowing death) or positive killing in the first week of a defective child's life. The act of killing, though not considered homicide, was a miasma or pollution requiring purification; but allowing the child to die was acceptable. At the end of one week the father, having determined that the child could be embraced and cared for within the constraints of the *oikos* (household, economy), presented the child to the assembled clan for naming and membership.[3] In Plato's *Republic* (Book V), the crippled, sick, and deformed were to be abandoned if there was no hope of restoration or recovery. This response resonated with the Hippocratic ethic, which viewed the attempt to support hopeless lives as immoral, thereby prolonging suffering and dying.

But despite the power of this pagan tradition, it was the conviction of the Semitic Near East, especially the moral covenant of Israel, that became the dominant ethos of the Christianized Roman Empire. Inspired by Jesus' mercy on children and the sick, early Christian writers univocally condemned the exposure of children. In Book XVI of *The City of God*, Augustine challenged our impatience with deformity by reminding us of the providential design of the whole creation. Just as in the *Enchiridion* resurrection became the force that transformed all who were deformed, so here we are asked to view what we see as an aberration as the providential variation of creatures by which God enriches his creation. In a passage where he reflected on monstrous births and siamese twins he wrote;

God is the creator of all, and He Himself knows where and when any creature should be created or should have been created. He has the wisdom to weave the beauty of the whole design out of the constituent parts, in their likeness and diversity. The observer who cannot view the whole is offended by what seems the deformity or a part, since he does not know how it fits in, or how it is related to the rest ([3], p. 662).

The Augustinian and Early Christian ethos is quite accurately portrayed in the modern placard: "I know I'm Somebody 'cause God don't make no junk." In the post-Renaissance and Reformation eras, we witness the same dialectics of concern and neglect. In ancient Ireland, the Down's syndrome child was called 'Dinne LeDia' (Gift of God). There is also the custom of "turning to the wall" and allowing death. In medieval Germany, although we frequently see the reverence for sickly lives as a divine call, the disordered child was often seen as a changeling, a daemonic trick. When asked about a grotesquely abnormal child from Dessau, Luther advised that the child be flung into the river to test the spirits by the watery ordeal, saying that homicide could be risked on the grounds that "he was entirely of the opinion that such changelings were merely a lump of flesh, a massa carnis, and that there was no soul in them"([15], v. 45, pp. 396–397). If a creature could be designated desouled or bedeviled, it seems the ethics of sanctity and life were suspended and one could justify either abandonment or positive killing. Paul Althaus, a commentator on Luther's ethics, cautioned us not to draw inferences for contemporary questions of infanticide from a moral system colored by "primitive dualism and mythological concepts of the devil"([2], p. 96).

Not only was strange birth construed as spiritual power from above or below, in the late medieval world-view it was seen as a portent of the future. In the search for etiology and meaning, in a 1523 treatise entitled *Der Papstesel*, Luther and Melanchthon interpreted the discovery of a monster found floating on the Tiber River as an act of God signalling the demise of the papacy ([14], p. 397). In 1569, the birth of twins conjoined at the chest was read by the physician Jacques Roy as a sign that Catholicism would survive the Huguenots ([14], p. 397).

Superstitious and supernatural etiologies slowly yielded to a more reasoned yet complex explanation as, for example, was offered by the 16th century French surgeon Paré:

There are reckoned up many causes of monsters; the first whereof is the glory of God, that his immense power may be manifested to those who are ignorant of it . . . Another cause is that God may punish men's wickedness . . . Another cause is the injury of hereditary diseases . . . Monsters are also occasioned by the craft and subtlety of the Devil ([14], p. 397).

One of the first great scientific observers of birth anomalies was the devout Zwinglian naturalist Albrecht Von Haller. In *Icon es Anatomieae*, (1743), he studied a set of Siamese twins joined at the chest and upper abdomen. Since anatomically distinct nerve trees proved distinct wills, and the single heart proved that 'anima' did not reside in the blood, Haller concluded that "this twinning was not a deformity but perhaps a new type of living creature and a proof of the manner in which divine wisdom can realize new human forms that are complete in their own ways" ([10], p. 61.) Our modern Western ethos was shaped by naturalism and supernaturalism, by the Catholic Mediterranean emphasis on accepting nature and subservience to transcending authority and the Protestant Nordic emphasis on human dominion over nature and private judgment. These, I contend, were elaborations of the primal psychic dispositions of awe and fear, control and manipulation.

In our search for understanding and direction in such problematic births, we may attribute the event to either divine or daemonic action, to retribution or premonition, to natural causes or mutation. We may attack or acquiesce to nature. As I have pondered the why and wherefore of the Danville family's ordeal, it appears that through the trauma of two parents and two children our whole society is vicariously groping for its own understanding of life and death, health and disease, normality and abnormality. As in past cultures, our society declares its values and meanings through symbolic events such as this birth. Though today we construe the event more as a teratogenic accident than a metaphysical omen, we are, like the ancients, forced to interpret the event within a framework of meaning. The theological meanings we bring to events shape the decisions we make. Now, however, there is a new dimension of responsibility.

THE NEW FACTOR: PRESCIENCE AND POWER

Unlike all of our predecessors, we can no longer innocently plead blind fate or acquiesce to 'nature's course'. Now we know things before they come about and can profoundly modify the outcome of natural process. Indeed, our power is a part of nature. For instance, that which our ancestors called the 'Holy Idiot' or the Mongol is to us a Down's syndrome (trisomy-21) child, a chromosomal aberration, an abnormality that can be detected before birth. Recently a medical journal reported the case of a mother carrying twin fetuses, one of whom had Down's syndrome. Arguing that the family could not care for a retarded child, the mother requested that the 'affected' fetus be killed in the womb and the 'normal' baby be brought to term ([22], p. 59).

Could not the Danville family contend similarly that, if they could have had a glimpse into their fetal window, found the Siamese pair and aborted the creature, that there would have been no controversy; indeed, society might have expected that action? But on this side of the birth canal, releasing life becomes a major public threat. It became so grievous a crime that State's Attorneys and public agencies compounded the family agony by seizing custody and bringing accusations of murder.

Should we knowingly consent to the birth of a defective child? This question was raised by one of the leading Catholic moralists of our time [11]. Tort for wrongful life cases may, in the future, test whether we have the legal right to knowingly proceed with the birth of a defective child. H. Tristram Engelhardt, a leading biomedical philosopher, asks whether there is valid jurisprudential concept in what is called "the injury of continued existence" [7]. The foreknowledge we have acquired in modern technology presents an awesome responsibility. Where knowledge of injury exists, where it is known that harm will only intensify and no amelioration is available (e.g., Tay-Sachs disease detected via antenatal diagnosis), is there a sense in which we become accomplices to the evil if we do not terminate the pregnancy? If the Siamese twins will not survive without profound diagnostic, surgical, and life-support interventions, is there not a sense in which we can be accused of compounding the affliction if we initiate these measures? Perhaps feeding, hydration, and warming are basic responsibilities. But what kind of feeding: intravenous, nasogastric, hyperalimentation? What of antibiotic treatment, resuscitation, oxygen and respiratory therapy? Where on the continuum of life supports do we pass from measures that are ordinary, pain relieving, and life prolonging, to those that are extraordinary, which compound suffering and prolong death?

The Greeks thought that reality was constituted out of four basic elements: earth, water, air, and fire. Perhaps we should accede to a perennial wisdom and speak of a fundamental obligation to provide newborns with food, fluids, air and warmth; and, when it comes to the sophisticated range of other technological life supports, we should carefully consider whether we are conserving life or the dying process.

The deepest springs of moral insight available to our civilization are the Hebrew and Christian scriptures. Here the fall from innocence is symbolized by the acquisition of knowledge. Here we learn that our creator makes us free and accountable creatures. Here shame and guilt signal the fact that we are inescapably responsive, responsible beings.

THE ABORTION ANALOGY

As we seek to delineate responsibility in this case, we begin by drawing moral inferences from other areas. For example, we look to personal and public values concerning abortion. If we search for deformity in fetal diagnosis and terminate such pregnancies, can the abortion analogy be used to help decide about defective newborns? In unpublished essays, William Bartholome, the pediatrician-ethicist, argues 'no'. He points to the danger of our reasoning from the licit practice of birth control, to the morally equivocal practice of early termination of any unwanted pregnancy, to the questionable practice of selective feticide and neonaticide based on quality of life judgments. Bartholome argues that this is wrong, not on 'right to life' grounds but on grounds of fundamental justice and equity. To consider some lives qualitatively inferior, to withhold equitable care from the handicapped, therefore claiming that they possess less claim to protection, is to assail the basic moral requirement of equality.

While I agree with this logic, I find it morally unconscionable and psychologically unhealthy to know and not to act. To discover disease and debilitation and do nothing about it is irresponsible. We must recall the Genesis announcement of the ascent into knowledge and the fall into sin and responsibility. When we have the capacity of foreknowledge and prevention, we must act responsibly in the light of that knowledge.

Selective abortion for fetal disease offers an analogy that supports a 'let die' posture in this case. Life bears down with sufficient pain. We need not knowingly compound its burden. We should do all we can to prevent, detect, and correct birth defects. We must come to the aid of the sick with genetic medicine and fetal therapy; sometimes with moral courage we must terminate those conceived lives that bear profound and grievous injury. Today in public policy we ask: "When does life begin?" "Does life begin at conception?" "Shall public funding be used for prenatal screening for spina bifida and, subsequently, for abortion?" Of course life begins at conception; no thoughtful scientist or moralist would argue otherwise. But these questions do not address the real issues. The point is we have been given foreknowledge and power, freedom and accountability by God. We are now responsible with a terrifying yet wonderful freedom; we cannot offer the excuses of fate and inevitability.

It is at this precise point of arbitration over life and death that we must remind ourselves of the irresistible and pervasive malevolence in the heart of man. Our wick is short, our staying power weak, our caring capacity fragile. We stand, some say, on the brink of an age that will be characterized by constant contempt for others, disregard for the weak and helpless, and unyielding demands for constant self-gratification. The biblical communitarian ethos of our civilization is yielding to the libertarian. As we discuss public transportation some argue cynically,

"If you can't afford a car you shouldn't travel." We may move to genocide, fratricide, suicide – even holocaust. At the Wailing Wall of Jerusalem, 5000 survivors of the Holocaust were reminded by Elie Wiesel:

Something went wrong with our testimony; It was not received. Look, look at the world around us; suspicion again, violence everywhere, hatred everywhere, state-sponsored terror, racism, fascism, fanaticism, antisemitism ([29], p. 4).

We live in an age when life seems pitted against life. Indeed, as the value of life vision and commitment has eroded in our culture, we have chosen more and more a life style of hedonistic self-gratification, nihilism, and an apocalyptic disregard for life, the earth, the future. As one writer has said, our lust for life may be transmuting into a lust for destruction [16].

THE "DO NO HARM" ANALOGY

If the dialectics of compassion and contempt do indeed animate our moral dispositions, we do well to examine the capacities for 'doing harm' that reside in everyone, often under the guise of 'doing good'. The ancient moral codes, both semitic (e.g., covenant code of Israel, Hammurabi) and naturalistic (e.g., Hippocratic deontological writings), caution us against doing harm to another. Indeed, this moral command precedes the beneficence imperative (*Primum non nocere*). When is prolonging life harmful? When does continued existence constitute an injury? How shall we calculate the burden of harm against the bestowal of life and health? Which persons are involved in the avoidance of harm and the achievement of health? Our moral traditions would lead us to be suspicious of gestures that seek to spare others harm or do things 'for their own good', because such altruism is often disguised self-interest. Our ethics will seek the unadulterated good of the specific person(s) involved and thus place great weight on their own assessment of their situation and their consent. Our religious heritage will not allow us to equate, in a superficial way, pain with evil or health with good. Our ethical heritage will also prompt us to see our common solidarity and corporate destiny. We do suffer and die in companionship with one another just as we live and thrive together. All moral determinations should attend to these facts of our existence and thereby to the legitimacy and limitation of the 'do no harm' analogy.

THE NAZI-NUREMBERG ANALOGY

Recognition both of what is in the heart of man and the structural power of the demonic in our world prompts us to be morally cautious in allowing, and certainly in assisting, the death of injured newborns. Our hesitancy at this point and our erring on the side of life must forever be shaped by the experience of the Nazi Reich and the instruction of the Nuremberg medical trials. In the early 1930s, Karl Binding published a pamphlet entitled 'Die Freigabe der Vernichtung lebensunwerten Lebens' (Permitting the Extermination of Life Not Worth Living). In 1938, the father of a deformed child asked Hitler if he could kill the boy. Hitler referred the matter to Brandt to look into and then authorized physicians to carry out the euthanasia. By the spring of 1939, the killing of mentally deficient and physically deformed children had become commonplace ([26], pp. 282–283). In the first weeks of the anguish in Danville, the parents were often reminded, by letter, of this precedent.

The Nazi analogy is both sobering and dangerous. Of course, the memory of this atrocity must forever bind our conscience, but there are discontinuities between the cases. The underlying motive of the Nazi death program was certainly not euthanasia – the merciful consideration of suffering persons. The goal was race purification and the elimination of what were considered to be subhuman populations. When, then and now, economic considerations, concern for resources, and ability to muster up caring capacity and redirect energies to sustain the non-rehabilitatable sick are invoked, the analogy haunts us in condemnation.

But if we take the euthanasia taboo of this memory and join it with our technical power to indefinitely prolong life, even just the vegetative filament of existence, we may come to inflict even greater injury on those who suffer. It will then take the enforced death-prolongations in the semi-life of many Karen Quinlans and Baby Does to remind us that we have gone too far.

MORAL CONSIDERATIONS: LIFE, LIBERTY, HAPPINESS

Three themes of moral discourse help us come to terms with this case, motifs of philosophical and legal parlance. These themes are derived from our religious and moral heritage. Therefore, they relate to both the personal and societal analysis and adjudication of the Danville case and others like it.

Life – The Danville twin case occurred at a moment in political history characterized by a significant societal value shift. We live in a day of reassertion of a 'right to life' public philosophy. Henry Hyde, an Illinois congressman, has succeeded in the national legislature with various pro-life, anti-abortion initiatives. Our law-making leadership has considered a "life begins at conception" clarification of the 14th Amendment. Phyllis Schlafley, an Illinois laywoman, has promulgated a view on family life and women's destiny that has gained such wide currency as to successfully stymie the passage of the Equal Rights Amendment. The Reagan Administration has declared itself opposed to abortion and has pressed Baby Doe and Baby Jane Doe guidelines. Dr. Everett Koop, a Philadelphia pediatrician and Surgeon General of the United States, has for years expressed a right to life, anti-abortion message in the context of the broader theme of historic catastrophe and decline of the Christian West. His films, with colleague pastor Francis Schaefer, on the plight of the human race are known to millions. Koop, like Dr. William Kieswetter of Pittsburgh's Childrens' Hospital, is a distinguished surgeon with experience with Siamese twins. These men share an evangelical-fundamentalist theological persuasion. Dr. Koop has expressed grave reservations about the probity of neonatal anti-dysthanasia (allowing defective newborns to die). This becomes clear in his responses [13] to the Hopkins Down's syndrome case and the Duff and Campbell review of Yale University cases where children with severe defects were allowed to die ([5], pp. 890–894).

The focus on the right to life and sanctity of life applies also to the Danville family. The ordeal has reoriented their lives, redirected their life energies, and taken its toll on the family structure. Now that only one of the twins will likely survive, what will his life be like?

As we ponder the theme of defending life, it might be proposed that the birth of severely deformed children insults and assaults the lives of families and that self-defense is justifiable. Although this notion must be pursued with utmost care, it seems relevant to the discussion. In contrast to the dominant theme of new life as divine blessing, there is in Jewish ethics a thread that sees the fetus, particularly the distorted fetus, as an aggressor against the life of the mother [8]. Roman Catholic medico-morality has also pondered the case of the baby whose birth demands the death or injury of its mother [4]. All recent ethics will save the mother. Whether the right to life refers also to the vitality and viability of a family remains a crucial issue to consider.

When I discussed the Danville twin case among the fellowship of the

Hastings Institute (Institute of Society, Ethics and the Life Sciences), many of my colleagues in medicine, nursing, philosophy, theology, and ethics felt that the initial decision of doctors and family not to begin life-support – even feeding and hydration – was justifiable in light of the jeopardy the birth presented to the family and the drawn-out suffering it implied for the children. Joseph Fletcher, whose writings on genetics, abortion, and care of defective newborns are widely known, felt that withholding treatment could be justified on the basis of the overriding harmful effects on the family and on many persons if the lives were prolonged. In sheer ethicometrics, the costs greatly outweighed the benefits.

Alternatively, Paul Ramsey argued that it was wrong not to feed and hydrate such newborns. The principle of the covenant of life with life mandated support, although he found extraordinary measures (e.g., resuscitation) questionable. A critical determination for Ramsey was whether or not the twins were dying. Could they be separated? Could one be saved? The answer to those questions would determine the moral status of particular life-saving or death-hastening actions. Ramsey also felt that the ultimate legal adjudication of the case should occur at two levels. One proceeding should render a decision on the issue of euthanasia. Another deliberation should consider penalties.

Willard Gaylin, John Fletcher, and others regretted that this case ever moved into the public arena. It should have been handled in the confidentiality of the family-medical team relationship, with consultation of an ethics committee, and with collegial discussion in order to develop clear, unequivocal decisions to which all persons involved were party and agreed. Consensus should have been sought. In the face of moral uncertainty and lacking consensus, sustaining life is a community obligation and the right to life as personal entitlement must be preeminent.

Liberty – Next to the value of life, the most widely invoked topic in medical ethics today is liberty. Gerald Dworkin [6], Mark Siegler [23], and many others have used the criteria of freedom, self-determination, and parental prerogatives as leitmotifs for moral judgment. To whom does the decision to prolong or protract the life of these children belong? Do the parents, the physicians, the state or the courts have jurisdiction? We commit most decisions about procreation and family life to the parents. Or, better stated, we challenge and usurp the oversight of the family only in situations of obvious neglect, abuse, or brutality. Does this case belong under the rubric of right to privacy (a derivative of liberty), or is it a concern of community justice?

Parental authority is a theme that supports the view that this case should never have passed into the public domain. The decision, admittedly profound and tragic, should have transpired in the privacy, confidentiality, and discretion of the parent-physician relationship. The blunders of communication or quandaries of conscience that drew it into the public limelight are understandable and forgivable, but as one legal colleague has said, "This should not go into the courts; they have no superior wisdom to adjudicate these searching questions. Bad cases – bad law."

Happiness – The final theme that has been helpful in pondering the case is happiness. By this I do not mean the banal superficial notion of comfort and complacency current today for which we use the label happiness. The deeper meanings of felicity, compassion, justice, and blessedness of which the Beatitudes, the charter of human happiness, speak have definite bearing on this case. In a broadcast at the time of the Baby Jane Doe case, Vatican radio condemned newborn euthanasia, which "distinguishes between lives which have meaning because they are useful, efficient and joyous and those to which all meaning has been denied because they are judged useless, inefficient and without joy" ([24], p. 20).

Happiness is not a facile matter of delights and a sense of usefulness, rather it is fulfillment that becomes possible in an environment of caring. What does this mean for parents who in care have drawn away and begun to grieve both the disappointment and the loss of this, their only offering of ongoing life to this world, their own flesh and blood? What does it mean to demand that they now remain attached, or worse yet, that they are not to be entrusted with this offspring? Although custody has been restored and although both parents still attend the children, the threat of court intervention still exists.

Family, the basic covenant of life, is the care-giving and life-giving fabric that patterns, binds, and weaves each of us into a history and a future. It is the paradigm and the representation of the divine embrace of our life. It is only within covenants of care, where happiness is a prospect because hope, not despair, prevails, that life and liberty are possible. Where children are unwanted and neglected and no nurture is present, only frustration and violence are possible. If we acknowledged this fact, perhaps we would not magnify this and other singular cases out of proportion, but might begin to work on the real childhood moral crises of our society such as the starvation death of children *en masse* around the world, the fact that even in America a major cause of retardation is maternal and infant malnutrition, and the fact that 40 per cent of children born in Chicago do not have legal or otherwise accountable fathers. If human happiness and well-being are to flourish, we must reactivate the intimate communities of caring such as the churches and neighborhoods and thus relieve the public agencies, which should only be expected to serve those who fall through the cracks.

CONCLUSION

In conclusion, though life, liberty, and happiness may serve as helpful normative criteria to work through this case, an ultimate question mark appears in our moral calculation when we ponder the humanity and plight of cases such as these. The children are human. Like us, they have usually been given a name. Healy, in his review of Roman Catholic moral theology, reminds us that Siamese twins are to be baptized, either conditionally or absolutely ([12], p. 25). They possess souls; they bear the divine image. They are ours; they are like us; they are God's heritage; and, in His inscrutable will, they have transected our lives for a meaning, certain though indiscernible. They are monstrous in the literal sense of that word; they are guides into ourselves, beyond ourselves and out to the edge of the future which is God's prolepsis, His becoming among us: "I am who I will be." (Exodus 3: 14). Like Elephant Man, they remind us, in our condescension, whose life it is anyway. Like those in extremis throughout the ages, they plead to us to uphold them, yet do no harm. What this means in terms of saving or letting die, of probing, investigating, operating, separating, engaging or withdrawing remains for us, parents and guardians, doctors and nurses, friends and advisors, judges and jurors to determine in courage and grace. We must watch over one another with generosity and gratitude.

Carl Sandburg continued his walk through the sideshows of the circus. Along the way, there was a deep-chested, barefooted man without arms. He handed Sandburg a note with an offer to write his name on a card he could keep, for only ten cents. "I said, 'I would if I had the ten cents. All I've got is a nickel.'" The man took the nickel in his left foot, put a pen between his toes, and wrote 'Charles A. Sandburg.' "It was the prettiest my name had ever been written. His face didn't change. All the time it kept that quiet look that didn't strictly belong with a circus. I was near crying. I said some kind of thanks and picked up my feet and ran" ([21], pp. 182–153).

University of Illinois, College of Medicine
Chicago, Illinois, U.S.A.

NOTES

[1] This case was widely discussed in the Illinois and national media. See, for example, [7].
[2] The root monstrare, to show forth or demonstrate. It carries a symbolic meaning of conveying some significance beyond the immediacies of the event.
[3] For summaries of the practice of infanticide in the Greco-Roman world, see [28] and [19].

BIBLIOGRAPHY

1. Amundsen, D. W.: 1978, 'Medical Ethics, History of: Ancient Near East', *Encyclopedia of Bioethics*, Macmillan, New York.
2. Althaus, P.: 1972, *The Ethics of Martin Luther*, Fortress, Philadelphia, Pennsylvania.
3. Augustine: 1972, *The City of God*, D. Knowles (ed.), Middlesex, United Kingdom.
4. Connery, J. R.: 1978, 'Abortion: Roman Catholic Perspectives', *Encyclopedia of Bioethics*, Macmillan, New York, pp. 9–13.
5. Duff, R. S. and Campbell, A. G. M.: 1973, 'Moral and Ethical Dilemmas in the Special Care Nursery', *New England Journal of Medicine* **289**, 890–894.
6. Dworkin, G.: 1970, *Darwinism, Free Will and Moral Responsibility*, Prentice-Hall, Englewood Cliffs, New Jersey.
7. Engelhardt, H. T., Jr.: 1975, 'Ethical Issues in Aiding the Death of Young Children', in M. Kohl (ed.), *Beneficent Euthanasia*, Pantheon, Buffalo, New York.
8. Feldman, D. M.: 1978, 'Abortion: Jewish Perspectives', *Encyclopedia of Bioethics*, Macmillan, New York, pp. 5–9.
9. Haffter, C.: 1968, 'The Changeling: History and Psychodynamics of Attitudes to Handicapped Children in European Folklore', *Journal of the History of Behavioral Sciences* **11**, 55–61.
10. Haller, A.: 1972, 'Albrecht Van Haller', *Dictionary of Scientific Bibliography*, Scribners, New York, pp. 61–66.
11. Häring, B.: 1975, *Ethics of Manipulation: Issues in Medicine, Behavior Control and Genetics*, Seabury Press, New York.
12. Healy, E. F.: 1956, *Medical Ethics*, Loyola University, Chicago, Illinois.
13. Koop, C. E. and Schaeffer, F.: 1983, *Whatever Happened to the Human Race*, Good News Press, New York.
14. Lipton, M.: 1971, 'History and Superstitions of Birth Defects', *Journal of the American Pharmaceutical Association* **11**, 395–399.

15. Luther, M.: 1955, *Luthers Works*, Fortress, Philadelphia, Pennsylvania.
16. Mailer, N.: 1970, *Of a Fire on the Moon*, Beacon, Boston, Massachusetts.
17. 'The Moral Dilemma of Siamese Twins', *Newsweek*, June 22, 1981, p. 40.
18. Otto, R.: 1959, *The Idea of the Holy*, Pelican, London, United Kingdom.
19. Piers, M. W.: 1978, *Infanticide*, Norton, New York.
20. Reynolds, V. and Tanner, R.: 1983, *The Biology of Religion*, Longman, London, United Kingdom.
21. Sandburg, C.: 1952, *Always the Young Strangers*, Harcourt and Brace, New York.
22. 'Saving One, Dooming Another', *Time*, June 20, 1981, p. 59.
23. Siegler, M. and Jonsen, A.: 1982, *Clinical Ethics*, Macmillan, New York.
24. 'Vatican Condemns Mercy Killings', *Chicago Sun Times*, December 14, 1983, p. 10.
25. Vaux, K.: 1981, 'Danville's Siamese Twins Test Society's Deepest Beliefs', *Chicago Tribune*, June 28, pp. 1–2.
26. Veatch, R. M.: 1978, 'Death and Dying: Euthanasia and Sustaining Life, Public Policies', *Encyclopedia of Bioethics*, Macmillan, New York, pp. 278–286.
27. Virgil: 1961, 'Aeneid XII', vv 1056–1061, in L. Gedda, *Twins in History and Science*, Thomas, Springfield, Illinois.
28. Weir, R. F.: 1984, *Selective Nontreatment of Handicapped Newborns*, Oxford University Press, New York.
29. Wiesel, E.: 1981, 'Wiesel at the Wailing Wall', *New York Times*, June 19, p. 4.

INFANTICIDE IN A POST-CHRISTIAN AGE

The papers by Darrel Amundsen [1], Gary Ferngren [4, 5], and Kenneth Vaux [9] provide an overview of a very important segment of Western intellectual history: reflections on moral obligations to defective newborns. Amundsen gives an account of how infanticide was appreciated by our intellectual antecedents in the ancient world. Ferngren then brings us to the modern era by examining the contributions of the Christian synthesis, which supplanted the views of classic times. The difficulty is that ours is in great measure a post-Christian age. Large-scale states such as the United States not only encompass Buddhists, Hindus, Taoists, Confucians, deists, and atheists in addition to Christians and Jews, but the very character of such states reflects an ever-increasing neutrality towards the special Judeo-Christian assumptions of the West. One needs critically to assess the extent to which Judeo-Christian assumptions may guide secular policy with regard to the treatment of defective newborns.

This is not to suggest that much of the Judeo-Christian heritage does not survive. However, the moral canons of that heritage appear justifiable for a large-scale secular pluralist society not on their own terms, but only insofar as rational arguments can be offered to justify particular tenets, or insofar as policy influenced by or in accord with such tenets is chosen through democratic processes that do not foreclose the rights of dissidents. Which is to say, the pagans have triumphed. To appeal to a general rational justification is to take seriously a peculiar aspiration of the Greeks: their interest in setting cultural peculiarities aside so as to frame arguments in the anonymous terms of reason. To appeal to general democratic processes under which the participants retain rights to privacy and dissent is to endorse the view that public authority comes from the consent of the governed, an understanding that has its roots in the Anglo-Saxon heathen past which shaped common law. Much of the contemporary culture-shock for Christians in the West and for Moslems

R. C. McMillan, H. T. Engelhardt, Jr., and S. F. Spicker (eds.),
Euthanasia and the Newborn, 81–86.
© *1987 by D. Reidel Publishing Company.*

in the East derives from the character of limited secular democracy
which has led to radical changes in the acceptance of contraception, the
rights of women, and the provision of abortion. The question of infanticide rises against this background of changes and shifts in moral assumptions and the tensions which they have engendered.

SOME PRELIMINARY DISTINCTIONS

To address the moral issues raised by Amundsen, Ferngren and Vaux,
one will need to distinguish among different senses of infanticide: active
infanticide in which some positive action is taken that will kill an infant,
versus passive infanticide, where an infant dies through the omission of
certain acts that could have saved it. In addition, one will need to divide
each of these categories in terms of whether the infanticide is intended
or simply foreseen. Each category raises its own questions, for some
have held that it is improper to intend the death of another, and others
have held there is a moral difference between killing versus letting die,
whatever one's intentions. As Amundsen shows, in ancient times it was
licit actively to kill infants in Rome and passively in Greece. For
example, Amundsen notes Table IV and its injunction that fathers
ought quickly to kill deformed infants. The pagans could directly intend
death since there was nothing intrinsically immoral in killing one's child
under such circumstances. The Christians, however, since they regarded
children as the gifts of God, could not directly intend to take God's gift
of life. At most, they could see their duties to save an infant defeated
either by costs or through redefining the object involved. The first,
defining the circumstances which defeat obligations to treat, has been an
approach traditional to Roman Catholicism. Many of its moral theologians have focused on how major psychological and financial costs
involved in treating a very severely deformed child can defeat the usual
obligations to save a child's life. One may not intend to kill a child. But,
as such moral theologians recognized, and as indeed all individuals
must, no duty of beneficence is absolute. If the burden is sufficiently
great and the chance of succeeding sufficiently slim, the *prima facie* duty
to save another is defeated [2].

   Vaux' treatment of Luther offers the other classic option for Christians, namely, to conclude that a very severely deformed infant is not an
infant at all, but a monstrosity. As both Amundsen and Vaux acknowledge, Augustine was not sympathetic to this approach. However, it is a

plausible approach, at least for certain very extreme cases, such as anencephalic children. When no or little brain is present and there is no possibility of sentient life, not to mention personal life, it would be a moral misunderstanding to try to sustain such an infant, even if it could be done cheaply and effectively. There is no person in the body to be benefited. This appears to be a part of the argument framed by the Roman Catholic moral theologian Richard McCormick [6]. Indeed, everyone or nearly everyone should be willing to accept at least passive and unintended infanticide in certain very extreme cases.

THE STATUS OF INFANTS

With certain important qualifications, the child under Roman law could be regarded as a product of the father and as an entity under his power. In contrast, the child for the Christian is a gift of God, which itself receives life as a gift, placing the family and others under special fiduciary obligations. However, if Christian understandings do not provide appropriate policy for a secular state, the question arises of the extent to which the public policy of such a state should approach to the understandings of ancient Rome and Greece.

To some degree, we have avoided a return to the policies of our heathen antecedents by making children wards of last resort of the state under the doctrine of *parens patriae*. However, we will need to set limits insofar as we do not wish to abrogate all notions of parental sovereignty. Public policy in a post-Christian age will require, on the one hand, recognizing the interests of society in protecting children, yet, on the other hand, respecting the family which has produced the child, since the child can no longer be officially recognized as a gift of God. To a significant degree, current arguments focus on the extent to which the *paterfamilias* doctrine should survive as a notion of family sovereignty. Insofar as any element of family sovereignty remains regarding treatment decisions about newborn children, it becomes the burden of the state (since it is the state which is intruding) to show that the parent's actions are improper, not the parents' burden to show that they are acting properly. Who has the burden of proof, and how heavy that burden is, will of course be decisive. In a peaceable, secular, pluralist society, it would appear difficult not to recognize a certain element of familial sovereignty.

This is particularly the case, given the arguments of Vaux about the tension among moral goods. In many of the difficult cases, it is very hard to sustain the position that parents are obliged to treat in all circumstances. The more considerable the costs involved, the more an adequate understanding of what should be done will be dependent on appreciating the suffering and pain of the child and the family within the context of the particular family and its moral convictions. It is only in this way that one can determine how devastating the costs will be. This will involve consulting with the parents, since significant elements of the costs are personal and psychological. Which is to say, the more the personal, psychological, and economic costs escalate, the more plausible it becomes that parental decisions to refuse treatment should carry significant weight.

One would think that this position would be one consonant with general Christian views. To pursue the goal of saving particular infants' lives at any costs is to embrace an idolatrous understanding of life. If Christians do indeed believe in an after-life, there must be more important things to do than invest major sums in the treatment of children when the costs are significant and the likelihood of success far from certain. Which is to say, one would think that one could frame a strong Christian moral argument in favor of passive infanticide. And of course, such an argument exists already in the traditional distinction between ordinary and extraordinary treatment, between that treatment which is appropriate and that treatment which is inappropriate because it involves an inordinate burden upon the family or society [8].

DISCRIMINATING AGAINST THE HANDICAPPED

The Christian viewpoint also gives, as John Paris has suggested [7], a basis for a moral justification of discriminating against those infants born with severe mental and physical handicaps. In those cases where an extraordinary burden is involved, one may cease treatment. However, one is not obliged to cease treatment. It follows then, with regard to the class of infants whom one is excused from treating because that treatment would be very costly and success unlikely, that one may choose to treat those who, if they did survive, would survive with few handicaps and not to treat those who, if they did survive, would have significant mental and physical handicaps. One would only be forbidden to discriminate on the basis of likely future mental and physical handicaps with respect to those infants whose treatment would not constitute an inordi-

1ate psychological or financial burden. One may not discriminate where
one is obliged to treat. But with respect to those infants whose treatment would constitute an inordinate burden, one may morally (even if
not legally) discriminate.

This conclusion should not be either novel or shocking. When it comes
to supererogatory courageous acts, one may morally freely choose whom
to save or not to save. One may save one's family and let strangers die.
Or in this case, one may decide to save at great expense a child likely to
be normal, but not one whose future physical and mental handicaps
would constitute even further psychological and economic burdens, in
addition to the inordinate costs involved in saving the child's life.

A LOOK TO THE FUTURE

Amundsen, Ferngren and Vaux succeed in introducing us to our modern difficulties in understanding the status of infants in a post-Christian
age. We must in framing policy for a secular state consider what our
obligations to infants ought to be, without relying uncritically upon the
Judeo-Christian heritage. We will need to examine what the costs and
benefits would be, for example, of reinstituting something similar to
Solon's law, so as to permit parents to allow to die, and to die painlessly,
severely deformed infants whose treatment would be extraordinarily
costly. One might still hold that active infanticide would have too many
adverse social costs. Perhaps such costs could properly include the
special psychological trauma involved in actively taking the life of an
infant. The most we might wish to support would be the discontinuation
of all treatment and the use of heavy sedation. In any event, we will
need to examine at what point parents are allowed to decide: "The costs
are too much; we will let this child die and try to conceive again."

As Vaux has suggested, the Christian moral perspective includes ways
to allow parents to make such decisions, even if in an indirect fashion.
The Christian viewpoint made accommodations because the costs of
treatment in certain cases were so high that selective passive infanticide
was likely to be accepted by all out of desperation. We are now faced
with the more general task of reexamining these issues in an age that
owes much to the moral insights of the Judeo-Christian heritage, but
whose public policy cannot be justified by simple appeal to that heritage. We will need to ask what rational men and women ought to accept
with regard to a policy of selective infanticide for severely defective

newborns. We will need to bear in mind the testimony of the past, which Amundsen provides, namely, that societies are able to distinguish between letting die (or killing quickly) newborns who have not yet been formally enrolled in all the rights of persons, versus killing children who have been enrolled. There appears to be a human capacity to distinguish between infanticide and the murdering of children. This is as one would expect. Given the great loss of infant life under natural conditions there are likely to be special abilities to distance oneself emotionally from early infant death in a way that would not undermine moral commitments to older children.

A mature policy will need to take into account insights from the Judeo-Christian heritage, experiences from our pagan past, and the modern disciplines of a secular bioethics. We are only beginning to understand what it means to think through the use of expensive medical technologies within the context of a secular, pluralist society. Much serious intellectual work will be required to fashion decent and justifiable policies with regard to the treatment or non-treatment of defective newborns.

Baylor College of Medicine
Houston, Texas, U. S. A.

BIBLIOGRAPHY

1. Amundsen, D.: 1987, 'Medicine and the Birth of Defective Children: Approaches of the Ancient World', in this volume, pp. 3–22.
2. Cronin, D.: 1958, *The Moral Law in Regard to the Ordinary and Extraordinary Means of Conserving Life*, Pontifica Universitas Gregoriana, Rome.
3. Engelhardt, H. T.: 1986, *The Foundations of Bioethics*, Oxford University Press, New York, chapters 4 and 6.
4. Ferngren, G.: 1987, 'The *Imago Dei* and the Sanctity of Life: The Origins of an Idea', in this volume, pp. 23–45.
5. Ferngren, G.: 1987, 'The Status of Defective Newborns from Late Antiquity to the Reformation', in this volume, pp. 47–64.
6. McCormick, R.: 1974, 'To Save or Let Die: The Dilemma of Modern Medicine', *Journal of the American Medical Association* **229**, 172–176.
7. Paris, J. J.: 1983, 'Right to Life Doesn't Demand Heroic Sacrifice', *The Wall Street Journal*, November 28, 30.
8. Pope Pius XII: 1958, 'The Prolongation of Life', *The Pope Speaks* **4**, 393–398.
9. Vaux, K. L.: 1987, 'Danville's Siamese Twins: Religio-Moral Perspective in the Case of Defective Newborns', in this volume, pp. 65–80.

SECTION II

TREATMENT OF NEONATES: REGULATION, LEGISLATION, AND THE RIGHTS OF PARENTS

NANCY M. P. KING

FEDERAL AND STATE REGULATION OF NEONATAL DECISION-MAKING

BACKGROUND AND OVERVIEW

The Baby Doe controversy, which has so engaged the public interest in recent months and is still far from being finally decided, has focused attention once again on the problems of proxy decision-making, especially for infants. My paper will begin by tracing the recent history of federal and state intervention in medical decision-making for severely ill and handicapped newborns. Next I will describe a legally sound medical decision-making framework, with parents as the appropriate decision-makers, and conclude by demonstrating how the decision-making models favored by the federal government and state laws fall short of providing to parents the authority properly conferred upon them by law.

The Bloomington Case

In April of 1982, a baby identified as 'Infant Doe' was born in Bloomington, Indiana, with Down's syndrome and esophageal atresia with associated tracheoesophageal fistula.[1] The infant's parents, apparently believing that his other handicaps were so severe that survival was not in his best interest, refused to authorize surgery that would repair the fistula and permit the baby to be fed by mouth. The hospital sought court authorization to perform the procedure, but the courts upheld the parents' decision.[2] Infant Doe died six days after birth. On November 7, 1983, the United States Supreme Court refused on mootness grounds to review the Indiana ruling, and left the decision intact [10].

Federal Intervention

Baby Doe's death attracted Presidential notice; Mr Reagan immediately instructed the Secretary of the Department of Health and Human

R. C. McMillan, H. T. Engelhardt, Jr., and S. F. Spicker (eds.),
Euthanasia and the Newborn, 89–115.
© 1987 by D. Reidel Publishing Company.

Services (DHHS) to notify hospitals that discrimination against handicapped infants was forbidden by federal law. The notice issued by DHHS to hospitals stated:

It is unlawful for a recipient of federal financial assistance to withhold from a handicapped infant nutritional sustenance or medical or surgical treatment required to correct a life-threatening condition if: (1) the withholding is based on the fact that the infant is handicapped; (2) the handicap does not render the treatment or nutritional sustenance medically contraindicated [2].

The DHHS Office for Civil Rights (OCR) then established a procedure to investigate suspected cases of discrimination. DHHS' authority was based on Section 504 of the Rehabilitation Act of 1973,[3] which forbids discrimination against 'otherwise qualified' handicapped persons in the provision of federally funded programs and services. That legislation, though it has been fraught with complexities in other settings, appeared to be the Administration's best enforcement tool.

(1) *The Baby Doe Regulations*. Regulations intended to implement the policy expressed in the directive and notice were issued in March of 1983. They required the posting of a 'Baby Doe Hotline' notice giving a phone number to call to initiate OCR investigation. In apparent belief that a significant number of babies were being routinely denied clearly beneficial treatment, DHHS issued the regulations as interim final rules to take effect in two weeks – a fast track that required special justification in order to survive scrutiny under the Administrative Procedure Act. The evidence upon which the regulations were based appeared to consist primarily of a television videotape about several similar cases and a few small studies of actual and hypothetical decision-making about seriously ill newborns, most of which dated back to the early 1970s.[4]

(2) *American Academy of Pediatrics v. Heckler*. The American Academy of Pediatrics and two children's hospital associations (along with a large number of *amici curiae*) immediately challenged the regulations in federal district court. Judge Gerhard Gesell's decision [1] declared the regulations in violation of the Administrative Procedure Act because they were issued without adequate consideration of the relevant factors, including the risks created by disruption of hospital routine by the OCR investigation, the rights and preferences of parents, current medical standards, the scope and applicability of Section 504, and the recommendations of the President's Commission for the Study of Ethi-

cal Problems in Medicine and Biomedical and Behavioral Research. Moreover, the government had demonstrated no true emergency justifying waiver of standard Administrative Procedure Act notice procedures.

New proposed rules were published on July 5, 1983 [19]. The preamble to the new rules addressed some of the issues about which Judge Gesell had expressed concern – the applicability of Section 504, the rights of parents, the evidence upon which DHHS had relied, etc. – and called for comments on a number of other questions. To the rules themselves were added provisions for intervention by state child protective agencies and an appendix that attempted to explain the standard by which discrimination against handicapped infants was to be measured. According to the appendix, only 'medically contraindicated' treatments were unnecessary, and any decision based on grounds other than legitimate medical judgment would subject the recipient institution to loss of all federal funding.

In essence, therefore, the revised regulations were vitually unchanged. Faced with the threat of further litigation from the same groups, at the end of the 60-day comment period, DHHS published final rules [16] that in some respects were very different.

(3) *The Infant Care Review Committee.* The final Section 504 regulations, which were preceded by some 28 pages of detailed analysis of comments and defense of the government's position, provided for the establishment by recipient hospitals of Infant Care Review Committees (ICRCs) to assist in the decision-making process. These committees, closely modeled on the review option advocated by the President's Commission in its report *Deciding To Forego Life-Sustaining Treatment* [41] and by the American Academy of Pediatrics,[5] were not *required* by the regulations, but were 'encouraged'. State child protective agencies were encouraged to consult with committees that exist at hospitals where discrimination has been reported, and to model their investigatory guidelines after those adopted by DHHS. DHHS' guidelines,[6] however, were equivocal regarding the effect of the existence of such a committee on its investigation and enforcement policy. The guidelines stated: "Unless impracticable, whenever a recipient hospital has an Infant Care Review Committee, established and operated substantially in accordance with [regulations], the Department will . . . solicit the information available to, and the analysis and recommendations of, the ICRC" ([18], p. 1654). The guidelines also provided that on-site investiga-

tion will begin with a meeting with the committee. The regulations themselves stated only: "In seeking to determine compliance with this part . . . by health care providers that have an ICRC established and operated substantially in accordance with this model, the Department will, to the extent possible, consult with the ICRC" ([18], p. 1652). The hotline and investigatory mechanisms remained otherwise the same. Thus, although DHHS seemed to endorse the committee concept with enthusiasm in its commentary, which is without legal effect, the choice of highly tentative language in the regulations themselves left hospitals with little guidance as to how much difference the presence of a committee will actually make when a hotline complaint is received.

The model committee described in the regulations has three functions: policy development, concurrent review of specific cases, and retrospective chart reviews. When engaged in concurrent review, the committee is to ensure that parents have been fully informed not only of their infant's condition and prognosis but also of the existence of public and private agencies, parent support groups, and other sources of services and assistance in the area. One committee member is also to be designated as special advocate for the infants; the special advocate's role is to argue for full medical intervention on the infant's behalf.

The committee is to follow the parents' wishes whenever they wish to continue life-sustaining treatment, unless such treatment is medically contraindicated. When the family refuses consent, if the treatment is not medically contraindicated in the committee's judgment, the committee is to recommend that the hospital bring the case to court or to a child protective agency.

The committee's prospective policy-making role could be of considerable importance; through their committee, hospitals could develop treatment guidelines for specific categories of cases. Development and promulgation of such guidelines could bring together information on the most effective available medical technology, community resources, and the perspectives of interested groups, providing occasion for comprehensive examination of and education about important issues in decision-making about handicapped infants, and minimizing the chance that decisions might be based on lack of knowledge or on poor communication.

The ICRC concept was a new addition to state and federal regulatory options regarding decision-making for newborns. Few ethics committees existed before these regulations,[7] and subsequent state and federal statutory schemes for neonatal decision-making have been modeled after DHHS' ICRCs.

Baby Jane Doe

Around the time of the promulgation of the final regulations, another Baby Doe was having an important influence on the federal decision-making role.

Baby Jane Doe is a microcephalic, hydrocephalic spina bifida baby who was born on Long Island in October, 1983. When her parents decided, after extensive consultation with physicians and clergy, not to authorize surgery for the spinal lesion, the hospital concurred in their decision. The case was not initially reported through the federal Baby Doe Hotline; instead, an out-of-state lawyer with a reputation for aggressive action in right-to-life cases somehow received information about the case and brought it to the government's attention. The hospital refused DHHS access to the infant's medical records, in violation of the investigatory schemes set up in the regulations; the Department of Justice then brought suit in federal district court in New York to gain access to the records. Judge Leonard D. Wexler denied the request, and went on to explain that a hospital which honors a parental decision not to consent to surgery for a handicapped child cannot be charged with discrimination against that child, because the hospital "lacks the legal right to perform such procedures, unless there is consent by either the child's natural guardians (i.e., her parents), or by some legally appointed guardian" ([30], p. 614). Because hospitals cannot act without the consent of the child's guardian, if they fail to perform surgery it is not because the child is handicapped but because its parents have not consented.

It might, however, be argued that the parents, in refusing to consent to the surgical procedures, made a decision which, had it been made by a recipient of Federal financial assistance, would have been violative of the act and that [the hospital], in carrying out such a decision, violates the act, and should not be allowed to hide behind the decision of the parents. Such an analysis . . . would be invalid. . . . The failure of [the hospital] to perform the surgical procedures cannot possibly be regarded as a violation of the rehabilitation act ([30], p. 614).

The Court of Appeals for the Second Circuit affirmed Judge Wexler's decision [29], but on grounds other than the parental autonomy rationale on which the lower court had relied. Instead, the appellate court examined the legislative history of the Rehabilitation Act and decided that Congress had never intended it to apply to the circumstances at issue. By holding that Section 504 could not support regulations applied to medical decision-making, the court set the stage for the American Medical Association's (AMA's) recently successful lawsuit, *American Medical Association v. Heckler*, to void the regulations and preclude the federal government from promulgating any similar regulations under that authority [2].

On June 9, 1986, the Supreme Court upheld the decision in the Baby Jane Doe case, finally declaring that the federal government lacks the power to enforce treatment guidelines through regulations promulgated under Section 504. *Bowen v. American Hospital Association*, 54 U.S.L.W. 4579 (1986).

Federal and State Statutes

There was thus only one avenue remaining to the federal government whereby it could affect decision-making for and medical treatment of handicapped infants. That route lay through the state agencies responsible for the reporting and prevention of child abuse, and it was soon tried.

Federal legislation – The Child Abuse Prevention and Treatment Act of 1974 [7] and the Child Abuse Prevention and Treatment and Adoption Reform Act of 1978 [8] – provides funding for state social services programs that address the problem of child abuse. Two different bills proposing amendments to this legislation were passed by the House and Senate; the final version, approved by a joint House-Senate conference, was signed by the President at the close of the Ninety-eighth Congress.[8] The amendments add a 'medical neglect' provision to the statutory definition of child abuse and neglect, and provide that the withholding of certain "medically indicated treatment from disabled infants with life-threatening conditions" constitutes medical neglect.[9]

The amendments must be implemented by DHHS guidelines for states to use in developing programs.[10] States must have such programs in place one year after the passage of the amendments, or they will lose the funds provided to them under the statute. Therefore, states wishing to retain their federal funding will enforce their own child abuse statutes, appropriately amended, against hospitals, physicians, and parents suspected of medical neglect.[11]

Use of the system of state child abuse laws in this way solves the problem raised by Judge Wexler in the Baby Jane Doe case. Although hospitals and physicians may not be technically guilty of medical neglect for refusing to act without parental consent, under the child abuse reporting laws they have an independent obligation to report any instances of medical neglect to the state agency.[12]

The bigger problem, however, is not solved by a new federal definition – or, for that matter, by any of the state statutory definitions of medical neglect in the handful of states that have considered or passed similar legislation independent of the federal law.[13] That problem is the meaning and scope of any medical neglect provision. On the one hand, there is no reason to suppose that any treatment readily identifiable as neglect is not already covered by state laws merely because it is 'medical'. Parental refusal to provide medically indicated treatment is by this argument no different from failure to feed or clothe the infant, and nothing is added to the child abuse law that could not have been identified as neglect without such an amendment.

On the other hand, the definition of 'medically indicated treatment' may have been intended by Congress to narrow the scope of permissible medical decisions for infants. Indeed, the Child Abuse Amendments were intended as a solution to the same perceived problem the Baby Doe regulations were drafted to solve. In order to determine whether the federal regulations issued pursuant to Section 504 and the Child Abuse Amendments with their new regulations actually intrude on decision-making prerogatives that properly belong to the parents, we must examine the legal tradition of decision-making for infants.

APPROPRIATE DECISION-MAKERS AND APPROPRIATE DECISIONS

In drafting the original Baby Doe regulations, DHHS paid little attention to the role of parental decision-making in the care of severely handicapped newborns. In responding to what was apparently viewed as a pattern of medical decision-making that clearly ignored the best interests of the infants, DHHS placed the federal government squarely in the state's traditional role: the protector of the infant's best interests whenever the parent – usually assumed to be adequately filling that role – is perceived deficient in so doing. Once the determination is made that the state should step in, parents will in fact have no further say in decisions about their infant's care.

In reality, of course, much controversy has always surrounded even this familiar *parens patriae* principle. Its boundaries and the standards employed for determining parental fitness to decide are subject to extensive debate and disagreement. The uses of the principle in medical decision-making for handicapped newborns are even more fraught with difficulty, and the government's role in this setting deserves searching examination. The state's decision to take on the parental role requires a double justification: It must be shown that (1) parents cannot or will not make acceptable decisions, and that (2) the state in its turn can do better. Because the Federal regulations, rather than operating on a case-by-case basis, would hold *a priori* that parents of an entire category of infants cannot appropriately decide, the justification must be considerable.

The Nature and Origins of Parental Autonomy

In the Anglo-American legal tradition, a parent's authority to make decisions for his or her infant does not stem from any *independent* right or interest belonging to the parent or family. Parental authority is derived solely from the recognition (or assumption) that parents are the best determiners of their infant's best interests. When the infant is deemed incapable of exercising his or her decisional right, that right can be delegated to the parent, whose decisions are likely to reflect congruence of interests with those of the infant and a subjective appreciation of his or her needs.[14]

Essentially, therefore, the parent's authority is that of a proxy or substituted decision-maker, rather than some separate and intrinsic right to impose parental values on infants. Do parents have any special claim, then, to serve as proxies for their infants? If so, does that claim still have validity for decisions substantially affecting their infants' survival, as in decision-making for handicapped newborns?

Legal and historical precedents accord great deference to family values and parental choice when the question of decision-making on behalf of persons *de jure* or *de facto* incompetent arises. This deference has several sources and justifications. The first is pragmatic: Parents and family are usually more able than any other decision-maker to know the incompetent person well enough to make a substituted decision that reflects as accurately as possible his or her preferences, likely choices, or desires formerly expressed when competent. The court's decision in the Karen Ann Quinlan case [23] exemplifies this reasoning.

This subjective 'substituted judgment' standard cannot be applied, of course, in decision-making for newborns, because their personalities are not developed sufficiently to enable a decision-maker even to create likely choices from expressed preferences. Instead, family values and lifestyle choices can be implemented through an 'identity of interest' standard, on the assumption that minor children share or will come to share the values and beliefs their parents teach them. This standard relies for its fair application on a decision-maker who has the same stake in the matter at hand as the incompetent, and who can thus be depended on to press the incompetent's interests fully in the course of pursuing his or her own.[15]

Whereas the substituted judgment standard can be applied by proxies other than family members, or even by courts fully informed about the incompetent person,[16] the identity of interests standard can only be applied by a proxy who actually shares and can promote the incompetent's interests. In decision-making for newborns, the parents will almost always be the only available candidates for this role.

The second justification for deference to parental autonomy reinforces this practical empirical reality with what is perhaps best labeled a philosophical tenet of the political system: The right of private persons to be free, in certain aspects of their daily lives, from governmental interventions. This right has various constitutional and quasi-constitutional labels. In the past it was often termed a 'liberty interest'; more recently, it has become known as the 'right of privacy'.

Conceptually, the privacy right can be envisioned as creating a sphere of protected activity. Governmental authority – for example, the police power to legislate for the public health and safety, or the *parens patriae* power to act on behalf of persons whose interests are not otherwise protected – can operate freely to affect those actions and interests of families that are well outside the protected sphere of privacy. As the governmental intervention becomes more intrusive, moving closer to the zone of privacy, progressively greater justification is required. Penetration within the privacy zone itself, wherein are located fundamental rights to engage in activities like marriage, procreation, child-rearing, and health care decision-making, among others, cannot be accomplished unless there exists a compelling governmental interest in the intrusion. Parental, family and individual decisions about raising and educating children [20, 26, 32], contraception [12, 13, 27], and abortion [11, 25] are among the activities that have been held to be within the province of the privacy right and thus constitutionally protected.

The Limits of Parental Autonomy

The privacy right, practical reality, and societal tradition firmly establish parents and family as the appropriate decision-makers for severely ill newborns. But because the parental decision-making right is not free-standing, deriving instead from the infant's best interests, it is not an absolute right. Our privacy analysis provides the model for identifying when that right will be overridden and a governmental decision-maker will be substituted for the parent. The parent as an acceptable decision-maker can be replaced by the state if the state can identify a compelling interest of its own that conflicts with the parental right. The infant's best interest – that is, the infant's interest in life, health, and safety – is such a compelling interest. The state may protect this right of the infant if the parents fail to do so, since it is that right from which the parent's right is derived in the first instance.

Thus, the parents as appropriate *decision-makers* may be replaced if, and only if, they make an inappropriate *decision*. As the Supreme Court has held, parents do not have the right to make martyrs of their children [22]. Nonetheless, an important tension exists in a decision-making structure that grants to parents great deference merely in recognizing their decision-making role, yet gives to the state the power to examine every decision in order to identify and interfere with all those decisions of which it disapproves. There are many ways in which inappropriate decisions can be identified; how the government chooses to do so is crucial, because some methods preserve much family privacy, while others do not. Whatever means is used, the standard applied by a governmental decision-maker will always be the same: the objective standard of the child's best interests.

(1) *Parents and the States.* The least intrusive means of identifying inappropriate decisions is through the courts. This sounds paradoxical, because the courtroom experience itself is highly disruptive; but, in the ordinary process of the common law, only the most obviously bad

parental decisions will be examined. Most family choices will remain private, unreported, or even unseen.

Should the government determine that certain kinds of parental decisions are more at risk of being bad decisions than others, a somewhat more intrusive mechanism can be put into place. Child abuse and neglect statutes, and the social services agencies that enforce them, are examples of such a mechanism. The statutes provide a system for reporting and investigating suspected abuse, and set certain standards whereby experts – child protective services workers – can make a preliminary determination of whether a parental choice is appropriate. The social service system can then intervene in various ways before the question gets to court, and can present evidence to the judge regarding the 'correct' decision to make. It is within this system that the new federal definition of neglect of congenitally impaired infants purports to operate.

(2) *Parents and the Federal Government.* Finally, the state can determine – as the federal government at first attempted, in effect, to do in the Baby Doe regulations – that the risk of inappropriate decisions is so high that parents should no longer be considered the appropriate decision-makers in certain category of cases. Let us backtrack a moment to be sure we understand how this came about. We said earlier that parents enjoy decision-making authority because of the identity of their interests with their child's, and that they can lose that authority by virtue of a decision that is not in the child's best interests, objectively considered. Now, the bad decision can come about for one of two reasons: (1) the parent may be ignorant of what is best for the infant, or incapable of providing it; or (2) the parent may have interests of his or her own that are not identical to the infant's and thus may be unable to further the infant's interests because they conflict with personal interests.[17] A bad decision by a parent, then, might just be a bad decision, or it may be evidence that the parent is not the appropriate decision-maker in the first place, according to the identity of interest standard.

Does the reason the state views the decision as bad make any difference in decision-making for handicapped newborns? The answer is yes, and the difference is crucial. Let us return briefly to our least intrusive monitor of parental decisions: the courts. Establishing the parents as appropriate deciders whose decisions are subject to judicial scrutiny (and may be changed if inappropriate) has important consequences for the way those decisions are examined by courts. We said earlier that once it is determined that a decision is bad, the courts, the states (through social services agencies), and the federal government all use the same standard to reach a new decision: the objective best interests of the child standard. But first it must be determined that the decision is bad. If the same objective standard is used, the process is reduced to a single step: determining whether what the parent decided is what the court (or agency or government) would do. This is easy and neat – and it completely eliminates all of the deference to parental autonomy that logically flows from the application of the identity of interests standard, since it does not use that standard at all.

Deference to Parental Choice – What It Really Means

What the courts in fact do is slightly different – just different enough to have great significance for families. What they do is what the Indiana courts did in the original Baby Doe case: Courts examine the parents' decision not to see whether it is the right one, but whether it falls within the realm of possible decisions permitted to an appropriate decision-maker. This is precisely what deference to parental and family values means: The recognition that there is almost always more than one possible choice, each reflecting a response that is reasonable under the circumstances though not necessarily the choice that would be made by a different decision-maker.

Judge John G. Baker, the Indiana Superior Court Judge who decided the Bloomington Infant Doe case, submitted to DHHS a comment on the proposed regulations that perfectly explains the standard by which the particular decisions of appropriate deciders are to be viewed:

> The question in the Infant Doe case was, when parents are confronted with two competent medical opinions, one suggesting that corrective surgery may be appropriate and the other suggesting that corrective surgery and extraordinary measures would only be futile acts, does the law allow the parents to select which medical course to follow? It was the decision of the Indiana Court that the law provided the parents with the responsibility of choosing which medical course to follow without governmental intervention ([18], p. 1630).

The flaw in the Infant Doe decision did not lie in the choice of this deferential review standard. It is correct to leave to the parents a choice among acceptable alternatives. Unfortunately, however, insofar as can be determined, the court and the parents had before them medical evidence suggesting that non-treatment of easily correctable defects was an acceptable alternative for Down's infants. This is, at best, rarely the case. It will not be possible to come to a firm judgment about the decision so long as the records are sealed; clearly, however, the government responded to what was probably a bad outcome by changing the only obviously correct aspect of the case: the standard used to test parental decisions. The result is much like killing the messenger who brings bad tidings: Not only is the act unjust in itself, but it discourages others from coming forward to perform a needed task.

When the federal government wrote the Section 504 Baby Doe regulations, as well as the proposed regulations for the Child Abuse Act amendments, it identified the entire realm of medical decision-making about impaired newborns as at great risk of bad parental decisions. The most defensible explanation for this determination would be that the infant's interest in life itself conflicts irreconcilably with *any* parental decision in favor of non-treatment, so that the identity of interests standard is simply inapplicable to all non-treatment decisions. (Certainly there is no margin of error in decisions that result in death; in other circumstances, children may grow up to ratify their parent's decisions, thus disproving the possible conflict of interest, but no such checking mechanism exists here.) Therefore, by this argument, parental decisions will be respected only when they are correct.[18] In some cases, of course, even non-treatment decisions will be correct; when death is imminent, the infant's actual interest in life is small and may be outweighed by the risk and intrusiveness of treatment or the likelihood of suffering.[19] For example, non-treatment of spinal lesions in anencephalic babies is acceptable, but this determination, so the argument goes, is to be made by the government – never by the parents.

Nevertheless, even this most plausible explanation for governmental intrusion into these difficult decisions is ultimately indefensible. Despite the very real risk that some parental and family interests may not be entirely congruent with those of the infant, parents in fact rarely make choices that can fairly be called incorrect. The clear consensus of legal authority is that the decision belongs to the parents unless it is shown to be wrong – that is, to fall outside the realm of decisions that can be viewed as a reasonable interpretation of the child's best interests. This position amply supports the kind of case-by-case intervention that the courts and social services agencies provide, but is not compatible with the approach taken by either the original federal regulations or the ones proposed under the federal child abuse amendments. The final regulations promulgated under the child abuse amendments appear to be significantly different in this respect – at least in spirit – from earlier versions. We will examine those regulations more closely below. It remains very possible, however, that the new regulations could require states to exert intrusive decision-making authority in order to preclude loss of federal child abuse funds.

But we said that the reason parents *retain* this decisional power is that they rarely decide wrongly. How can a determination like that be made? The government has the burden of proof on the matter: that is, the duty to show that bad decisions that wrongfully allow handicapped infants to go untreated and die are prevalent enough to justify taking away parents' power to decide. One problem in making such a showing is that the number of cases in which any hard decision, good or bad, is made may be very small. The number of handicapped infants about which difficult decisions must be made is not large. Only approximately 4000 Down's syndrome babies are born per year in the United States; perhaps 20 of these will also have life-threatening surgically correctable defects. The number of children born with neural tube defects each year is perhaps 6000. That number includes anencephaly, meningomye-locele, and many other lesser defects, and in only one percent of those cases is there likely to be ambiguity regarding what course of treatment should be pursued. In most cases the defect is so severe or so minor as to afford no difficulty in deciding on appropriate treatment.[20] Another, much larger category of seriously ill newborns does exist, however – the premature infant, of whom nearly one-quarter million are born each year. Premature infants, in whom handicaps and potentially life-threatening treatable conditions are much more closely interlaced than they are in spina bifida or in Down's babies with other defects, present a more difficult analytical problem that appears to have been insufficiently anticipated by the regulators.[21] Whatever handicapping condition is examined, most authorities consider, as the President's Commission reports, that almost all decision-making regarding seriously ill newborns adheres to proper standards ([41], p. 223). We must therefore examine how those standards should be determined: that is, the relationship of parental decision-making to medical authority.

Determining the Range of Acceptable Decisions

Much of the criticism of the Baby Doe regulations came first from physician groups and focused principally on the regulations' attempt to curtail physicians' decision-making discretion. One physician commentator in the *New England Journal of Medicine* described the regulations as attempting

a remarkable distinction between medical decisions and decisions concerning the well-being of the patient, regarding the latter as outside the physician's purview but within the purview of the government. Oddly enough in this day of celebrating holistic medicine, the Administration seems to advocate that physicians not consider the whole patient, but rather act as highly skilled technicians whose job is to repair parts of the body ([1], p. 659).

The mandate of the first set of proposed regulations that all infants receive 'customary medical treatment' was widely perceived by physicians both as vague and as infringing upon their medical judgment.[22] The final Section 504 regulations required the provision of 'nourishment and medially beneficial treatment' (as determined with respect for reasonable medical judgments) ([18], p. 1651), but the guidelines and examples offered appear to restore little of the discretion the earlier versions of the regulations had removed.[23] The language of the child abuse amendments and their new regulations, which require provision of 'medically indicated treatment', seems to hark back to the vague terms of the proposed regulations. Though there is little legislative history on the language choice, the hearings in Congress about the amendments addressed the same broad concerns that had been considered by DHHS at the beginning of the controversy.

Concern for the physician's power *vis-à-vis* the state obscures concern for how parents fit into the balance. In fact, the American Hospital Association (AHA) suggested that the Section 504 regulations conflicted with the Supreme Court's abortion decisions, not because the regulations ignored family autonomy, but because they all but eliminated the *physician's* judgment. The AHA's reasoning is interesting: It views the abortion cases as giving prominence to the *physician's* judgment in declaring abortion to be a matter between a woman and her doctor ([33], pp. 5–6). This is an unfamiliar perspective on *Roe v. Wade*, but it is an accurate one: In the abortion cases, the physician is accorded a prominent, gate-keeping role that comports with the medical expertise required for abortions. This role has no equivalent in most of the other areas of family autonomy discussed earlier, that is, childrearing, education, lifestyle choices, and the like. Therefore, to make fully credible the argument that parents are the appropriate decision-makers, we must examine whether the physician ought not to be the decision-maker in circumstances where medical knowledge is required – that is, we must ask what medical judgment means in Baby Doe cases.

For an answer we return to the first step of the two-step process of decision analysis employed by the courts. First the court determines whether the decision is really inappropriate. Because parents have not been ousted as decision-makers in general, this is not the same as determining what the court itself would decide; instead the court looks to whether the decision falls within the realm of decisions acceptable under the circumstances. How is that realm to be defined?

Recall that the parents are chosen as decision-makers because they are believed best able to act in the infant's best interests. As a consequence, the outer limits of parental autonomy are dictated by the objective best interest standard. But because a decision in the infant's best interests confirms the appropriateness of the parent as decision-maker, what is acceptable is *not* limited to the single decision the court would make. Instead, any decision is acceptable that can reasonably be considered to be in the infant's best interests under the circumstances. As Judge Wexler put it in the Baby Jane Doe decision, the court must determine whether "the parents in question are in fact acting upon a reasonable interpretation of the child's best interests" ([30], p. 616 (footnote omitted) (And he found that they had so acted.)).

As long legal experience with reasonableness standards has shown, such a term can be broadly or narrowly applied. The jury determines the appropriateness of parental decisions, and it is precisely this kind of social judgment – the balancing of societal consensus about child-rearing with respect for parental autonomy – for which the jury system is best suited. Where the decision-making process or at least some aspects of it require expert knowledge, juries will still decide what decisions are acceptable, but they must decide on the basis of that expert knowledge. In decision-making for newborns, as in other medical contexts, the choice must be among 'competent medical opinions' – the language used by the judge in the Bloomington Baby Doe case.

When competent adults make decisions regarding their own health care, they are legally free to choose *any* course, provided that it does not infringe upon other parties' important rights and interests (for example, such a decision may not injure others or require them to act in derogation of their own values). Thus, competent individuals may, under many circumstances, make health care choices that are entirely unacceptable to the medical profession.[24] However, medically unacceptable choices – that is, choices which no medical professional is willing to consider appropriate under the circumstances – are generally outside the realm of acceptable decisions for handicapped newborns ([41], pp. 213, 219). This is necessary because establishing such medical parameters represents the only truly fair and feasible way of ensuring that parents are indeed acting in accordance with their infant's best interests. This does not constitute a delegation of decision-making authority to physicians, but it permits the parents to make any of a number of decisions, rather than mandating the one course of action an individual physician would choose. Instead, it corresponds precisely to the jury's establishment of parameters of socially acceptable choices where no expert knowledge is involved, embodying the same decision to trade off a degree of family autonomy against the risk that unusually or potentially dangerous parental decisions are not being made in good faith upon adequate information.[25] When the federal government prescribed the Baby Doe regulations, then, it attempted to circumscribe not the discretion of physicians, but that of parents.

The Effects of Federal Intervention

Do the Section 504 regulations – or the regulations accompanying the child abuse amendments – actually circumscribe parental decision-making? The regulations require that medically beneficial treatment be provided, as determined according to 'reasonable medical judgment'. If parental discretion is already appropriately circumscribed by reasonable medical judgments, then the only way the regulations can further limit that discretion is to declare that at least some of what would, but for the regulations, be considered reasonable medical judgments are not in fact reasonable under the regulations. This is precisely what the Section 504 regulations attempt to do.

Suppose that DHHS had declared, by statue or in its Section 504 regulations, that certain treatment options considered reasonable by the medical profession were nevertheless discriminatory and that therefore hospitals and physicians could continue to practice that way if they chose, though they would lose federal funding. That position would be legally defensible, unless the loss of funding were so extremely coercive a sanction as to preclude hospitals and doctors from daring to practice as they wished ([39]; [18], p. 1641). The focus of our analysis would then shift to whether or not there was discrimination in fact, and the government's position would be somewhat analogous to the effort to control hospital costs. For example, if an insurance company declares a certain procedure too expensive for reimbursement under a particular policy, the company is not questioning medical judgment but simply refusing to pay for medically acceptable but costly treatment options. However, the insuror's decision that a procedure is too costly is a crucially different, considerably less complicated determination than the decision that a given treatment choice is discriminatory. In practical terms, DHHS' problem in the Section 504 regulations remains the same regardless of the language in which it is couched: There is simply insufficient social consensus to label the treatment options in question discriminatory.

Handicap is not susceptible of line-drawing as cost is – or as sex, age, racial identity, and other potentially discriminatory determining factors are. The problem of determining what an otherwise qualified handicapped person is for the purpose of the Rehabilitation Act is severe in every other context in which the Act has been applied;[26] it was compounded in the regulations because an evaluation of handicap is part of the very determination of what options are medically acceptable. Each determination is necessarily individual and dependent on circumstances – whether the medical problem is Down's syndrome or the thornier issue of extreme prematurity. Indeed, the decision of the Court of Appeals relied specifically on this difficulty, stating that " the comparatively fluid context of medical treatment decisions" made Section 504 very hard to apply: Where the handicapping condition is related to the condition(s) to be treated, it will rarely, if ever, be possible to say with certainty that a particular decision was 'discriminatory'".[27] To mandate what DHHS defines as 'medically beneficial' treatment in all instances thus constitutes centralized decision-making of the sort most likely to lose sight completely of the needs of the individual newborns involved in each case.

Parental Autonomy and Ambiguous Cases

The final Child Abuse Amendment regulations appear at first to be very different, in tone and in effect, from the proposed regulations and the now dormant Section 504 regulations. Whether they are truly different will not be discernible except in their enforcement, but examination of their provisions and their preamble is nonetheless enlightening. The crucial question is: How do these regulations deal with the most difficult, ambiguous cases faced by parents?

First, the regulatory preamble states clearly that the Department intends to continue to press the validity of the Section 504 regulations by seeking certiorari to the Second Circuit Court of Appeals from the Supreme Court; it also asserts that the two sets of regulations are completely compatible and should both be in place and in force. ([5], p. 14885). However, the preamble goes on to present these regulations' scope and purpose as much more limited than previous versions.

Most notable is the preamble's forthright statement on the role of parents:

The decision to provide or withhold medically indicated treatment is, except in highly unusual circumstances, made by the parents or legal guardian. Parents are the decision-makers concerning treatment for their disabled infant, based on the advice and reasonable medical judgment of their physician (or physicians). . . .

We want to emphasize that it is not the CPS agency or the ICRC or similar committee that makes the decision regarding the care of and treatment for the child. This is the parent's right and responsibility. . . . The parents' role as decision maker must be respected and supported unless they choose a course of action inconsistent with applicable standards established by law ([5], p. 14880).

Perhaps less conspicuous, but more powerful, is a discussion placing the amendments squarely within the context of the existing child abuse and neglect statutory and regulatory scheme in precisely the way discussed earlier:

The new law and its legislative history make clear that Congress understood and intended that 'medical neglect' is a form of "child abuse and neglect" within the meaning of the Act and the present regulations, and that the "withholding of medically indicated treatment from disabled infants with life-threatening conditions" is a form of medical neglect. . . . [These new regulations] simply define[e] 'medical neglect' as the failure to provide adequate medical care, and. . . state[e] that medical neglect includes, but is not limited to, the withholding of medically indicated treatment from disabled infants with life-threatening conditions ([5], p. 14881).

Thus, the final regulations claim to do no more than reinforce and clarify the existing child abuse and neglect scheme for this small included category of child neglect cases. The preamble's regulatory impact analysis explains carefully and in detail how small the impact of these regulations will be:

[T]he role of these rules in the larger context of medical care for infants is minor. . . . [V]irtually all such infants now, and in the future, will receive 'state of the art' medical care, often at great expense, quite irrespective of the new statutory provisions of this rule. . . . [O]nly a very small fraction of births involve any serious question of survival. Of these, only a fraction would not be treated appropriately under current medical practice, and would involve even a potential allegation of medical neglect. These considerations suggest that the potential number of cases which the statute might impact is not large. The number differentially affected by any particular wording of the rule itself would be far smaller ([5], p. 14886).

It is tempting to wonder why regulation is still considered necessary if its impact is expected to be so small. The answer may perhaps be found in the history of the regulations' approach to cases where, in the words of the President's Commission's report on treatment refusal for severely ill newborns, an infant's permanent handicaps "are so severe that continued existence would not be a net benefit to the infant" ([41], p. 219).

Both the Section 504 regulations and the proposed child abuse amendment regulations appeared to deny parents the opportunity to refuse treatments that would permit their infant to survive a year or two but would fail to relieve – or would itself result in – severe and permanent retardation, paralysis, and pain.[28] The proposed regulations put forward, in addition, a number of 'clarifying definitions' meant to elaborate on the instances where treatment need not be provided ([6], pp. 48166–48167).

Those clarifying definitions proved immensely controversial. As pointed out in the preamble to the final regulations, many comments on the proposed regulations objected strongly to those definitions as exceeding Congressional intent. One such comment came from the six principal sponsors of the child abuse amendment; they asserted in particular that the regulatory requirement that death be 'imminent' was specifically rejected by the Conference Committee that negotiated the amendment's final language ([5], p. 14879). All of the diagnostic examples were deleted and 'imminent' was (somewhat grudgingly) replaced by this statement:

[T]he Department continues to interpret the Congressional intent as not permitting the 'merely prolong dying' provision to apply where many years of life will result from the provision of treatment, or where the prognosis is not for death in the near future, but rather the more distant future ([5], p. 14891).

Moreover, here and elsewhere in the guidelines and preamble, DHHS has attempted to emphasize that more specificity is unnecessary because it is expected that each decision will be made conscientiously in the light of all the medical circumstances of each case and with the exercise of 'reasonable medical judgment' – a term repeated with great frequency throughout, in an attempt to bolster physicians' confidence that the practice of medicine will not be infringed upon by the regulatory scheme. All of these changes do seem to suggest that the impact of the final regulations upon parental rights and medical judgment will be considerably less adverse than that threatened by previous versions. Nonetheless, DHHS continues to regard as impermissible any determination that includes in the weighing of harms and benefits the quality of the infant's life – except where "the treatment itself involves . . . significant pain and suffering for the infant that clearly outweighs the very slight potential benefit of the treatment for an infant highly unlikely to survive" ([5], p. 14892). Thus, neither parents nor 'reasonable' physicians are permitted to opt for nontreatment in that category of ambiguous and wrenchingly difficult cases where some might decide that continued existence is not in the infant's best interest.

The President's Commission takes the position that where real ambiguity exists, because of both factual uncertainty[29] and the problem of balancing harms and benefits ([40], pp. 220–223), the choices of fully informed parents should be honored, whether their decision is to treat or not to treat ([51], p. 218, Table 1). According to the federal government, however, such ambiguity does not exist. The regulations would eliminate parental discretion in this category of cases by refusing to recognize a non-treatment option.

Nevertheless, both the government and the President's Commission recognize that there are futile therapies. Earlier regulatory materials specifically discussed treatment, for example, for anencephalic or cephalodynic infants or those with certain other severe anomalies. (See, [41], p. 219: [18] p. 1654.) The final regulations do not use examples to elaborate on their discussion of treatments that, according to reasonable medical judgment, are 'futile', or 'virtually futile . . . and . . . inhumane', in terms of the infant's survival ([9]; [5], p. 14888). But any attempt to present such terms as 'purely medical' or objective determinations must fail; it seems undeniable that value factors and net benefit determinations play some role in defining certain treatments as futile or as merely prolonging the act of dying in these cases. Thus, it seems equally impossible for the government to deny that similar factors affect all other medical benefit determinations besides. Blanket determinations to treat suffer from a failure to face these inextricable value questions, which has been labeled the 'technical criteria fallacy'.[30]

CONCLUSION

Courts can, should, and sometimes do offer parents of handicapped
newborns a range of options, and uphold their choices in ambiguous
cases. After much negotiation on many fronts, the federal government's
role in decision-making for these infants is downplayed somewhat from
its initial interventionist posture. The child abuse amendments appear
to do little more than emphasize and clarify the state social services
system's role in medical neglect in the hospital setting. Even the posture
of the model Infant Care Review Committee guidelines has changed
somewhat: the guidelines are clearly and explicitly labeled purely advisory. No institution need have an ICRC; its form, composition, and
operation are stated to be entirely flexible; it is asserted that having one
or not having one will make absolutely no difference in terms of
anyone's legal responsibilities; and – most important – the ICRC's role
as advisor and policymaker is emphasized. Even when the ICRC acts in
specific cases, it is only to 'counsel' a course of action [17].

Does all this appearance amount to a real change, either in federal
policy or in the states' likely implementation of it? Probably not. The
ICRC is still expected in the new regulations, as it was earlier, to make
its own determinations as to whether it agrees with the parents' or the
physicians' treatment decision in particular cases. (See [17], p. 14896;
[18], p. 1653; see also [14], p. 48172.) This is an unacceptable substitution of the ICRC's judgment for the family's that may bring more
cases before the courts. As we have seen, the proper role for a decision-
maker other than the parents is only to determine whether a particular
decision – even one with which it might disagree – is reasonable, unless
some real showing of unfitness demonstrates that the parents' decision-
making discretion should be displaced and another's decision substituted. Second, the federal policy does not now recognize – and never
has recognized – the validity of parental discretion in ambiguous cases.
The final regulations are much less specific and particular than earlier
formulations in establishing this position, and it is possible, if not likely,
that in the enforcement process a greater number of ambiguous cases
will in practice be left to parents; however, the regulatory changes were
not at all aimed at such a result.

It remains to be seen how the decentralized implementation of these
guidelines and regulations through state social services systems will
work. Despite the purely advisory status of the ICRC, many hospitals

have been moving toward putting committees in place, and will almost certainly continue to do so. Whatever form they take, ICRCs have a valuable role to play – one that will probably not be outweighed by the risk they potentially pose to parents' decision-making rights. Committees will probably see few cases, and will probably make few controversial pronouncements. Still, the possibility does exist that parents may be left feeling as though their decision has come before a panel of strangers, without even the fairness guarantees offered by the courts.

Perhaps it is too much to expect the crucial matter of the ambiguous cases to be correctly resolved by federal regulation. It is not easy for the courts to resolve it either; indeed, even the courts have not always succeeded in protecting the well-established right of competent, nonterminal adults to choose death over a painful and diminished existence. It is not easy for any of us to recognize that there are difficult and painful choices that cannot, indeed should not, be avoided by drawing bright lines and making hard and fast rules. Nonetheless, parents do have the legal right and the moral authority to decide for their infants, even – indeed especially – in the ambiguous cases the very existence of which the federal regulations seek to disavow. No federal or state governmental authority should be able to deny parents that dignity – or that responsibility.

The University of North Carolina
Chapel Hill, North Carolina, U.S.A.

NOTES

[1] For further medical information, see [40].

[2] The court records in the case are sealed and the decision is unreported. Dr. Joanne Lynn of the President's Commission for the Study of Ethical Problems in Medicine and Biomedical and Behavioral Research reports that the court heard only medical evidence from the physician who had advised the parents to refuse surgery (personal communication, Jan. 25, 1984), but the presiding judge stated that the parents were given two acceptable medical options. See [18], p. 1630.

[3] No otherwise qualified handicapped individual in the United States, as defined in Section 706(7) of this title, shall, solely by reason of his handicap, be excluded from the participation in, be denied the benefits of, or be subjected to discrimination under any program or activity receiving Federal financial assistance [24].

[4] See the discussion in [19]. Among the studies cited were [34] and [43].

[5] See [41], Appendix F. Only 17 of 602 hospitals had such committees as of 1983.

[6] The guidelines appear as Appendix C to the regulations ([18], 1953–1954).

[7] See [41], Appendix F. Only 17 of 602 hospitals had such committees as of 1983.

[8] The President signed the Child Abuse Prevention and Treatment and Reform Act Amendments [9] on October 11, 1984. The Amendments had a long and tortuous history, beginning with great differences between the original House bill, H.R. 1904 (see H.R. Report 98–159, 98th Congress, 1st session), and the Senate version, S–1003. The version that ultimately passed the Senate was much closer to the House bill, see *Congressional Record-Senate*, S–9307–9329 (July 26, 1984), but the differences were still significant enough to convene a joint House-Senate conference. The conference committee reached agreement in September, 1984, and the final version quickly passed in Congress. See *Congressional Record-House*, H–10327– 10339 (September 26, 1984), and *Congressional Record-Senate*, S–12382–12392 (September 28, 1984). The AMA still opposes the amendments and is likely to challenge them once they are implemented and enforced. See [37].

[9] New Section 4 (b) (2) (K) of the Act. The amendments define "withholding of medically indicated treatment" as "the failure to respond to the infant's life-threatening conditions by providing treatment (including appropriate nutrition, hydration, or medication) which, in the treating physician's or physicians' reasonable medical judgment, will be most likely to be effective in ameliorating or correcting all such conditions." The exemptions from this definition are when the infant is chronically and irreversibly comatose and when treatment would merely prolong dying; not be effective in ameliorating or correcting all of the infant's conditions, would be futile and inhumane, or would be virtually futile in terms of the infant's survival and inhumane under the circumstances. Section 3(3) of the Act, 42 U.S.C. 5 102 (1984).

[10] On December 10, 1984, interim regulations [6] and guidelines [14] appeared in the *Federal Register*. Final regulations [5] and guidelines [16] were published in the *Federal Register* of April 15, 1985.

[11] Existing regulations require the state to define abuse and neglect "in accordance with" the federal definition, but stipulate that use of identical language is not necessary so long as the state's definition is "the same in substance" ([4], Section 13401.14).

[12] Although federal law only requires that states "provide for the reporting of known and suspected instances of child abuse and neglect" (42 U.S.C. Section 5103 (b) (2) (B)), virtually all states require reporting, at least by professionals and institutions. See [6], p. 48162.

[13] See e.g., [3, 15]. Similar legislation has been proposed in Connecticut (S.B. 453), California (S.C.R. 75), Indiana (S.E.A. 418), and North Carolina (H.B. 1029, defeated).

[14] There is a vast body of legal literature setting forth the exegesis of parental autonomy. One of the best collections of writings on the question is [36], especially chapters by Alexander M. Capron, Joseph Goldstein, and Margaret O'Brien Steinfels.

[15] Most common applications of this standard are in property law and civil procedure, to determine whether the actions of persons who appear to have financial and related interests in common with another can in addition be treated as actions by the other. Examples include virtual representation of incompetent persons in trust law, third party consent to searches and seizures of commonly held property, and representation of a class by individual members of that class in class action lawsuits. See Capron, "The Authority of Others to Decide about Biomedical Interventions with Incompetents", in [34], p. 115.

[16] This was attempted by the court in [28].

[17] "Parents should be the surrogates for seriously ill newborns unless they are disqualified

by decision-making incapacity, an unresolvable disagreement between them, or their choice of a course of action that is clearly against the infant's best interests" ([41], p. 6).

[18] Correctness is, of course, a matter of the judgment of the reviewing body, though it may ostensibly be objective.

[19] The Quinlan court put forward this sliding scale analysis: "We think that the State's interest [in the preservation of life] weakens and the individual's right to privacy grows as the degree of bodily invasion increases and the prognosis dims" ([23], p. 644).

[20] These figures are derived from [41], pp. 198–203, and Dr. Joanne Lynn, personal communication. Most sources of statistics on handicapped infants do not attempt to distinguish ambiguous cases from children who are so mildly or severely affected as to preclude legitimate debate over appropriate treatment.

[21] According to personal communication by Dr. Joanne Lynn. See the final regulations' discussion of the comments on handicapping conditions in [28], pp. 1636–1637.

[22] See, e.g., [32]; testimony presented by the American Academy of Pediatrics before the Senate Subcommittee on Family and Human Services, April 6, 1983; [45].

[23] See discussion at [18], p. 1637, and the guidelines on p. 1654. See also discussion at text accompanying notes 27–29.

[24] "Every human being of adult years and sound mind has a right to determine what shall be done with his own body" ([24], p. 129). See generally [42].

[25] "By far, most cases involving judicial inquiry into parents' medical choices for their children have occurred in situations in which parents have opted for unconventional 'medical' care for their children . . ." ([43], p. 2137 n. 67).

[26] See the extensive discussion of Section 504's legislative history in [29], and cases cited therein, on the definitional problems.

[27] See the majority opinion in [29], rejecting the dissent's attempted analogy between handicap and race.

[28] See discussion at [28], p. 1637, and the examples in [6], p. 48164.

[29] The preamble to the Section 504 regulations discusses the impact of known possible complications of treatment, and interprets Section 504 as requiring treatment if it is *likely* to achieve its intended result, but does not address the obvious corollary that reasonable medical judgment might differ regarding that very likelihood. The problem of factual uncertainty is particularly severe in treatment of premature infants (see [41], pp. 220–221), a category not initially considered by the regulators but addressed later in the child abuse amendment regulations. See Note 20.

[30] See [44]. This term became current in the course of the controversy over British physician John Lorber's criteria for selection of treatment vs. nontreatment in children with spina bifida. See, e.g., [38]; [41], pp. 221–223.

BIBLIOGRAPHY

Cases, Statutes, and Regulations

1. American Academy of Pediatrics v. Heckler, 541 F. Supp. 395 (D.D.C., 1983).
2. American Hospital Association v. Heckler, American Medical Association v. Heckler, 585 F. Supp. 541 (S.D.N.Y. 1984), aff'd, F. 2d (2d Cir. Dec. 27, 1984), *petition for cert. filed* (Mar. 27, 1985).

3. Arizona Revised Statutes Annotated, 36–2281–2283 (West Supp. 1983).
4. Child Abuse and Neglect Prevention and Treatment Program, 45 CFR Part 13840 (1984).
5. Child Abuse and Neglect Prevention and Treatment Program; Final Rule, 50 *Federal Register* 14878 (April 15, 1985).
6. Child Abuse and Neglect Prevention and Treatment Program; Proposed Rule, 49 *Federal Register* 48160 (December 10, 1984).
7. Child Abuse Prevention and Treatment Act, Pub. L. 93–247, 42 U.S.C. 5111 *et seq* (1976).
8. Child Abuse Prevention and Treatment and Adoption Reform Act of 1978, 29 U.S.C. 794 (1978).
9. Child Abuse Prevention and Treatment and Adoption Reform Act Amendments of 1984, Pub. L. 98–457, 42 U.S.C. 5101 *et seq.*(1984).
10. Doe v. Bloomington Hospital, Indiana Ct. App. (Feb. 3, 1983), *cert. denied*, 104 S.Ct. 394 (1983).
11. Doe v. Bolton, 410 U.S. 179 (1973).
12. Eisenstadt v. Baird, 405 U.S. 438 (1972).
13. Griswold v. Connecticut, 381 U.S. 479 (1965).
14. Interim Model Guidelines for Health Care Providers to Establish Infant Care Review Committees: Notice, 49 *Federal Register* 48170 (Dec. 10, 1984).
15. Louisiana Revised Statutes Annotated, 40:1299.36.1 – 36.3 (West 1983).
16. Meyer v. Nebraska, 262 U.S. 390 (1923).
17. Model Guidelines for Health Care Providers to Establish Infant Care Review Committees, 50 *Federal Register* 14893 (April 15, 1985).
18. Nondiscrimination on the Basis of Handicap; Procedures and Guidelines Relating to Health Care for Handicapped Infants, Final Rules, 49 *Federal Register*1622 (Jan. 12, 1984).
19. Nondiscrimination on the Basis of Handicaps Relating to Health Care for Handicapped Infants, Proposed Rules, 48 *Federal Register* 30846 (July 5, 1983).
20. Pierce v. Society of Sisters, 268 U.S. 510 (1925).
21. President's Directive of April 30, 1982, and Notice to Health Care Providers, Office of Civil Rights, Department of Health and Human Services, 47 *Federal Register* 26027 (May 18, 1982).
22. Prince v. Massachusetts, 321 U.S. 158 (1944).
23. In re Quinlan, 70 N.J. 10, 355 A. 2d 647, *cert. denied*, 429 U.S. 922 (1976).
24. Rehabilitation Act of 1973, Section 504, as amended, 29 U.S.C. 794 (1976).
25. Roe v. Wade, 410 U.S. 113 (1973).
26. Schloendorff v. Society of N.Y. Hospitals, 211 N.Y. 125, 129, 105 N.E. 92, 93 (1914).
27. Skinner v. Oklahoma, 405 U.S. 438 (1942).
28. Superintendent of Belchertown State School v. Saikewicz, 373 Mass. 728, 370 N.E.2d 417 (1977).
29. U.S. v. University Hospital of State University of New York, 729 F.2d 144 (2d Cir. 1984).
30. U.S. v. University Hospital of State University of New York, 575 F. Supp. 607 (E.D.N.Y. 1983), *aff'd*, 729 F.2d 144 (2d Cir. 1984).
31. Wisconsin v. Yoder, 406 U.S. 205 (1972).

Articles and Books

32. Angell, M.: 1983, 'Handicapped Children: Baby Doe & Uncle Sam', *New England Journal of Medicine* **309**, 659.
33. Carlson, R.: 1983, 'The 1983 Supreme Court Abortion Decisions: Impact on Hospitals, a Conflict with Baby Doe?', *Health Law Vigil* October 14, 5–6.
34. Duff, R. and Campbell, A.: 1973, 'Moral and Ethical Dilemmas in the Special-Care Nursery', *New England Journal of Medicine* **289**, 890–894.
35. Fleischman, J. and Murray, T.: 1983, 'Ethics Committee for Infants Doe?', *Hastings Center Report* **13**, 6.
36. Gaylin, W. and Macklin, R. (eds.): 1982, *Who Speaks for the Child?*, Plenum Press, New York.
37. Krieger, L.: 1984, 'Conferees Adopt Senate "Baby Doe" Legislation', *American Medical News*, Sept. 21.
38. Lorber, J.: 1974, 'Selective Treatment of Myelomeningocele: To Treat or Not to Treat?', *Pediatrics* **53**, 307.
39. Note: 1983, 'Defective Newborns and Section 504 of the Rehabilitation Act: Legislation by Administrative Fiat?', *Arizona Law Review* 25, 709.
40. Pless, J. E.: 1983, 'The Story of Baby Doe', *New England Journal of Medicine* **309**, 664.
41. President's Commission for the Study of Ethical Problems in Medicine and Biomedical and Behavioral Research: 1983, *Deciding to Forego Life-Sustaining Treatment*, U.S. Government Printing Office, Washington, D.C.
42. President's Commission for the Study of Ethical Problems in Medicine and Biomedical and Behavioral Research: 1983, *Making Health Care Decisions*, U.S. Government Printing Office, Washington, D.C.
43. Todres, D. *et al.*: 1977, 'Pediatricians' Attitudes Affecting Decision-Making in Defective Newborns', *Pediatrics* **60**, 197–201.
44. Veatch, R. M.: 1977, 'The Technical Criteria Fallacy', *Hastings Center Report* **7**, 15.
45. Weir, R. F.: 1983, 'The Government and Selective Non-treatment of Handicapped Infants', *New England Journal of Medicine* **309**, 661.

MARGERY W. SHAW

WHEN DOES TREATMENT CONSTITUTE A HARM?

INTRODUCTION

As an intern rotating through pediatrics, I performed the admission work-up one evening on a cute and chubby four-month-old boy who was semi-comatose.[1] I quickly determined that he was gravely ill with high fever, intermittent seizures, slight cyanosis, and nuchal rigidity. I called the resident and we worked frantically for the next eight hours to save his life. He kept slipping away and we brought him back. Our working diagnosis was acute meningitis, bacterial in origin. We performed a spinal tap and then ordered a portable chest X-ray, blood tests (including a type and cross-match), and cultures and sensitivities from throat, blood, and spinal fluid. Then we performed a 'cut-down' so that we could administer intravenous fluids and medications quickly, started IV glucose-and-saline with high doses of broad-spectrum antibiotics, and used ice packs to bring down his fever. He needed digoxin, vaso-pressors, and finally cortisone to sustain him in his struggle to survive against overwhelming odds.

I told his parents that he might not live through the night. Several times during the night his breathing was labored and stertorous; at other times it was so shallow we thought it had stopped altogether. Even though he was receiving oxygen, he became more cyanotic. But somehow he managed to stay alive (or we managed to keep him alive) through the night, and by the time the attending pediatrician arrived for morning rounds, the infant's temperature had dropped, his blood pressure was up, and his condition was 'stable'. He congratulated us for performing a great job and there was a feeling of pride when we saw the relief on the mother's face.

Over the next several days his condition improved from 'critical' to 'serious'. He responded poorly to external stimuli but I didn't consider it significant, considering how ill he had been. His name was Peter Yamm

R. C. McMillan, H. T. Engelhardt, Jr., and S. F. Spicker (eds.),
Euthanasia and the Newborn, 117–137.
© 1987 by D. Reidel Publishing Company.

117

and the nurses affectionately referred to him as 'our little sweet potato'. Before the end of the week I had rotated from pediatrics to general surgery, scarcely giving little Peter a second thought. Now I was preoccupied with gall stones, peptic ulcers, hernias, and thyroid nodules.

Several years later, as an associate professor at the medical school, I was conducting research on blood groups in children with Down's syndrome, hoping to be the first person to map a human gene on chromosome no. 21. This research took me to a state hospital to obtain blood samples on patients with Down's syndrome institutionalized there. After obtaining finger-prick blood samples from three children playing in the corner of a cheerfully painted four-bed room, I was ready to move to the next room when I noticed a gangly boy lying in a bed near the door. He was curled up in a fetal position, staring at nothing, slobbering and grunting. The nameplate above his bed read 'Peter Yamm'. I was in such a state of shock to see the fruits of my midnight labors as an intern that I stopped drawing blood from the other patients and drove home.

After talking about this jolting experience with my husband and a former fellow intern, I went back to the state hospital the next day to read Peter's chart. As I had suspected, he had never returned home when he was discharged from the hospital but was admitted for permanent institutional care after his close brush with death. This was the first time I asked myself the question, "When does treatment constitute a harm?"

In order to discuss the question – when does treatment constitute a harm – it may be helpful to first define types of treatment and harms. Next, I will try to identify some of the sociological and scientific elements that have contributed to our concern over the issue of defective infants – why we are being inundated in the professional literature with questions surrounding the treatment of handicapped newborns, and why we are calling conferences to address these questions.

This discussion will be limited to possible legal responses to the dilemma society faces in fashioning appropriate behavior for the treatment or withholding of treatment of seriously defective neonates. These include criminal law sanctions against those who fail to provide care, statutory law protecting persons who choose not to accept medical care, and tort law responses to disagreements among the principal actors in the drama – the health professionals, the parents, the infant, and the state. Both intentional and nonintentional (negligent) tort actions are possible. Finally, I will summarize our present ability to prevent the birth of handicapped children and comment on the future promises of recent scientific advances to decrease further the frequency of handicapping conditions, thus ameliorating our confrontation with the difficult issues before us today.

DEFINING TREATMENT AND HARM

Some Preliminary Definitions

Before attempting to answer the question – when does treatment constitute a harm? – we should first attempt to define treatment and, second, define harm. This discussion will be limited to the medical treatments of defective newborns, and the legal harms to the infant and its parents.

Types of treatment – *Curative* treatment is one that will provide a cure for the condition, returning the infant to a normal homeostatic state without further intervention. An example of cure is antibiotic treatment for infection. Closely allied to curative treatment is *corrective* treatment. This would include surgical repair of congenital anomalies such as patent ductus, club foot, cleft palate, or ileal atresia. *Palliative* treatment alleviates symptoms but does not deter the natural course of the disease. Digoxin for congestive failure and dialysis for renal failure constitute palliative therapy. *Prophylactic* treatment is given to prevent disease, such as antibiotics for an immune-compromised individual or a milk-free diet for an infant born with galactosemia. Finally, *supportive* treatment is given to increase comfort, such as narcotics for pain, mobilization to prevent bed sores, and intravenous or enteric feeding to maintain nutrition. These categories of treatment are not mutually exclusive but they help to analyze the types of treatment that may be given to, or withheld from, a defective newborn.

Kinds of legal harm – Several kinds of legal harms might accrue from giving or withholding treatment. *Physical pain and suffering*, which is legally compensable, is of greatest concern. The degree of discomfort may be worsened or lessened by treatment; the pain induced by treatment may be short-lived, as in post-surgical pain, or it may be long-lasting, as in dialysis. The natural pain and suffering of the disease or defect may be prolonged if the treatment merely extends life without reversing the course of the disease. *Mental and emotional pain and suffering* may be more likely to be recognized by the courts as applicable to the parents than to a young infant who does not have the cognitive skills to remember or anticipate physical pain. Nevertheless, it is important in our analysis because both family members and the health professionals endure a great deal of anxiety and emotional pain and suffering in making decisions about the treatment of defective newborns. *Economic loss* is the third category of harm that is recognized in the law. It is spread between the family and society in varying degrees.

When is Treatment Harmful to the Infant?

Oppressive and invasive treatment can be harmful if it produces more pain than no treatment. If an infant is subjected to multiple diagnostic procedures, corrective operations, and drugs with side effects, and if, after these heroic measures, death occurs anyway, a great deal of pain and suffering could have been spared by giving only palliative and supportive treatment.

Treatment is harmful if the quality of life after treatment is worse than it would have been without treatment and the child survives in either case. It is also harmful if it allows a child to live who would have otherwise died and the child is handicapped to such an extent that there is little or no opportunity to enjoy life. A life in coma or in such a retarded state that there is no cognition or sapience is generally considered by adults to be not worth living and certainly should not be considered worthwhile for infants who might have a much longer life expectancy to suffer in a vegetative or diminished state.

Intervention can also be harmful if it prolongs the process of dying. Unless there is a reasonable expectation that the quality of life will be improved, whether or not the child dies, treatment should not be instituted. Trisomy-13 and trisomy-18 with multiple birth defects and severe retardation are examples of conditions that are known to be fatal in the first one or two years of life and often within weeks or months after birth, and there is no known treatment except surgical intervention to correct certain defects and provide palliative and supportive therapy. To repair a congenital heart defect in a child who is expected to die within a few months of other causes could be considered treatment that constitutes a harm.

When Does Treating the Infant Harm the Parents?

The parents may be harmed economically and emotionally in every situation that would harm the infant. In addition, they could be devastated if the child survives to enjoy some little pleasure such as being held or fed, but is otherwise utterly dependent throughout life and is unable to recognize others and to give or acknowledge love. Such parents and their other children are given no hope of respite from a life-long burden of caring for the child. The family suffers economically, through medical and nursing expenses, and through the child's lack of productivity at an age when it would have been independent of the parents, had it been normal.

How Should the Parents' Needs be Balanced Against the Infant's Needs?

Suppose it were possible to arrest a normal child's development at a tender age and that child would continue to live a normal life span. Because no one would wish to have the duty of caring for a six-month-old infant for the rest of its life without hope of development or independence, keeping such a child alive would impose an arrest of development on the parents as well. Parenting is expected to come to an end after two decades of a child's life, and it gradually diminishes much sooner than that. If it does not, the parents are not allowed to develop their own full potential. If the law requires the parents to accept the burden, then it chooses in favor of the child's diminished capacities over the parents' normal capacities. Because we do not require people to be altruists, even though that may be beneficial to society, we should not require parents to sacrifice their well-being entirely in favor of the child. If the parents are emotionally incapable or unwilling to bear the tremendous burden that the defective child thrusts upon them, the state should accept their burden and relieve the parents of their duties without punishment. Parents differ in their stamina, their parenting capacities, and their anger. If faced with a burden without hope of relief, they should not be required to become martyrs for their defective child.

SOCIETAL DEVELOPMENTS CONTRIBUTING TO LEGAL CONFRONTATIONS

In the early 1960s public attention was drawn to the battered child syndrome [42], and for the first time in this country society began to seriously question the wisdom of the policy of the state's noninter-vention into family affairs. Heretofore, parental authority and control over their children were nearly absolute and children were treated as chattels of the parents [51]. Concerns about child abuse led to criminal statutes and family codes outlining the legal duties and obligations of parents toward their children, with sanctions for failure to provide food, shelter, education, and medical care [46]. Termination of custody is a possible outcome if the parents cannot be rehabilitated, and in out-rageous cases prison sentences may be imposed upon the parents, particularly if the battering resulted in death of the child [16].[2]

At the same time that state intervention into family affairs was growing, scientific advances were contributing to a better understanding of birth defects and hereditary disease. Cytogeneticists discovered that a chromosomal aberration was responsible for Down's syndrome and for many other conditions of greater severity, involving both physical defects and mental retardation. Biochemical geneticists were elucidat-ing the enzyme deficiencies in inborn errors of metabolism. These dis-coveries gave rise to widespread neonatal genetic screening, such as for phenylketonuria (PKU), mandated by state legislatures [49]. This form of state intervention was accepted because dietary treatment of PKU had been developed that would prevent mental retardation. Then in the late 1960s the technique of amniocentesis and prenatal diagnosis of chromosomal and biochemical abnormalities was introduced [44].[3]

Concurrently with child law development and greater scientific under-standing of the causes of physically and mentally defective infants, the famous trilogy of cases, *Griswold* [9][4], *Eisenstadt* [7][5], and *Roe v. Wade* [23][6], was decided by the U.S. Supreme Court, giving parents the fundamental right to decide not to have children by protecting con-traceptive use and abortion under the constitutional umbrella of repro-ductive privacy. This allowed parents who were at high risk for having genetically abnormal children to choose to have healthy children and circumvent the birth of defective ones [41].[7]

New developments in tort law quickly followed these expanded reproductive rights. Parents brought wrongful birth suits, alleging that their right *not* to have children was denied them when sterilization operations failed, when pregnancy was not diagnosed in time for an elective abortion, or when physicians had failed to warn them of increased risks of birth defects and genetic disease and failed to offer them diagnostic prenatal tests [47]. The courts at first refused to allow a cause of action because of the pervasive belief that "every child is a joy and a blessing" [2], and "who can put a price tag on a child's smile?" [30]. The Blessings Theory soon gave way to the Benefits Rule, whereby the harms the parents suffered by having an unwanted child were mitigated by the benefits of the child's society [22].[8] Inevitably, some of these wrongful birth cases involved defective children, and courts slowly began to accept the concept that children could be burdens to their parents rather than blessings or benefits. Today, most courts recognize wrongful birth claims made by the parents of both healthy and defective children and they award just compensation to parents if, through another's negligence, they were deprived of their right not to become parents [47].

Less striking is the gradual development of the tort of wrongful life, giving children (rather than the parents) a right to claim that they should not have been born in a defective state [48, 50].[9] Only two states have so far recognized this cause of action on behalf of the child ([10], [32]), but it is my opinion that acceptance will slowly become more widespread [21].[10]

These four societal developments – rapid scientific discoveries, a constitutional right to control reproduction, wrongful birth and wrongful life torts, and state intervention into family affairs in child abuse and neglect cases – have laid the foundation for the increasing legal concerns, tensions, and dilemmas over the treatment of defective newborns.

Parents are claiming a right to make decisions on behalf of their infants, and to allow them to die without corrective, prophylactic, or supportive therapy, under the principles of family autonomy, family privacy, and freedom of religion. Physicians, on the other hand, who had typically made these crushing decisions for the parents in a benevolent and paternal way, began to include parents in the decision-making process. This increase in shared responsibility came about because of the rapid development, in case law, of the doctrine of informed consent, [26][11] and the rise in medical malpractice claims. Thus the stage was set for governmental intervention when health professionals and parents disagreed.

LEGAL RESPONSES TO CONFLICTS OVER WITHHOLDING TREATMENT FROM DEFECTIVE NEWBORNS

Criminal Liability

At the present time, parents and physicians who decide to withhold treatment, allowing the infant to die, and hospitals that condone such behavior may be criminally liable under various state statutes [33, 38, 46]. There are no exceptions written into these homicide laws that would afford them a measure of protection. Although they are rarely prosecuted, this cloud hangs over them and vigorous prosecuting attorneys do, occasionally, bring charges.

What is the nature of the criminal charges? The most serious is first degree murder, where malice is required. In one adult euthanasia case one judge has written, "[I]f any life at all is left in the human body, *even the least spark*, the extinguishment of it is as much homicide as the killing of the most vital human being" ([28], p. 364).

Other cases have held that mercy-killing, which does not require malice, is equally punishable [6 , 19 , 27 , 31]. Still others are brought under the rubric of attempted murder, aiding and abetting, accomplices, or accessories to the crime [33, 38].[12] A lesser charge of involuntary manslaughter is also possible under some state statutes [3]. Finally, all states have child abuse and neglect statutes, requiring physicians and nurses to report such incidents to the police or to welfare authorities [46]. Failure to do so is a misdemeanor.

None of the criminal statutes include any exceptions that would allow active or passive euthanasia of defective newborns. But because so few cases are brought to the attention of authorities, it would seem to reflect that there is a great moral ambivalence toward treating defective neonates. Thus, criminal liability does not seem to be an appropriate solution to these cases and it certainly does not promote the concept that withholding treatment in certain cases may be a desirable end in itself.

Statutory Law

An alternative to liability under homicide and other criminal statutes is for the legislature to provide guidance for physicians and parents as to when treatment may be withheld or withdrawn. Many courts have asked the legislature to act, but few have done so. An exception can be found in North Carolina [18, 36]. The North Carolina legislature has enacted a statute that provides for the withdrawal of extraordinary means of treatment of a terminally ill, incompetent person when there is an absence of a declaration by a living will. It makes no mention of whether this would apply to decisions made on behalf of defective newborns, apparently contemplating those situations where a formerly competent adult is now incompetent, but there is nothing in the language of the statute that would prohibit such an interpretation.

Under the North Carolina approach, extraordinary treatment may be withheld or stopped when certain conditions are met. The statute defines extraordinary as any medical procedure or intervention which would only serve to postpone death artificially by sustaining, restoring, or supplanting a vital function. In order to meet the requirements of the act, the patient's condition must be terminal, incurable, and irreversible. Withholding or discontinuing extraordinary treatment is then permissible at the request of the spouse, guardian, or the majority of first degree relatives, in that order. If none of these persons is available, then the physician may use his or her own discretion.

Since it is unlikely that most legislatures will attempt to resolve the controversies surrounding the case of defective newborns, statutory law is an unlikely solution, but as will be shown in the ensuing discussion, the common law applied by our civil court system is well-equipped to afford relief to those who have a conscientious desire to act in the best interests of the handicapped infant.

Nonintentional Torts – The Tort of Wrongful Continued Existence

Most of the legal concerns with the care of defective newborns has been the crime or tort of withholding or withdrawing treatment, thereby causing death. Here we will examine the possibility that there can be a wrong committed and a subsequent legal remedy for one who has been harmed by being kept alive. If it is wrong for a physician to treat infants aggressively who have no reasonable hope of surviving or who have no reasonable hope of developing a cognitive and sapient state, then the harm could be called the tort of wrongful continued existence [39].
Tort actions for interference with death – All elements of a tort action must be shown by a preponderance of the evidence on behalf of an infant plaintiff in order to sustain a holding of wrongful continued

existence. These are: (1) a duty to permit death to occur; (2) a breach of that duty; (3) a legally cognizable injury; (4) a showing that the injury was proximately caused by the breach; and (5) a measurement of damages [45]. Although it is never possible to predict a court opinion in advance, it is quite likely that a cause of action for wrongful continued existence would meet formidable obstacles, similar to those enunciated by the courts in wrongful life cases [48 , 50].

First, there must be a duty on the part of physicians and other caretakers to allow the infant to die. The argument for such a duty would rest on a correlative right – the right to die. Courts have frequently articulated a "right to die" for incompetent, terminally ill patients and for comatose patients with no reasonable hope of returning to a cognitive and sapient state [13 , 14]. One court has upheld the right of a fully conscious patient to be removed from a respirator because his condition was hopeless and irreversible even though his condition was not terminal [25]. The right to die is based on two legal doctrines: the right to privacy and the right of personal autonomy or self-determination as enunciated in informed consent cases.

Duty, Breach, and Injury – A physician's duty in medical malpractice cases arises from an expected standard of care based on skill, knowledge, and experience, and by comparison to professional standards set by other physicians in similar circumstances [45]. Thus, if it is common medical practice to allow an anencephalic baby, or one with trisomy-18, to die by providing only comfort, water, and sedation, then a physician who puts the infant on a respirator, starts IV or gastric feedings, and administers medications to prevent circulatory collapse, or interferes with the process of dying by resuscitation, might be found to have breached a duty to let the infant die. If those measures were successful, causing existence to be extended, even if only for days or weeks, then the infant, through a guardian's complaint, could claim injuries of prolonged pain and suffering, increased medical costs, and an invasion of the right to privacy, by interference with the right to die.

Proximate Cause – In order to sustain a cause of action for wrongful interference with death, if duty, breach, and injury have been demonstrated by a preponderance of the evidence, an additional hurdle must be overcome. The parents or guardian who brought the suit on behalf of the infant must show a causal connection between the breach and the injury. In legal terms this is called proximate cause [45]. Proof may be difficult if damages are sought for pain and suffering because the discomfort may merely be the natural result of the condition rather than induced by the intervention. Increased *intensity* of suffering may be absent unless the diagnostic and therapeutic procedures caused extra pain, but increased *duration* of suffering would be present. There should be no difficulty, however, in proving that the economic loss through increased medical bills was proximately caused by the breach.

Defenses – Numerous objections to a tort action for wrongful continued existence could be raised. It might be argued that there is *never* a duty to allow a patient to die because this would be anathema to the professional code of ethics. But the corollary is that a "right to die" is empty of meaning if that right imposes no duties on others. Arguments found in wrongful life cases, doubtlessly, would be raised, i.e., that it is impossible to compare the utter void of nonexistence with life with defects [48 , 50]. Similarly, one could claim that existence *per se* is not a legally cognizable injury. This argument has been rebutted in several wrongful life cases that were upheld by finding that the infant both *exists and suffers* [10 , 32]. Thus, the metaphysical quandary that courts place themselves in by stating that nonexistence is unknowable to man and a value cannot be placed on nonlife, can be circumvented by placing the emphasis on the suffering rather than on existence itself. If the only way to reduce or alleviate suffering is to allow death to occur, then it should be a legal wrong to prolong that suffering and postpone death. Perhaps a better phrase would be the "tort of wrongful continuation of suffering" rather than the "tort of wrongful continued existence".

The courts may also use public policy arguments to disallow a cause of action for wrongful existence by stating that such a policy would undermine the principle of the sanctity, reverence, and preciousness of life. Recognition of the tort of continued existence would also require physicians to withhold treatment based on quality-of-life decisions. But if most reasonable adults would prefer death to a prolonged and painful life, then substituting that judgment for an infant would not be unreasonable.

Damages – The measure of damages would not be based on prolonged life *per se*, as for food, clothing, and shelter, but would be based on the special damages of the cost of medical and nursing care during the period that the suffering was prolonged. Damages for physical pain and suffering are assessed by juries in other types of legal cases and could also be done in the context of wrongful continued existence.

Tort actions by parents – Alternatively, a cause of action could be brought by the parents themselves, rather than by the child. The parents could complain of lack of informed consent to treat the child against their wishes or of invasion of family privacy and family autonomy in treatment decisions resulting in extra medical costs and emotional pain and suffering. Wrongful birth suits brought by parents have been much more successful than wrongful life suits brought by infants. It should be noted, however, that in wrongful birth suits the parents claim a tortious interference in their reproductive decision-making, an argument which would not be available to them in wrongful continued existence actions. Thus, it is not clear that parents' claims would also be more successful in the latter context than those brought by the infants themselves.

Tort actions for existence in a vegetative state – Thus far we have examined only those cases where life is prolonged or death is postponed and the suffering caused by interference with death is the basis of the tort. What about cases where death would not naturally follow, but there is continued existence in a vegetative state? If this resulted from aggressive treatment where the child's condition was worse after the medical intervention than if no treatment had taken place, then it would be necessary to show that an ordinary, reasonable physician could have predicted that the treatment might be more harmful than nontreatment. Most such cases would have resulted either from ordinary medical negligence or from lack of informed consent by failing to disclose to the parents the risks of treatment and the alternative choice of no treatment. No new cause of action would be needed. Damages awarded in such cases would allow for continued life-long care. It is less likely that emotional pain and suffering would be recognized for a damage award if there were no cognition or sapience. Courts would feel more comfortable with these cases because of precedents already set in malpractice law. Physicians would likely raise the emergency defense, which allows treatment without informed consent, and it would be incumbent on the parents to show that no emergency existed when treatment was undertaken. An action by the parents for their emotional pain and suffering would fall under case law set by bystander precedents [5]. Tortious invasion of the parents' privacy and family autonomy in treatment decisions would probably be more likely to be recognized in jurisdictions using the *reasonable patient standard* of informed consent than those that use the *professional standard* of disclosure if the family was excluded from the decision-making process.

Tort actions for existence in a diminished state – The most difficult cases to analyze, and the type which in some ways is the most tragic, is the situation where an individual with severe physical handicaps and deformities has an appreciable amount of mental development and an average life expectancy. Such a person may wish to claim a wrongful existence for having had life-threatening defects repaired during infancy that prevented death. An example of such a situation might be an infant born with multiple congenital anomalies and mild mental retardation where a congenital heart defect had been repaired and further deterioration of mental capacity was prevented by shunting the hydrocephaly, but other problems, such as limb malformations, kyphoscoliosos, paraplegia and loss of bladder control, persist. Such a person is utterly dependent on others for existence and is aware of the stigmatization and discrimination of the handicapped imposed by our social norms. Individuals vary in their fight to make life meaningful and some have a low threshold for anger and depression. Some will make an adjustment to their disabilities while others will give up and commit suicide. Still others may want to seek legal redress for the mental and physical pain and suffering brought on by their continued existence.

For several reasons, courts would be unlikely to recognize such a complaint. First, it would be difficult to identify a right to die in the case described. It does not fit the description of terminal illness, irreversible coma, or non-cognitive existence. Second, even though the court may find that a wrong was committed by repairing the heart defect by showing that a reasonable physician, using ordinary medical judgment, would not have recommended surgery, the damages might be mitigated, or even denied altogether, because of the Benefits Rule [33]. This rule requires that the opportunity to find some enjoyment of life would outweigh the harm committed or the right to die. Also, the court may find that there is no legal right to be born as a whole, functioning human being. This case might be decided on the precedents set by the 'dissatisfied life' cases under the rubric of 'wrongful life'. Such cases have not met with success in the courtroom [35]. But arguments could be made that it is a 'diminished life' case rather than a 'dissatisfied' one.

There are a number of reasons why tort law, a civil action between private parties, is preferable to governmental intrusion by criminal suits in these difficult life-and-death decisions in the neonatal period. It preserves a respect for family privacy and autonomy and encourages physicians to include the parents in the decision-making process and to honor the parents' wishes unless their reasons for requesting the withholding of treatment are egregious or irrational. It would also curtail heroic treatment and expensive life-prolonging measures that escalate the costs of keeping infants alive over weeks or months when the prognosis is dim or hopeless. In some of these cases the infant is little more than an experimental subject for testing aggressive treatment regimens.

Physicians may feel that they are in double jeopardy if they believe that treatment is mandated by governmental regulations but they are also liable in tort for worsening an infant's condition or prolonging death when the parents do not give informed consent. Courts should consider this dilemma when they are reviewing statutory and agency law that promotes governmental intervention in these intensely delicate and private matters. Since it is unlikely that guidelines drawn up by ethics committees or statutes designed by legislatures will provide comprehensive coverage for the myriad situations that arise in the newborn intensive care unit, it seems preferable to retain a rebuttable presumption that parents know best.

Tort actions brought by the child against the parents – So far we have discussed the wrong of continued existence in the medical malpractice context for which we have found precedents in wrongful life, right-to-die, informed consent, and invasion of privacy cases brought against health professionals and hospitals. It is much more problematic that a cause of action brought on behalf of an infant against its parents would be recognized by the courts. Tort actions brought against parents in wrongful life cases have been uniformly unsuccessful in the courts [20, 35].

Recently, however, a California appellate court, in upholding a wrongful life action, enunciated *in dictum*, that

[I]f a case arose where, despite due care by the medical profession in transmitting the necessary warnings, parents made a conscious choice to proceed with a pregnancy, with full knowledge that a seriously impaired infant would be born, that conscious choice would provide an intervening act of proximate cause to preclude liability insofar as defendants other than the parents were concerned. Under such circumstances, we see no sound public policy which should protect those parents from being answerable for the pain, suffering and misery which they have wrought upon their offspring. [4].

If such a tort were ever recognized, it could be logically extended to parents who insist on heroic measures to keep an already-born defective infant alive who otherwise would die. Such a case could arise when physicians advised against treatment that would be futile except to prolong a defective existence.

Soon after the California opinion was announced there was a public outcry and the legislature moved quickly to disallow tort actions brought by children against their parents for allowing them to be conceived or born.[13] Apparently the court was not in tune with society's sentiments or public policy. But we cannot say that public policy will not change in the future concerning wrongful life or wrongful continued existence cases. If parents are ever held accountable, it is likely that the courts would insist on a stricter standard of negligence than mere preponderance of the evidence. Because family autonomy, family privacy, and promotion of family harmony are jealously guarded by the courts, we might expect that a clear and convincing evidentiary standard would be required before a child could prevail against its parents. The United States Supreme Court has held that before parental rights can be terminated in child neglect cases the clear and convincing test of parental unfitness must be met [24].

Another way of evaluating the appropriateness of parental decisions to treat or to withhold treatment can be drawn from analogies to child abuse cases. California has adopted a 'reasonable parent' standard when allowing parents to discipline their children by inflicting physical harm [8] and several other states have followed this precedent. In the context of treatment of defective newborns, one would look to the decisions of other parents when evaluating the reasonableness of a particular case. Again, the court should allow wide latitude in parental decision-making and should not uphold a child's allegations of wrongful continued existence without clear and convincing evidence that the parents' decisions lay far outside the social norm.

Another reason that the child might fail against its parents can be found in the doctrine of intrafamilial immunity which disallows lawsuits between family members. This doctrine has been eroded over the past few years both in the context of interspousal immunity and parent-child immunity. Only three states retain unqualified parental immunity for all tortious acts against their children [1].[14]

In summary, it is quite unlikely that an infant would prevail against its parents. If we look to the blood transfusion cases among Jehovah's Witnesses for guidance, we see that the state can override the parental wishes on behalf of the child [11, 12, 15, 29, 34]. But these cases can be distinguished because they involve the state's interest in keeping a child alive rather than a state's interest in allowing a child to die.

Intentional Torts

The discussion thus far has centered around medical malpractice actions brought by parents or children against physicians, and negligence actions brought by children against their parents. Another branch of tort law – intentional torts – should also be considered.

The most common intentional tort is assault and battery, although invasion of privacy is also classified as intentional. The reason for discussing the distinction between intentional and nonintentional (negligence) torts is that in the former the damage awards can be much greater, expert evidence is not required, and malpractice insurance is not available.

The tort of battery can be simply defined as 'unconsented touching' [45]. Any treatment without consent, unless it falls under the emergency exception or is allowed by statute, constitutes battery. From knowledge of how neonatal intensive care units operate, it can be safely assumed that technical battery is the norm rather than the exception. Parents are often unavailable, or if available, are not consulted before treatment is instituted. Not all of these treatments are emergencies. But for practical reasons, battery is seldom alleged in such situations.

In the early informed consent cases, there was much discussion about whether treatment without informed consent constituted battery [17]. Even though malice is not an element of battery (battery can be done benevolently), the courts distinguished between no consent at all and lack of informed consent, making the former a battery and the latter an act of negligence [17]. Thus, if the parents have given no consent at all, battery could be alleged for instituting treatment of a defective newborn. However, for policy reasons, it is unlikely to be used as a means of legal redress.

THE PREVENTION OF HANDICAPPED CHILDREN

It is my contention that, although we will never realize the idealistic goal of bringing all children into the world in a mentally and physically sound condition, we can approach that goal asymptotically. It is now possible, with our *present methods* of prenatal diagnosis, to nearly eradicate neural tube defects, chromosomal disorders, hemoglobinopathies, inherited sex-linked recessive disorders, and many inborn errors of metabolism.

Alpha-fetoprotein (AFP) testing can be used as a paradigm for the prevention of neural tube defects (NTD) such as anencephaly, mye-lomeningocele, spina bifida, hydrocephalus, and related conditions. All pregnant women could be screened for increased maternal serum AFP by a simple and inexpensive test [52]. An elevated level is found in approximately one in every 15 pregnancies. A repeat test will exclude about half of these as false positive tests. If an elevated level is found in two successive maternal serum samples, then an ultrasound scan is performed to rule out the presence of twins or erroneously reported gestational age. Of those that remain, an amniotic fluid sample will further eliminate false positive tests, leaving one per thousand fetuses with NTD. If these mothers undergo selective abortion the frequency of NTD at birth could be reduced from 3000 such births per year in the United States to perhaps fifteen or fewer. This could result in two positive outcomes: (1) the agonizing decision of treatment or non-treatment of these cases at birth would virtually disappear since society could afford to treat vigorously all of these children whose destiny is not death in spite of treatment, without overburdening our health care resources; and (2) such handicapped children might be given an ele-vated, rather than a reduced, social status because of the rarity of their tragedy. It is difficult for us to be very concerned with 3000 NTD births per year, but if there were only 15 cases we might become more sensitive and empathetic to their plight, treating them as very special members of society who need our protection. The outpouring of responses following President Reagan's recent plea for a liver donor for an infant with hepatic failure is an example of the emotional and financial support available from the public when rare medical emergen-cies arise.

Two recent medical advances which are presently in the experimental stage will greatly influence the prevention of handicapped children in the near future. These techniques have been applied successfully in clinical situations and they will be incorporated into standard prenatal care within a few years. The first is called CVB (chorionic villi biopsy) [43]. This allows diagnosis of fetal defects during the sixth to ninth week of pregnancy and can be used for all conditions presently discovered by amniocentesis except for neural tube deffects. Many parents will find it more acceptable to selectively abort a defective fetus during the first trimester rather than waiting until the sixteenth to eighteenth week of gestation when quickening has occurred and the mother's enlarging abdomen makes the fact of pregnancy publicly known.

The second diagnostic technique, which is becoming rapidly applied to *all* genetic diseases, even those that cannot be presently diagnosed by identification of the abnormal gene product, is the use of genetic markers called RFLPs (restriction fragment length polymorphisms) to determine whether a disease gene is hitchhiking with a marker gene [37]. Recently, the Huntington disease gene was mapped to chromosome no. 4 because it was closely linked to an RFLP located there [40]. This technique allows all Mendelian conditions to be identified prenatally, regardless of the pattern of inheritance, and even though the defective gene product is unknown. So far, about 75 percent of the human genome has been mapped with over 700 RFLP markers and the entire genetic material will probably be mapped before the end of the decade. Some optimistic geneticists are predicting complete coverage within two to three years because of the rapid discovery of new markers.

It is becoming apparent that quality-of-life choices will be made for the fetus during routine prenatal care and the burden of birth defects will succumb to scientific advances, just as infectious disease was dramatically reduced after the development of vaccines and the widespread use of antibiotics. Somatic gene therapy is on the horizon and will be tested within the next year or two, but germinal gene therapy is a more distant goal, which will probably not be explored in human beings for at least a decade. Animal experimentation has already shed light on the feasibility of germinal gene therapy. But until we learn better how to prevent birth defects, genetic disorders and environmentally-induced handicaps, we must continue to wrestle with the day-to-day decisions concerning the treatment or nontreatment of defective newborns.

The University of Texas Health Science Center
Houston, Texas, U.S.A.

NOTES

[1] Identification characteristics, including the name used, have been changed to protect the anonymity of the patient.
[2] In *Johnson v. State* (1840) [16], a mother's criminal conviction for repeatedly beating her child was reversed on appeal, in order to protect the family unit.

[3] For extensive discussions of the application of amniocentesis to prenatal diagnosis, see Milunsky [44].

[4] In *Griswold v. Connecticut* (1965) [9], the U.S. Supreme Court held that state statutes prohibiting the use of contraceptives by married couples unconstitutionally infringed on their right to privacy in reproductive decision-making.

[5] In *Eisenstadt v. Baird* (1972) [7], the Supreme Court extended to unmarried persons the right to use contraceptives without state interference.

[6] In the famous abortion case of *Roe v. Wade* (1973) [23], the Supreme Court held that, with limited exceptions, abortion before fetal viability is constitutionally protected.

[7] An outstanding example is the Tay-Sachs screening program among Ashkenazi Jews whereby married couples can be tested to determine whether they are carriers of the Tay-Sachs gene and, if both are carriers, all fetuses can be tested for the disease, allowing the parents to selectively abort defective fetuses and bring normal and carrier fetuses to term. See, e. g., Kaback [41].

[8] The Benefits Rule, as it appears in the Restatement of Torts (1930) [22] states: "Where the defendant's tortious conduct has caused harm to the plaintiff or to his property and in so doing has conferred upon the plaintiff a special benefit to the interest which was harmed, the value of the benefit conferred is considered in mitigation of damages, where this is equitable" ([22], Section 920).

[9] Tedeschi claims that since damages are compensation for injuries, the child who claims he should never have been born lacks standing to sue because but for the tort, he would not be here to complain ([50] p. 529). He also maintains that it is impossible to compare defective existence with no existence at all ([50] p. 530). See also the discussion of wrongful life in Shaw ([48] pp. 104–111).

[10] Since the delivery of this paper on 10 May 1984 in Macon, Georgia, a third state, New Jersey, has recognized the tort of wrongful life. See *Procanik v. Cillo* (1984) [21].

[11] Judge Benjamin Cardozo, later a Supreme Court Justice, laid the cornerstone for the doctrine of informed consent in *Schloendorff v. Society of N. Y. Hospital* (1914) [26], when he wrote, "Every human being of adult years and sound mind has a right to determine what shall be done with his own body."

[12] See, e. g., Va. Code, Section 18.2–22 (1975) [33]. See also extensive discussion of possible criminal liability in the pediatric context in Ellis ([38] pp. 393–423).

[13] Cal. Civ. Code, Section 43.6 (West 1982) reads in part:
 (a) No cause of action arises against a parent of a child based upon the claim that the child should not have been conceived or, if conceived, should not have been allowed to have been born alive.
 (b) The failure or refusal of a parent to prevent the live birth of his or her child shall not be a defense in any action against a third party, nor shall the failure or refusal be considered in awarding damages in any such action.

[14] See cases in Cases and Annotations (1981)[1].

BIBLIOGRAPHY

Cases, Statutes, and Regulations

1. Annot: 1981, 'Liability of Parent for Injury to Unemancipated Child Caused by Parent's Negligence – Modern Cases', A.L.R. 4th, 1066, at Section 13, 1113–1125.
2. Ball v. Mudge, 64 Wash. 2d 247, 250 391 P.2d 201, 204 (1964).
3. Biddle v. Commonwealth, 206 Va. 14, 141 S.E. 2d 710 (1965).
4. Curlender v. Bio-Science Laboratories, 106 Cal. App. 3d 811, 165 Cal. Rptr. 477 (1980).
5. Dillon v. Legg, 68 Cal. 2d 728, 69 Cal. Rptr. 72, 441 P.2d 919, 29 A.L.R. 3d 1316 (1968).
6. Eichner v. Dillon, 73 A.D. 2d 431, 426 N.Y.S. 2d 517 (1980), *modified*, 52 N.Y. 2d 363, 420 N.E.2d 64, 438 N.Y.S.2d 266 (1981).
7. Eisenstadt v. Baird, 405 U.S. 438 (1972).
8. Gibson v. Gibson, 3 Cal. 3d 914, 479 P.2d 648, 92 Cal. Rptr. 288 (1971).
9. Griswold v. Connecticut, 381 U.S. 479 (1965).
10. Harbeson v. Parke-Davis, 98 Wash. 2d 468, 656 P.2d 483 (1983).
11. In re B.B.H., 9 Fam. L. Rep. 2648 (Sept. 6, 1983).
12. In re President and Directors of Georgetown College, 331 F.2d 1000 (D.C. Cir. 1964).
13. In re Quinlan, 70 N.J. 10, 355 A. 2d 647 (1976).
14. In re Storer, 52 N.Y. 2d 363, 438 N.Y.S. 2d 266, 420 N.E.2d 64 (1981).
15. Jehovah's Witnesses v. King County Hospital, 278 F.Supp. 488 (W.D. Wash. 1967), *aff'd*, 390 U.S. 598 (1968).
16. Johnson v. State, 21 Tenn. 282 (1840).
17. Natanson v. Kline, 186 Kan. 393, 350 P. 2d 1093 (1960), rehearing *den'd*, 186 Kan. 186, 354 P.2d 670 (1960).
18. N.C. Gen. Stat., Section 90-322 (supp. 81).
19. People v. Conley, 64 Cal. 2d 310, 322, 411 P.2d 911, 918, 49 Cal. Rptr. 815, 822 (1966).
20. Pinkney v. Pinkney, 198 So. 2d 52 (Fla. Dist. Ct. App. 1967).
21. Procanik v. Cillo, U.S.L.W. 53, 2091 (1984).
22. Restatement of Torts, Section 920 (1930).
23. Roe v. Wade, 410 U.S. 113 (1973).
24. Santosky v. Kramer, 455 U.S. 745 (1982).
25. Satz v. Perlmutter, 362 So.2d (Fla. App. 1978), *aff'd*, 379 So.2d 359 (Fla. 1980).
26. Schloendorff v. Society of N.Y. Hospitals, 211 N.Y. 125, 105 N.E. 92 (1914).
27. State v. Ehlers, 98 N.J.L. 236, 240, 119 A. 15, 17 (1922).
28. State v. Francis, 152 S.C. 17, 60, 149 S.E. 348, 364 (1929).
29. State v. Perricone, 37 N.J. 463, 181 A.2d 751 (1962), *cert. denied*, 371 U.S. 890 (1962).
30. Terrell v. Garcia, 496 S.W. 2d 124, 128 (Tex. Civ. App. 1973, *writ ref'd n. r. e.*).
31. Turner v. State, 119 Tenn. 663, 671, 108 S.W. 1139, 1141 (1908).
32. Turpin v. Sortini, 119 Cal. App. 3d 690, 174 Cal. Rptr. 128 (1981), *rev'd*, 31 Cal. 3d 220, 643 P.2d 954, 183 Cal. Rptr. 337 (1982).
33. Va. Code, Section 18.2–22 (1975).

34. Wallace v. Labrenz, 411 Ill. 618, 104 N.E.2d 769 (1952), *cert. denied*, 344, U.S. 824 (1953).
35. Zepeda v. Zepeda, 41 Ill. App. 2d 240, 190 N.E.2d 849 (1963), *cert. denied*, 379 U.S. 945 (1964).

Articles and Books

36. Ackerman, J. W. and Pope, M. C.: 1982, 'Termination of Medical Treatment: A Judicial Perspective', *Journal of Legal Medicine* **3**, 211–243.
37. Botstein, D. *et al.*: 1980, 'Contruction of a Genetic Linkage Map in Man Using Restriction Fragment Length Polymorphisms', *American Journal of Human Genetics* **32**, 314–331.
38. Ellis, T. S.: 1982, 'Letting Defective Babies Die', *American Journal of Law and Medicine* **7**, 393–423.
39. Engelhardt, H. T., Jr.: 1975, 'Ethical Issues in Aiding the Death of Small Children,' in M. Kohl (ed.), *Beneficent Euthanasia*, Prometheus Books, Buffalo, New York, pp. 10, 47.
40. Gusella, J. F. *et al.*: 1983, 'A Polymorphic DNA Marker Genetically Linked to Huntington's Disease', *Nature* **306**, 234–238.
41. Kaback, M. (ed.): 1977, *Tays-Sachs Disease: Screening and Prevention*, Alan R. Liss, New York.
42. Kempe, C. H. *et al.*: 1962, 'The Battered Child Syndrome', *Journal of the American Medical Association* **181**, 17–24.
43. Kolata, G.: 1983, 'First Trimester Prenatal Diagnosis', *Science* **221**, 1031–1032.
44. Milunsky, A.: 1979, *Genetic Disorders of the Fetus*, Plenum Press, New York.
45. Prosser, W.: 1971, *Torts*, 4th ed., West Publishers, St. Paul, Minnesota.
46. Redden, W. C.: 1978, 'The Federal and State Response to the Problem of Child Mistreatment in America: A Survey of the Reporting Statutes', *Nova Law Journal* **2**, 13–74.
47. Robertson, G. B.: 1978, 'Civil Liability Arising From "Wrongful Birth" Following an Unsuccessful Operation', *American Journal of Law and Medicine* **4**, 141.
48. Shaw, M. W.: 1984, 'Conditional Prospective Rights of the Fetus', *Journal of Legal Medicine* **5**, 104–111.
49. Swazey, J. P.: 1971, 'Phenylketonuria: A Case Study in Biomedical Legislation', *Journal of Urban Law* **48**, 883–931.
50. Tedeschi, I.: 1966, 'On Tort Liability for "Wrongful Life"' *Israel Law Review* **1**, 513–538.
51. Thomas, M. P., Jr.: 1972, 'Child Abuse and Neglect Part 1: Historical Overview, Legal Matrix, and Social Perspectives', *North Carolina Law Review* **50**, 293–349.
52. Wald, N. J. and Cuckle, H. S.: 1979, 'Second Report of the United Kingdom Collaborative Study on Alpha-Fetoprotein in Relation to Neutral-tube Defects', *Lancet* **2**, 651–661.

STUART F. SPICKER

UNFOLLOWABLE LAW:
REFLECTIONS ON THE ESSAYS OF NANCY M. P. KING
AND MARGERY W. SHAW

HEALTH LAW

Professors King and Shaw have carefully and critically reviewed the significant factors that bear on legal proxy decision-making for severely impaired neonates, the status of tort law and its potential bearing on wrongful continued existence, as well as the role of governmental intervention and, at times, intrusion in such decision-making. Indeed, they appear to agree on a few basic principles that may well entail an agreement about certain policies, though these policies, regrettably perhaps, may not be in place at this very moment.

For example, although Shaw seems to focus her attention on the rights of physicians in the context of decision-making for seriously ill and deformed neonates [9], and King on the authority properly conferred by law on parents of such newborns, ([7], p. 104) both agree that, generally speaking, parents know what is in their infant's best interests (a point to be distinguished sharply from the fact that infants have no apparent interests of their own). King remarks that ". . . parents are the best determiners of their child's best interests" ([7], p. 104). The two attorneys generally agree, then, that in virtually all cases parents know what is in the best interests of their children, though admittedly in rare cases their decisions are 'egregious' and 'irrational' ([9], p. 130); they may also act wrongly, sometimes out of 'ignorance', or because they are simply 'incapable of providing' what is in their child's best interests ([7], pp. 99–102).

Given this general view – based on the empirical fact (yet an important one) that recent proposed legislation is probably applicable to a relatively small number of newborn cases – both King and Shaw appear to hold that decisions bearing on the future existence or nonexistence of a certain class of newborns should be taken on a case-by-case basis. Legal regulations, then – like the recently proposed re-construal of

R. C. McMillan, H. T. Engelhardt, Jr., and S. F. Spicker (eds.),
Euthanasia and the Newborn, 139–150.
© *1987 by D. Reidel Publishing Company.*

Section 504 of the Rehabilitation Act of 1973 (29 U.S.C. 293) in 1982,
[4] which was originally designed to address or redress discrimination in
the context of employment – they view as problematic, not only because
Section 504 was never designed for application in the context of neonatal intensive care, but because this Federal regulation would presume
to cover *all* cases, and, with such a wide application, would generate
wrongful action on the part of physicians, parents, and hospitals.

From the physician's viewpoint the dilemma is as follows: Physicians
in the neonatal units must either treat or not treat. If, in some cases,
they treat, then they are liable to legal action by parents (or someone on
behalf of the infant) for continuing to prolong the life of the newborn,
regarding which action the parents refused to give their consent. If they
do not treat, in some cases, then their hospital will be subject to a
financial penalty for failure to follow the law, in this case Section 504 of
the Rehabilitation Act. Thus the physician is either a defendant or
penalized through his/her affiliated hospital. This is the predicament
Professor Shaw alludes to in describing the physician's situation as one
of 'double jeopardy' ([9], p. 130).

From the perspective of the parents, the situation is quite different.
Here the matter, in the critical and ambiguous cases, is one of parental
authority and the intrusion by others (e.g., physicians, hospitals, judges,
the State, and/or the Federal government) into the private matters of
the family. Professor King reminds us of the very interesting, yet still
controversial, conclusion of the Superior Court of New Jersey in the
case *In re Quinlan*. Recall that that Court argued for a very unusual
principle in relating a patient's right to privacy with her medical status:
"We think that the State's interest contra weakens and the individual's
right to privacy grows as the degree of bodily invasion increases and the
prognosis dims" (355 A.2d. at 644). The contrary corollary could be
formulated as follows: We think that the State's interest pro (in the
preservation of life) strengthens and the individual's right to privacy
diminishes as the degree of bodily invasion decreases and the prognosis
is encouraging. This or a similar formulation is the one that underlies a
government's stance when it elects to override the decision of Jehovah's Witnesses parents who refuse to give their consent to provide their
infant with a plasma transfusion, based on religious grounds. The issue
here, of course, is the matter of progressive governmental intervention
or perhaps intrusion into parental decision-making. King and Shaw
remain focused on this key issue. Shaw remarks that it is intrinsic to

Anglo-American tort law to preserve a respect for family privacy and autonomy, but is not so much an advocate of unabridged parental authority as she is of unencumbered physician autonomy. For tort law, she says, also "encourages physicians to include parents in the decision-making process and to the honor parents' wishes unless their reasons for requesting the withholding of treatment are egregious and irrational" ([9], pp. 129–130).

The worry here, however, is not over the views of Professors Shaw and King. Rather, we should be aware of the not fully consistent position of the President's Commission for the Study of Ethical Problems in Medicine and Biomedical and Behavioral Research. In the now famous Chapter Six, 'Seriously Ill Newborns', of the Commission's report, *Deciding to Forego Life-Sustaining Treatment,* the Commission appears to advocate unencumbered parental decision-making, but also seeks to 'temper' parental authority ([8], p. 212). The Commission does state that in nearly all situations parents are the best decision-makers ([8], p. 214), and that "Americans have traditionally been reluctant to intrude upon the functioning of families. . ." ([8], p. 215). On the next page of the Report, the Commission's position is qualified – one should in fact override parental decisions when they decide on a course of action that is clearly against the infant's best interests ([8], p. 216). The introduction of the *best interest standard* here is seriously problematic, as King has shown ([7], p. 21). The Commission also maintains, without forwarding a sound argument, that 'special ethical duties' are owed to newborns with undeserved disadvantages. Furthermore, it maintains that there is a "general ethical duty of the community to ensure equitable access for all persons to an adequate level of health care" ([8], p. 7). But this last assertion clearly confuses the nondiscriminatory issue regarding these newborns – an issue which does not bear on the otherwise sensible "equitable access principle" in the context of a hospital's admission policy – with selection of newborns for treatment or non-treatment. By page 225, the Commission's confidence in parents wanes if it not entirely evanesces. The *parens patriae* doctrine begins to have great weight and the difficult matters such as decisions regarding (1) very low birth-weight babies on the edge of viability, (2) infants with multiple serious congenital anomalies, and (3) infants who are dying, are less and less the prerogative of parents ([8], p. 226). (In fairness, one Commissioner, Albert Jonsen, maintains that given the inadequate institutional care 'system' in the U.S. "the law must err on the side of its

strong presumption in favor of parental autonomy and family integrity"
([8] p. 228, n.101).) A key worry, then, is the issue of who makes
decisions in these difficult cases. It is incorrect to conclude, as John
Arras does, that the 'Who decides?' is merely a procedural and not a
substantive issue ([2], p. 25). What could be more substantive than the
nature of the freedom, rights, and obligations on the part of particular
human agents?

UNFOLLOWABLE LAW

The law is a system of social control. An unjust law, perhaps similar to
the one recently proffered from the 1973 version to 'apply' to grievously
afflicted infants, is often taken to be like counterfeit currency, which
causes trouble because it so closely resembles and may be taken for the
real thing; it therefore, being thought unjust, is taken to be non-genuine
law and not deserving of respect. Unfortunately, law can be, and quite
often is, unjust, unfair, and bad. Is it possible, then, for law to be
subject to moral assessment? That is, laws are perhaps not morally
neutral, but can be good or bad, just or unjust. Are there moral
standards independent of the law that can be brought to bear to judge
it? Are law and morality essentially connected in a special way? Furthermore, does the law itself carry within it the principles for its own moral
evaluation? It appears that there are significant conceptual connections
between law and ethics, not simply derived from their shared vocabulary of rights and obligations, responsibility and justice. To repeat, law
is a system of social control which is supposed to regulate conduct and
behavior. The law may do more than this but it can hardly do less. In
setting standards of conduct it is presumed that whatever the legal
requirement, it can be *followed* – that competent adults should be
capable of using it to guide their conduct. The legal requirement
imposed by the recent restatement of Section 504 of the Rehabilitation
Act of 1973 is supposed to be followable. If a putative legal requirement
cannot be used by those of us to whom it applies to guide our conduct,
then it is surely *defective*. When hospitals are told, for example, that
they are open to penalties for failure to comply with this law (in the
context of the neonatal clinic and NICU), and when the law itself is not
followable, perhaps we are correct in concluding that U.S. hospitals are
being treated unjustly, even if no actual cause of action is initiated (as it
appears is the case at this writing).

Here we have two problems: The Federal government's assertion that "The failure of a recipient of Federal financial assistance to comply with the requirements of section 504 subjects that recipient to possible termination of Federal assistance" (1) is *not consistent* with its claim to act to preserve human life because of its 'high' value, and (2) can be harmful to other hospital patients if funds are suddenly and actually terminated.[1] Furthermore, the Federal govenment has formulated inconsistent legislation so as to preclude it from being followable.

It is relatively easy to show that there is something out of joint in the Government's assuming the role of *parens patriae* on behalf of the seriously impaired newborn, and then placing a financial penalty on a hospital that allegedly failed to protect the newborn's life; the penalty seems rather lenient if such human life is held to possess such 'high' value. Furthermore, the termination of Federal assistance to a major U.S hospital could conceivably endanger the lives of other patients, who often rely on rather expensive intensive care and diagnostic evaluations while in the hospital. If the parents and physicians are alleged to *wrongly* decide to forego or withdraw treatment (to 'forego' includes withholding treatment), then why should the hospital be the sole responsible agent? Furthermore, such legislation can only serve to encourage parents of such seriously impaired newborns to either (a) give the infant over to a social welfare agency, should it survive, thus abandoning it and *a fortiori* all rights to determine its fate and future, or (b) take the infant home as quickly as possible in order to have it end its life outside of the hospital's jurisdiction, leaving the newborn and its parents without assistance at perhaps the time they need support and communication from health professionals the most. But more importantly, the proposed legislation (updated to cover cases of anomalous births of grieviously afflicted infants) is not in fact followable; and it should come as a surprise that more attorneys and physicians have not come forth to testify to this important fact about this particular legal 'Notice'.

Dr. Norman Fost, a professor of pediatrics, is, however, one of the few who points out that the notion of 'handicap' alone is not a "sufficient criterion for distinguishing justified from unjustified deaths" ([5], p. 7). Furthermore, one could argue that the notion of 'handicap' necessarily entails the notion of *loss of function,* whether that be taken to indicate loss of cognitive powers, senses, use of the limbs, or other losses. No newborn infant has developed to the point where we can properly speak of loss of function in any meaningful way, as we easily and correctly do when referring to children and adults. The diagnosis and subsequent prognosis that a given newborn *will eventually suffer* retardation, for example, is precisely a prognosis and a matter of factual uncertainty, not to mention that "the precise extent of retardation cannot be determined in early infancy" ([8], p. 202). So the language of the recent 'Notice to Health Care Providers' which iterated Section 504 to health professionals is unclear, unhelpful and misleading, adding to my thesis that such a 'Notice' is unfollowable. Again, as Dr. Fost points out, "it is not clear if or why a handicap can *never* be a justification for withholding treatment" ([5], p. 5), assuming that one is temporarily willing to allow the introduction of the term 'handicap' in the 'Notice'. But there is a second problem.

The use of the term 'handicapped' in this 'Notice' contains within it another danger: that those children and adults who actually bear handicaps will be viewed (or perhaps judged) in any way like these seriously ill newborns. In point of fact, it is important to 'neutralize' the way we discuss the anomalies of these newborns; for should we eventually determine a social policy that directs a decision that some of them should selectively be allowed to die (or be selectively terminated in sorrow and compassion), then no one would easily conclude that some 'slippery slope' is placed off-stage waiting to slide others away to their deaths. That is, it does not follow from any policy to terminate *some* severely impaired and ill newborns, or to simply allow *some* to die painlessly, that anything but fully-supportive and compassionate social systems will be provided for all the living children and adults who do indeed suffer from loss of functions of one sort or another. The treatment of non-newborns with Down's syndrome, for example, need be nothing short of the best available, given the resources of human time and material support. So the language of the 'Notice', in speaking repeatedly of handicaps, is inherently muddled. The moral course toward all neonates of various degrees of affliction is in no way assisted by the language of 'discrimination against the handicapped'.

Even more importantly, the 'Notice', and the law suggested which follows from it, is unfollowable in still another way: No sense can be made of the charge that newborn infants who are grieviously impaired can in principle be 'subject to discrimination' with respect to or in comparison with normal newborns. Here I am in full agreement with Professor King's point, that there is "simply insufficient social consensus to label the treatment options in question discriminatory" ([7], p. 106). The central point is that parents, physicians, and hospitals cannot "perpetuate discrimination" with respect to these impaired newborns, since to do so *would require that all morally relevant distinctions between normal and impaired newborns be absent.* But in fact morally relevant factors *are* present. These grievously impaired infants (neither the ones who will survive easily with routine treatment, nor the ones at death's door) who undergo chronic pain and suffering, who lack certain capacities at birth, whose prognosis is very dim for leading lives of even minimal value – these newborns can morally and justifiably receive treatment *different from* the others. The nondiscrimination clause in the recent 'Notice' forbids differential treatment only in the absence of morally significant differences between these newborns. But the newborns of whom we speak indeed suffer excessive burdens, pain being only one of them; for there are others – like the lack of a socially-viable future of even a minimal sort to warrant a valued human life. Therefore it follows that the non-discrimination principle of this law does in fact, ironically, *permit* non-treatment of the types of newborn cases we have here focused upon. The 'Notice' has in fact made possible the non-treatment of such ambiguous cases, as it does not really prohibit non-treatment. The law is unfollowable, then, in the most serious sense: it actually permits what it purports to disallow.

I should immediately add that as much as I am personally opposed to the spirit as well as the letter of this 'Notice', I am also dissatisfied (though far less so) with allowing parents unrestricted decision-making in these difficult cases. But we already have a reasonably adequate mechanism in the probate court system, under civil not criminal law, by means of which we can challenge, rarely one hopes, particular decisions of parents and/or physicians. This mechanism cuts both ways – the plea can also be made that infant Doe should *not* be treated, this being quite different from the charge that infant Doe should be treated. We seem to hear very little at the bench regarding the former plea. Future social policy in this domain, if we shall ever develop it, will surely have to make *that* charge equally likely in civil law courts.

If, then, it is the case that the 'Notice' we have been reviewing is unfollowable, and the putative legal requirements noted within it are *defective*, then it may be that penalizing hospitals is *unjust*. At least it appears that a moral claim about the injustice of this 'Notice' is warranted by the very standards of morality implicit in the law itself. To be sure, I have rested much of my argument on the unfollowability of the law; I equally admit that I have not as yet shown that there exists a necessary connection between the moral standard to be used in criticizing this or any law and the law itself. I am simply concerned with the way hospitals can be penalized (and this includes, indirectly their patients) and can run afoul of the unfollowable requirements of this law. What we can count on, however, is that this document (should it ever become a legal requirement, which is now more and more unlikely[2]) is defective. The sentences which constitute the law may indeed not tell us anything about what constitutes an injustice, for we cannot obtain simply from a reading of the law what is unjust. Rather, we need to know what constitutes an injustice. I must leave the matter of injustice to others more qualified to address this important issue in jurisprudence.

TOWARD SOCIAL POLICY

The joy for philosophers who attend to various issues which arise in the context of medicine and medical practice is that the difficult 'value of life' problems can and do often slide away as greater advances are made in biotechnology and scientific medicine. Let me explain.

Philosophy is properly capable of doing its analytic work in considering various *possibilities,* and not actualities. It is not a mere game (though something 'game-like' is present), but philosophers often begin an analysis with one of the following: "Suppose a world in which . . ." "Imagine a possible world such that . . .," or "Conceive, if you will, of a condition in which . . .". These expressions, and others like them, signal that only a possible world is being imagined or intuited for the consideration of some problem or distinction in need of further clarification. But given the 'world' of infirmity, sickness, deformity, and all maladies in general that are our fate in the natural lottery, but still in *this* world, moral issues in medicine, like those raised by Professors King and Shaw in the law/medicine interface, (e.g., "Ought we to end and the lives of certain newborns since to fail to do so constitutes a moral harm?") could be *empirically* resolved by having the troubles raised by these cases simply evanesce. This is the joy I mentioned. That is, if we could prevent (without doing harm or evil) the existence of newborns with serious life-threatening and/or debilitating conditions, I think we would all be pleased to do so. At the same time we should be reminded that for many prospective parents any new baby would be a blessing; for such parents it would be an infringement should they be inhibited from taking their newborn home. Some persons find continous joy in the family process, and they do not need others depriving them of the possibility of parental responsibility and commitment. In such cases where harm to the newborn is excluded, we usually find such a plea compelling.

Many of the problems raised by the care of defective newborns can now be avoided through prenatal diagnosis and interruption of pregnancy. State intrusions into parental and medical decision making are likely to encourage voluntary abortions, where there is high likelihood that the infant will be born with serious mental and physical conditions. In addition, one does not become pregnant in the hope of birthing and raising a very seriously deformed or congenitally malformed newborn. I believe this is the case even if we have become too quick to expect modern medicine to provide us only with a healthy baby. Even if we should be prepared to live and suffer serious burdens, as some noble minds tell us, it does not follow that we should not work to avoid having such burdens under adversity – I mean serious burdens to be borne not only by the infant itself but by parents, the community, and the state agencies which take over when parents refuse, as they presently have a legal right to do, to take their baby home. So though we might all tend to agree with this standpoint, we do not necessarily agree that ending the life of neonates (even through merciful acts of infanticide, given a setting where there would be no legal reprisal) is morally acceptable. Often we feel (or perhaps think) this way because someone stands to remind us that if their parents had so acted when they were born (regarding their disabilities noted at birth), they would not have survived. Such a 'counter-argument' usually includes the claim that, reasonably and rightly, this person has led a happy and useful life. But does such 'testimony' serve to convince us that all newborns should be maximally treated at birth, whatever the level of illness and however dim the prognosis, the exceptions being only those who *in extremis* are judged by medical criteria to have a very short life, all treatment literally futile?

This question compels us to consider future public policy with regard to the treatment/non-treatment of severely ill newborns. To be sure, there are already signs that we are moving toward the formulation of a social policy in this domain – we need only witness the attempt to impose that on our society by claiming that Section 504 of the Rehabili-

tation Act of 1973 applies to *all* neonates born in the 6800 U.S. acute
care hospitals. The complex process of forming and framing such a
social policy is not really touched by individual cases of newborns who
survive with serious illnesses. For the law being proposed – to sustain
the lives of all such neonates – is itself a potential source of moral evil,
whatever the relation that obtains between law and morality. Furthermore, no individual survivor, whose parents initiated appeals for continued treatment at birth, can serve to counter the concern of many to
establish a better social policy for parents, physicians, and hospitals.
The best illustration of this important *logical* point is found, perhaps, in
just such an episode as the one related by Glanville Williams, Professor
of English Law at Cambridge. After Williams' lecture on the evils of
British law against abortion (in our context it might well have been laws
against terminating treatment for some seriously ill newborn),

> a young man came to the platform and told me that he had nearly been an abortion
> himself. His elder brother was born defective, and when his mother became pregnant
> again she found a gynecologist who prepared to terminate the pregnancy. At the last
> moment she changed her mind. "And so," said the young man, "I was born." He waited
> expectantly for my comment. I replied, "I am very glad you are here". But then I added:
> "Nevertheless, should the circumstance of one's own birth affect one's attitude to future
> policy?" ([8], p. 157)

I think that the crux of the issue rests here with those who still oppose all
abortions and even all passive infanticides. From the fact of a few
successful lives (the decisions being made at birth), we can easily and
invalidly infer that it is right for all newborns to receive treatment,
whether or not their prognosis is worse than dim. Professor Williams
continues:

> Many events might have prevented my birth: for example, if the hotel in which my parents
> first met each other had been destroyed by fire or otherwise before their meeting, they
> would probably not have met and married and I should not have been born. But that is no
> reason why I should now oppose the demolition of this hotel or advocate that all hotels be
> fireproof. It is not a rational argument for or against adopting a particular policy in the
> future that if it had been adopted or not adopted in the past we should not be here. . . . In
> arguing social matters we must take our own existence as a datum ([8], p. 157).

In summary, the promulgation of Section 504 is a grievous social fact –
even if it is under serious challenge in the courts.[3] Yet, even if
successfully challenged by the medical profession, and even if unfollowable and incoherent, it may be in retrospect a rather bizarre step toward
a much needed social policy in this arena of the neonatal clinic. We can

perhaps only hope that the present Administration (through the Department of Health and Human Services) will, in its wisdom, appreciate the point that sometimes it is necessary to rise above one's principles.

University of Connecticut, School of Medicine
Farmington, Connecticut, U.S.A.

NOTES

[1] This sanction has since been rescinded; no longer are hospitals threatened that they will be deprived of federal funds. The matter has been shifted to state child-abuse statutes.

[2] Since this complex issue began, a series of events have occurred which bear on the outcome and final regulations. Though the Justice Department has appealed the Second Circuit Court's decision, holding that the federal government lacks the authority under section 504 of the Rehabilitation Act of 1973 to implement the Baby Doe regulations, new regulations have been written on the basis of Public Law 98–457: Amendments to the Child Abuse Prevention and Treatment Act (October 9, 1984). This law would bring the illicit withholding of medical treatment under state child-abuse laws. Although these regulations do incorporate some improvements over the previous ones, nevertheless they still involve a major intrusion into medical and parental decision making.

[3] On June 17, 1985, the Supreme Court granted *certiorari* in Heckler v. The American Hospital Association (an unpublished decision of the 2d Cir, on December 27, 1984), a decision that relied on the Stony Brook, New York case (U.S. v. University Hospital). This decision invalidated the use of the Rehabilitation Act regulation for regulations regarding handicapped newborns. (See N. King's essay, in this volume [7], Note 9, p. 112.)

BIBLIOGRAPHY

1. 'Amendments to Child Abuse Prevention and Treatment Act', Pub.L. No. 98–457, 98 Stat. 1749 (1984) (codified as amended at 42 U.S.C.A. 5101–5104 [West. Supp. 19851]).
2. Arras, J. D.: 1984, 'Toward an Ethic of Ambiguity', *The Hastings Center Report* **14** (2), 25–33.
3. Department of Health and Human Services: 1985, 'Child Abuse and Neglect: Prevention and Treatment Programs; Final Rule', *Federal Register* 50 (April 15), 14878–14901.
4. Department of Health and Human Services: 1984, 'Nondiscrimination on the Basis of Handicap: Procedures and Guidelines Relating to Health Care for Handicapped Infants', *Federal Register* 49 (8), Jan. 23, 1984, (45 *CFR*, HR, Part 84, pp. 1622–1645); also 48 *Federal Register* 9630 (1983); also 47 *Federal Register* 26, 017 (1982) (May 18, 1982).
5. Fost, N.: 1982, 'Putting Hospitals on Notice', *The Hastings Center Report* **12** (4), 5–8.

6. Heymann, P. B. and Holtz, S.: 1975, 'The Severely Defective Newborn: The Dilemma and the Decision Process', *Public Policy* **23** (4), 381–417.
7. King, N.: 1987, 'Federal and State Regulation of Neonatal Decision-making', in this volume, pp. 89–115.
8. President's Commission for the Study of Ethical Problems in Medicine and Biomedical and Behavioral Research: 1983, *Deciding to Forego Life-Sustaining Treatment*, U.S. Government Printing Office, Washington, D.C., pp. 197–229.
9. Shaw, M. W.: 1987, 'When Does Treatment Constitute a Harm?', in this volume, pp. 117–137.
10. Williams, G.: 1975, 'Euthanasia and the Physician', in M. Kohl (ed.), *Beneficent Euthanasia*, Prometheus Books, Buffalo, N.Y., pp. 145–168.
11. Williams, P. C.: 1982, 'Wrongful Life: A Reply to Angela Holder', in S. F. Spicker, J. M. Healey, and H. T. Engelhardt, Jr. (eds.), *The Law-Medicine Relation: A Philosophical Exploration*, D. Reidel, Dordrecht, Holland, pp. 241–252.

TOWARD NATIONAL PUBLIC POLICY
IN THE CARE OF
SERIOUSLY ILL NEWBORNS

JOHN M. FREEMAN

IF EUTHANASIA WERE LICIT,
COULD LIVES BE SAVED?

'Euthanasia', derived from the Greek, means a good or easy death. It has also come to mean acting or withholding action so that someone else will die under circumstances in which death would be a benefit to that person himself [2]. If death is sometimes such a benefit, why is euthanasia repugnant to so many people? One reason is that euthanasia has become identified with unjust killing or murder, and is thus widely condemned by Western religions. Another reason is that the adoption of a 'euthanasia' program by the Nazi regime in Germany tarred euthanasia with a stain that is hard to remove. Recent developments in medical technology demand, however, that we reconsider euthanasia because these developments make it possible to prolong life under circumstances in which many people, including patients themselves, acknowledge that life is not a benefit. Would legalizing euthanasia lead to another Holocaust? Or would legalization of active euthanasia permit the imposition of mechanisms for review and control which would eliminate some of the abuses of what is currently termed 'passive euthanasia'? More importantly, might euthanasia actually encourage physicians to embark on heroic therapies that might actually save lives?

Let us take a hypothetical case and explore several possible scenarios.

CASE 1

Scenario 1

Mr. Jones, a 55-year-old engineer, comes into the hospital for gall bladder surgery. He and his wife, a former nurse, have thought at length about death and had recurrent 'discussions' about prolongation of life. While he has not filled out a living will, Mr. Jones has clearly stated to his wife that he does not want to be kept alive for a prolonged period of time on 'those damn machines'. The surgery is done by Dr. Welby, an old and close friend of the family.

R. C. McMillan, H. T. Engelhardt, Jr., and S. F. Spicker (eds.),
Euthanasia and the Newborn, 153–168.
© 1987 *by D. Reidel Publishing Company.*

During surgery a problem occurs with anesthesia, and Mr. Jones suffers a cardiac arrest. After presumably only three or four minutes it is recognized, and the heart is restarted. While the residents close the incision, Dr. Welby comes out to talk to Mrs. Jones in the waiting room. He tells her about the problem and says, "I do not know how much damage was done to your husband's brain. It could have been considerable. I know your feelings and his feelings about putting someone on machines and, if you concur, I would just as soon not place him on a respirator."

Discussion

If, with the concurrence of Mrs. Jones, the physician elects *not* to put Mr. Jones on the respirator, he will die. Would not initiating the respirator be a morally good or at least acceptable decision?

The outcome would clearly be in concurrence with Mr. Jones' expressed wishes not to "be maintained on those damn machines". The decision would be made with the consent of the family, albeit with minimal time for reflection. It would avoid the potential of prolonged time on a respirator and the suffering of the family.

If one judges the morality of a decision by its outcome, it might be a good and moral decision *if* Mr. Jones were not going to wake up in good shape. But at this time is there any way of knowing that? Would it be a wise decision? Probably not, because there is no way of knowing how long the brain suffered a lack of oxygen and how much damage was done. The severity of the anoxic insult could be more clearly determined by the recovery over the next hours, days, or weeks. If Mr. Jones were put on the respirator, examined over the next twenty-four hours, and found to meet the clinical criteria of brain death, including a flat EEG, then the decision would have been good since Mr. Jones would indeed be dead by the current legal definition.

If Mr. Jones were put on the respirator and over the next several days showed no responsiveness, despite some electrical activity on the EEG, then the original decision not to treat might also have been an appropriate one, since it would avoid survival in a severely impaired state. If Mr. Jones were put on the respirator and over the next few days became responsive, but was demented and incapacitated, although sentient, the original decision still might have been a good one for the same reasons. If, however, Mr. Jones woke up with little or no brain damage, the original decision would have been a bad one for him since it would have deprived him of the life he desired.

At the time of the first decision, while Mr. Jones was still in the operating room, one cannot even venture a good guess, much less know the outcome. Who is present to oversee the decision made by the surgeon and the distraught family? Who will assure that a good decision or a right decision is made? There is, however, one advantage to this immediate decision. If Mr. Jones is not put on a respirator at this stage, it is virtually certain that he will not survive. Thus, the surgeon and the family can avoid all the adverse consequences of which the patient was so fearful.

Scenario 2

Let us turn to a different scenario with Mr. Jones. Dr. Welby finishes the operation, puts Mr. Jones on a respirator and sends him to the recovery room, then comes out to talk to Mrs. Jones. He carefully explains the events in the operating room and says, "Mrs. Jones, I'm terribly sorry, but I don't know how much, if any, damage has been done to your husband's brain. We will keep him on the respirator and do everything that is possible. A brain wave test will be done, which may give us some clue as to the amount of damage, but we will have to see how he recovers over the next few days." Mrs. Jones reiterates that her husband's greatest fear was that he would spend a prolonged amount of time on machines and drain his family of their life savings or, worse yet, that he would survive incapacitated and be a burden to himself and the family. Dr. Welby's response is, "Well, we will hope for the best and wait to see what happens."

Discussion

This is a much more standard scenario. Is it moral? Is it wise? Clearly, this is the community standard of care. It offers Mr. Jones the maximum opportunity to recover. But does it carry out his wishes not to survive severely incapacitated? That limbo state certainly is a possible, even a likely outcome – an outcome the patient clearly does not want. If the EEG turns out to be flat, Mr. Jones will probably die within the next thirty days, despite everything that can be done. Or, using the legal criteria of brain death, the respirator may be turned off when the EEG is flat. In either case, while the outcome may be more prolonged than in the first scenario, the family is not left with an undue burden. If in several days the EEG is not flat, Mr. Jones may recover fully, but, if he is unresponsive, is most likely to recover with an unknown, but possibly severe, degree of impairment. Should he be given that opportunity? Or should his family have the opportunity to say that neither he nor they want to take that risk and, therefore, that the respirator should be immediately discontinued? The longer he remains on the respirator, the more likely he is to survive severely impaired. This scenario offers both the optimal chance of a very good outcome, and the maximal chance for the worse possible outcome. Is it moral for the physician to make a decision to maintain him on a respirator without allowing the wife the opportunity to say 'No'? If Mr. Jones eventually begins to breathe on his own, we will lose our best chance for 'passive euthanasia'!

Scenario 3

It is now three days later. Mr. Jones shows some electrical activity on his EEG, but much slowing (evidence of severe brain dysfunction). He is on the respirator and has shown no signs of recovery – but no signs of deterioration either. Dr. Welby comes back to talk with Mrs. Jones and says, "Mrs. Jones, your husband has shown no signs of waking up. I am afraid that he has suffered severe and probably permanent brain injury. Patients who are going to make a good recovery usually show some response within this period of time. I recommend that we turn off the respirator and avoid the prolonged dying, of which your husband is so afraid. Since Mr. Jones seems dependent on the respirator, stopping it will be the most merciful way of allowing him to die. We are not killing him, we are merely removing the technology which is artificially pre-serving his life."

Discussion

Would this be a wise decision? It probably will accomplish both Mr. and Mrs. Jones' wishes. The probability of good recovery is small at this stage, but not nonexistent. The probability of death if one turns off the respirator is very high. By waiting three days, the physician has given Mr. Jones the best chance for a good recovery, but he has also increased the possibility of severely impaired survival without the respirator. Since

Mr. Jones does not meet the legal criteria for brain death, turning off the respirator is therefore probably illegal. But is it immoral or unethical? It meets the wishes of the patient and family, and the caveats about avoiding heroic and futile therapy. It is probably a common scenario.

Scenario 4

Mrs. Jones acquiesces, the respirator is turned off and much to everyone's dismay, Mr. Jones breathes on his own. Over the next three days he does not wake up, but is able to maintain blood pressure, heart beat, and spontaneous respirations. (This scenario is not unlike that of a recent court case in California [1].)

Scenario 5

It is now seven days after surgery, and Dr. Welby returns for discussions with Mrs. Jones. He says, "It looks like we are over the first phase. Mr. Jones is stable. We still have to feed him intravenously, but sooner or later we should be able to change that to tube feedings. He is breathing well on his own and no longer needs intensive care. We can transfer him to the ward and eventually to a nursing home." (Mr. Jones' worse fears have been realized.) Dr. Welby continues: "We will not do anything to prolong his life unduly. If he gets pneumonia, with your permission, we will not treat it. But fortunately or unfortunately, he shows no signs of pneumonia. We could discontinue his intravenous feedings, however, this would allow him to dehydrate slowly, and it may take many days for him to die."

Discussion

How can one make a decision for death at this point when there are no ready mechanisms by which death can be accomplished? The time for passive euthanasia and the events that would permit it have passed. There will be no good death. Mr. Jones will slowly dehydrate if the IVs are discontinued. If he gets pneumonia, a conscious effort will have to be made not to either diagnose or treat it – hoping that it will be lethal, but again with no guarantee. The time for a quick (good?) death has passed, and Mrs. Jones and the physicians have no way to accomplish Mr. Jones' fervent wish.

While I know of no physicians who have been placed on trial for death due to 'unrecognized' or untreated pneumonia, physicians from California were recently tried for murder for discontinuing intravenous fluids[1]. Who assures that decisions for or against these approaches to passive euthanasia are applied fairly, justly, and morally? Can these approaches, which produce a slow death, ever produce what could be considered a 'good death'?

Scenario 6

Let us return to the time of the first scenario. Dr. Welby comes out of the operating room for a discussion with Mrs. Jones. He tells her of the anesthetic mishap and that he does not know what the outcome will be. He states that the best course of action at this time is to provide maximal care for Mr. Jones, to put him on a respirator, to get the EEG and to see what happens over the next few days. He says, "Mrs. Jones, I think the possibility for Mr. Jones making a full recovery is small, but we should give him every chance. Despite everything we do, he may not make it. But, if he survives and is severely impaired, I can assure you that he will not suffer, and you will not have to suffer the prolonged agony of having your husband linger on in a vegetative state. As you and I have discussed with Mr. Jones several times, he does not want to survive in a severely impaired state. His wish to avoid this can be accomplished swiftly and painlessly by an injection. Our Euthanasia Committee understands these situations and will review the case to afford protection to everyone concerned. This way we are able to offer every patient the best chance for recovery and the best chance to avoid unacceptable outcomes."

Discussion

Here there is no question about embarking on therapy with concerns about not being able to stop. One can avoid the hypocrisy of not recognizing or not treating pneumonia should it occur, or the moral agony of watching someone starve or dehydrate, or struggle to breathe on his own. And yet, Mr. Jones can be offered all the protection of a carefully made and thoughtful decision, which allows adequate time to see the evolution of the disease or insult. The decision can be reviewed by an impartial committee constituted to assure that all of the patient's rights and those of his wife are protected from arbitrary or capricious decisions. Unlike most decisions to discontinue a respirator or decisions not to embark on therapy, these decisions could be made slowly, dispassionately, carefully, and with outside review.

COULD THE AVAILABILITY OF EUTHANASIA INDEED SAVE LIVES?

Licit euthanasia might improve decision-making in this and other relatively common situations. While decisions to discontinue therapy can often be made with thought and without inordinate pressure of time, decisions to embark on therapy often require speed with little time for considered reflection.

How often do physicians make less than a full initial effort because they think the outlook for 'good' recovery is small? How often do physicians stop after an initial effort out of concern for the future quality of life? How often do we find that we later regret that we 'did everything' when we see the patient remain unresponsive or severely impaired and resolve that the next time we will do less and avoid the disaster? Data are not available, and probably will never be, to answer these questions, but it is my guess that it happens not infrequently. Whatever its frequency, one should *always* be able to give maximal therapy whenever there is a possibility (however small) of a good outcome.

Should physicians faced with a life-threatening emergency ever consider the potential outcomes in their decision to initiate life-saving therapy? The answer is clearly no, since such consideration could never be informed or thoughtful under the pressures of time. But should patients and families be penalized because we have insufficient time to assure that our judgments (and theirs) in such situations are thoughtful and reasoned? Before high technology medicine, immediate intervention with life-saving techniques usually resulted in a life which could function independently – or else was ineffective, and the patient died. In that era we were unable to save many individuals for life on a respirator, or even to support a person until there was sufficient brainstem recovery to allow self-sustaining respirations with little cortical function. The methodology of total intravenous feeding or even prolonged maintenance of nutrition by tube feeding was not available. In order to survive for prolonged periods of time, people had to be sufficiently alert and aware to breathe on their own and to swallow (both to avoid aspiration and maintain nutrition). They had to be strong enough to overcome pneumonia (and other infections) once termed 'the old man's best friend'.

Today our technology permits us to circumvent each of these impairments that previously would have led to death, but new technology does not give us the ability to return the brain to function. Today, comatose individuals need rarely die of pneumonia or inadequate nutrition. The duration of their existence is largely determined by the level of the medical and nursing care given.

When efforts at maximal therapy are rewarded with satisfactory function, everyone is gratified. When, despite maximal therapy, death ensues, at least 'everything possible' was done. It is the limbo state that concerns patients, families, and physicians, the state in which a patient survives for a prolonged period of time in a condition unsatisfactory to himself and his family.

What constitutes such an unsatisfactory condition is a very individual matter. Clearly some families are very satisfied taking care of a loved one who makes little or no contact with his environment – others are not. Some individuals are satisfied coping as quadriplegics requiring total care – others prefer to be dead. Can we decide which is best? This first case is relatively easy because we have Mr. Jones' expressed wishes to guide us. Further, as a previously normal adult, we are better able to empathize with his condition and with his wishes and those of his family.

Decisions to end life are even more difficult when they have to be made by proxy for the infant, the mentally incompetent, or the comatose. Then we must be suspect of the motives of the family and the physicians, but these motives may also be born of genuine love and concern for the affected individual. We must be tolerant of wishes that might be different from our own [8]. I might prefer to be dead than quadriplegic. You might not. Does this make one of us right?

Let me turn to some examples in infants.

CASE 2

Ultrasonography, is now commonly used during pregnancy to establish gestational age and to detect abnormalities. Mrs. Smith, age 23 and healthy, is 24 weeks pregnant with her first child. A sonogram reveals that the infant's ventricles are large. What does the physician tell Mrs. Smith? 'Your infant probably has hydrocephalus, water on the brain.

We do not have enough experience to know if this will get worse and leave your infant with severe impairment, or leave your child normal or with only the need for a shunt at birth. Most infants with shunted hydrocephalus can do very well. A major determinant of your child's outcome may be the cause of the hydrocephalus, and we cannot determine that. If it was a viral infection, the chances of that virus having damaged the brain, in addition to causing hydrocephalus, are high. If the hydrocephalus is due to a small abnormality blocking the outflow of fluid, then, if the hydrocephalus does not become too severe, we can put in a shunt at birth, and your infant has a high probability of being normal. Some surgeons are placing shunts into the fetus in utero, but this experimental technique in no way assures a normal child. You have to decide soon, because now we could terminate the pregnancy. In a week or so this can no longer be done, and the infant will have to be carried to term."

Should Mrs. Smith decide to carry her child to term and run a substantial risk that the child will be retarded, but maintain the possibility of having a normal or treatable infant? Or should she terminate the pregnancy and try again? Would she make a different decision if she could be assured that a severely damaged child would not survive, but that at term a better assessment could be made and everything possible done for a child that had a chance of survival with a reasonable quality of life? Would the option of later euthanasia after appropriate thought, consideration, and review increase the chance of the mother carrying the infant to term? Would it increase the child's chance of survival?

CASE 3

Another woman presents at close to term having just had a sonogram showing an infant with massive hydrocephalus and a huge encephalocele. The sonogram shows other abnormalities, suggesting that the infant might have a syndrome in which the child dies shortly after birth of kidney disease. The child's head is far too large for a normal vaginal delivery. Should the physician recommend a caesarian section, which poses some risk to the mother, but affords the best chance for the child, or should the fluid be drained from the baby's head with a needle so that there can be a vaginal delivery – although the infant is unlikely to survive the birth process?

Since the infant may or may not have the syndrome, should we give the baby its best chance, and, if the infant is severely affected, assure the mother that its death will be painless and not entail prolonged suffering for either the infant or the family?

CASE 4

A child is born with a severe myelomeningocele, paralyzed below the chest (T10), with marked curvature of the spine and significant hydrocephalus. After considerable discussion over several days, the parents and physician agree that the quality of life for this child in his rural community without adequate facilities for the severely handicapped will be exceedingly poor. They agree not to close the back to prevent infection, not to shunt the hydrocephalus, and not to do anything 'heroic'. Is that an unreasonable decision? Everyone hopes the infant will die quickly. In two weeks the child appears critically ill with fever and seizures, but the meningitis remains 'undiagnosed' and untreated. Two weeks later he spontaneously recovers from his presumed meningitis, the back gradually heals over and the hydrocephalus worsens. Do we shunt the hydrocephalus to prevent future nursing problems, knowing that the infant is now probably worse off than when we initially decided not to treat? Or do we allow the infant to go untreated, allowing his head to grow to enormous proportions, ultimately to die in six months, or two years, or later? If everyone agrees during the newborn period that death would be a benefit for that child, why not provide the infant with a 'good death'? Who decides, and on what basis, that the infant's quality of life is so poor that death would be a benefit? Who reviews that decision to assure that it is not unreasonable? Conversely, how many severely impaired infants are treated only because, if untreated, they may not die 'quickly', and their death may not be 'good'?

While in this case we do not argue that euthanasia would save lives, we argue that at a time when all agree that death would be a benefit, passive euthanasia may not be humane, and may not work. If passive euthanasia is moral, but ineffective, might not active euthanasia assure a 'good death'? Would appropriate committee review, as proposed by the American Academy of Pediatrics [3], assure that the wisest and fairest decision for or against therapy is made? If there is concurrence that death is preferable to life for that infant, should we not be able to provide a 'good death'? Would such an option increase or decrease the number of survivors?

CASE 5

A child (or adult) has an inoperable brain tumor. After a surgical attempt at removal, she is given maximal radiotherapy, but the tumor recurs. Standard chemotherapy is attempted but is unsuccessful. After thoughtful discussions with the parents, the physician agrees to try a new experimental chemotherapy but to do nothing else heroic to prolong her life. The patient lapses into coma. Over several days her respirations become more labored and less frequent – twenty times per minute, later ten times per minute, finally three to five times per minute. The patient is gasping for air and blue from lack of oxygen. Since she is not responsive, we cannot tell if she is suffering, but the loving family at the bedside winces with each gasp. Should we give morphine for the 'pain' of which she does not complain, knowing that an 'unwanted' side effect will probably be cessation of respiration – if we give enough? Should we stop the steroids, which have been used to decrease swelling around the tumor, hoping that future swelling will end her agonal respirations? Or, rather than using these oblique techniques of passive euthanasia, should we be able to provide this individual and her family with a 'good death'? Should we use a simple, painless, quick-acting injection? Here, again, active euthanasia would not save lives, but would provide a better death.

OTHER CASES

Examples of emergency decisions where concern about outcome could alter therapy abound. They include: the newborn with obvious multiple malformations who requires resuscitation in the delivery suite; the child or adult who is brought to the emergency room, bradycardic and apneic; the individual brought to the emergency room decerebrate after severe head trauma; the patient on the ward who suffers a cardiac arrest and requires twenty minutes of external cardiac massage to reestablish heart beat and blood pressure. There is no time in these situations to consider carefully the ultimate outcome and quality of life if the patient survives. Should there be?

Discussion

Physicians currently deal with these situations in varying ways. For the individual dying a painful death, morphine or sedation is often used, partially for their primary effects on pain and discomfort, less often for their secondary effects on depressing respiration, but rarely in sufficient dosage to connect the drug dosage to death directly. Physicians maintain the fiction of passive euthanasia even while actively intervening.

There seems to be a growing consensus that there is no moral or legal requirement to continue or embark on medical or surgical therapies that only prolong the act of dying [9]. Yet, we are morally and legally prohibited from doing something active, which would relieve the suffering of that dying individual – from giving him or her a 'good death'.

There is growing discussion amongst the medical, legal, and ethical communities about the management of patients in a persistent vegetative state. There are individuals, such as in Case 1, who do not meet the criteria of brain death, but whose cortical functions have been so permanently damaged that they have and will continue to have little or no contact with the environment. Yet their brainstem functions are sufficient to allow respiration or maintenance of heart beat and blood pressure. These individuals are not dying and yet will not recover. They require no high technology but merely care and intravenous or tube feeding. Recent articles [4, 9], and a recent legal opinion [1] suggest that there is no legal or moral duty to continue treatment once it has proven to be ineffective. The court [1] found that the use of intravenous fluids were not traditional treatment, since they were not used directly to cure or address the pathological condition. Fluids merely sustain biologic function in order to gain time to permit other processes to address the pathology. In substance, the court found that since there was no treatment for the severe cortical damage and since there was no hope for spontaneous recovery from the damage, that maintenance of biologic functions was useless therapy and therefore not required.

If there is no necessity to maintain biologic function in the absence of cortical brain function, why then is it permissible to withdraw sustenance but not actively to end the biologic function in more humane ways?

In other situations, such as Case 2 or Case 3, physicians, together with parents, may elect to terminate a pregnancy to prevent the birth of a catastrophically impaired infant – even without certainty that the infant will be catastrophically impaired. They are willing to sacrifice a possibly normal infant to avoid the likelihood of a potential disaster. Would it not save lives to handle the disastrous situation when, and if, it occurs?

In other situations, such as the child with myelomeningocele (Case 4), physicians provide only 'ordinary' care, declaring that the diagnosis and management of meningitis or hydrocephalus would be extraordinary in those circumstances [7]. Still others operate on all of these infants to close the back and shunt the hydrocephalus prophylactically, because so few of the children die quickly or without prolonged suffering (at least for the caretakers). For such infants, the lack of availability of a good death leads to a lifetime of severe impairment for the child and the family. The decisions in these cases, even when thoughtful, are usually made by the family and the physician without the availability and protection of outside review [6]. When the decision is made not to treat, should there not be outside review or consultation? If death is deemed preferable, should a 'good death' not be feasible?

IF EUTHANASIA WERE LICIT

If euthanasia were licit, more individuals would be allowed a 'good death', a death with dignity, quick and without pain and suffering. If euthanasia were legal, perhaps embryos and fetuses now aborted, because of the possibility or probability of a severe defect, would survive if they were found to be free of the defect. If euthanasia were licit, perhaps more vigorous initial therapy could be used without the fear by physicians, family, and patients that the patient might be forced to survive in an unsatisfactory, limbo-like state. If euthanasia were licit, then controls could be imposed on the decision-making process to assure that the decisions were reasonable and tolerable – in contrast to the current secret, sometimes arbitrary, decision-making process that now goes on between a patient's family and the physician.

One major criticism of euthanasia is that legal killing could be used against categories of people, as was done during the Holocaust. That killing by categories as an instrument of policy has nothing to do with providing a 'good death' to individuals. That was not euthanasia, but rather a perversion of the term. I think of euthanasia as providing 'good' death, quickly and painlessly, in situations where death would be a benefit to the individual. I feel that if euthanasia were licit, its legalization could incorporate appropriate controls and review, controls that are lacking in our current decision-making process.

A second major criticism is that killing is a basic societal taboo. If that taboo were broken and killing of any sort sanctioned, it would be the thin edge of a wedge that would alter society. Further, since physicians are trained to treat disease and work on behalf of their patients, permitting euthanasia might fundamentally alter patient-physician relationships and abolish patient trust. These arguments, I believe, are paper tigers. We are not proposing to sanction killing, but rather to sanction active intervention to provide a good death in only those situations where death is the desirable outcome for the patient as determined by the physician *and* the family *with* outside review (see below). Patients and families would continue to perceive that physicians were working to help their patients, always working in the patient's best interest, and not preserving and treating meaningless existence over the opposition of patients or families.

With the growing concern of many individuals about the potential overuse of technology to preserve their lives, and physician concerns about termination of therapies, many states have enacted 'natural death' acts or durable powers of attorney to allow the patient's wishes that his life not be sustained indefinitely to be carried out. These are extensions of the patient's right to refuse medical care and to refuse life-sustaining therapy. In a sense they give the patient the right to 'passive' suicide. While suicide and aiding or abetting suicide are illegal, it is not clear why. In a carefully documented review, Engelhardt and Malloy [5] argue that in Texas, which had no law against suicide, there was no greater incidence of suicide or social disruption than in states in which suicide was illegal. They argue that Texas, which abandoned its law in 1973, should, in keeping with the tradition of individual liberty, return to allowing individual decisions about circumstances of death. They also recommend that Texas return to refusal to proscribe passively-assisted suicide. This, they say, would "return life and death decisions to the hands of those most concerned – those who would die" ([5], p.1037). It would be but a small step from passively-assisted suicide to actively-assisted suicide – to euthanasia with consent, consent that is voluntary or by proxy, with appropriate outside review.

PROCESS

I propose an ethics committee in each hospital – a committee that may soon be extant in response to the Report of the President's Commission and Department of Health and Human Services regulations. The composition of the committee should include representation from outside the medical community. Any situation where death would be considered a benefit by the patient or the family, any situation where active or passive euthanasia is considered desirable, would be reviewed by the committee. The wishes and desires of the patient, where available, should be given primacy. The desires of the family should be carefully evaluated when the family wishes an end to the patient's suffering. In no case should the family's desire for continued care be overruled. When the family wishes an end to the patient's suffering, the committee should carefully consider this request in light of the patient's disease, condition and prognosis. It should examine the family's motives and assure that this is a reasonable decision. The committee should act as the patient's advocate, being aware and sensitive to the fact that everyone will not advocate the same outcome in a given situation. Committee members should be tolerant of a diversity of positions [8] and assure that the decision to end a life is reasonable and directed to the patient's benefit – but the committee should not have dogmatic standards. The patient's physician should also act as the patient's advocate, being aware of the limits of his own prejudices and tolerant of diversity of opinion. When the physician is opposed to the family's or patient's desires for an end to suffering, outside consultation should be sought by the committee to assist in evaluation of the arguments.

Euthanasia should *never* be ordered by the physician or by the committee, but rather acquiesced to, on a plea by the patient or the relatives.

With these protections, and with periodic outside review of the committee's decision and decision-making process, we will have far greater protection than is currently available. Physicians can then embark on heroic therapies with appropriate consent without fearing; and without fear on the part of the patient and family, that the patient will be left in limbo. Thus I believe that if euthanasia were licit, lives would actually be saved, and those patients in a persistent vegetative state actually benefited.

The Johns Hopkins Medical Institutions
Baltimore, Maryland, U.S.A.

BIBLIOGRAPHY

1. Barber v. L. A. Co. Super. Ct. No. 69350 (Cal. C. App., Oct. 12, 1983).
2. Beauchamp, T. L. and Davidson, A. I. : 1979, 'The Definition of Euthanasia', *The*

Journal of Medicine and Philosophy **4**, 294–312.

3. Committee on Bioethics, American Academy of Pediatrics: 1983, 'Treatment of Critically Ill Newborns', *Pediatrics* **72**, 565–567.
4. Cranford, R. E. : 1984, 'Termination of Treatment in the Persistent Vegetative State', *Seminars in Neurology* **4**, 36–45.
5. Engelhardt, H. T., Jr. and Malloy, M.: 1982, 'Suicide and Assisting Suicide. A Critique of Legal Sanctions', *Southwestern Law Journal* **36**, 1003–1037.
6. Freeman, J. M.: 1984, 'Early Management and Decision Making for the Treatment of Myelomeningocele: A Critique', *Pediatrics* **73**, 564–566.
7. Gross, R. H. *et al.*: 1983, 'Early Management and Decision Making for the Treatment of Myelomeningocele', *Pediatrics* **72**, 450–458.
8. McDonnell, K. and Freeman, J. M.: 1984, 'Termination of Care in Defective Newborns', *Seminars in Neurology* **4**, 30–35.
9. Wanzer, S. H. *et al.*: 1984, 'The Physician's Responsibility Toward Hopelessly Ill Patients', *New England Journal of Medicine* **310**, 955–959.

JOHN C. SINCLAIR

HIGH TECHNOLOGY, HIGH COSTS, AND THE VERY LOW BIRTH-WEIGHT NEWBORN

There has been a recent and remarkable advance in knowledge, skills, and technology that allows for a considerably increased chance of survival for the very ill newborn infant. This phenomenon is best exemplified by the greatly improved outlook for the very low birth-weight infant treated in a neonatal intensive care unit. However, neonatal intensive care is very costly and questions have been raised both inside and outside the medical sector regarding the medical and economic justification of providing intensive care for babies born so early and so small as to be at or below the apparent limit of viability.

In this paper I will briefly review the growth in our capacity to provide neonatal intensive care, and then review the evidence regarding the efficacy and effectiveness of intensive care of very low birth-weight infants. In considering the economic costs of such care, I will outline the methods by which both costs and outcomes can be taken into account in an economic evaluation of a health program, and show the results in the case of intensive care of very low birth-weight infants. Finally, I will point to certain moral and philosophical questions which arise in the economic evaluation of health care programs and, more particularly, those which arise in the application of the results of such evaluation to future decisions about the provision of health care.

I will adopt the societal perspective in this paper. Therefore, I will not discuss those issues concerning costs and outcomes that pertain to medical management of the individual patient. Rather, I will attempt to identify and discuss issues of concern to society that arise in the context of health program evaluation and which pertain to the management of a whole group of patients – in this case, very low birth-weight infants.

GROWTH AND DEVELOPMENT OF NEONATAL INTENSIVE CARE

Hack *et al.* [15] defined four stages in the evolution of newborn care during this century:

R. C. McMillan, H. T. Engelhardt, Jr., and S. F. Spicker (eds.),
Euthanasia and the Newborn, 169–189.
© 1987 *by D. Reidel Publishing Company.*

TABLE I

Typical indications for admission of babies to neonatal intensive care

Low birth weight (whether due to prematurity or intrauterine growth retardation)
Birth asphyxia
Respiratory distress of any cause (e.g., hyaline membrane disease, meconium aspiration, pneumothorax)
Neonatal infections
Metabolic disturbances (e.g., hypoglycemia, electrolyte disorders, inborn errors of metabolism)
Convulsions or other neurologic disorder
Significant congenital malformations
Other significant neonatal disease (e.g., hemolytic disease, blood loss, infants of diabetic mothers, infants of mothers taking hazardous drugs, *etc.*)

(1) turn of century to mid-1940s: newborn care the responsibility of the obstetrician; basic principles as outlined by Pierre Budin [5].

(2) mid 1940s – early 1960s: many innovations in newborn care, most unsupported by clinical trials, but with a few notable exceptions, for example, in oxygen use [22] and temperature control [36]; several therapeutic disasters.

(3) early 1960s – early 1970s: beginning of neonatal intensive care. Rapid increase in basic and clinical research in perinatal and developmental medicine, together with technologic advances in microchemistry and bioengineering, leads to a surer scientific foundation (but also increasing complexity and cost) of neonatal care.

(4) early 1970s to present: increasing dissemination and application of existing knowledge through large-scale regional programs in perinatal/neonatal care.

Recommendations and guidelines for the organization and implementation of regional perinatal and neonatal programs have been published in Canada, the United States, and other countries. These recommendations recognize three levels of pregnancy risk, requiring stepwise increments in the complexity and cost of health services: Level I (about 85 percent of pregnancies), normal or low risk; Level II (about 12 percent of pregnancies), moderate risk; and Level III (about 3 percent of pregnancies), high risk. The proportion of live births requiring neonatal intensive care varies directly with the level of pregnancy risk; this proportion is about three percent in Ontario, Canada [1].

Typical indications for the admission of newborns to intensive care units are given in Table I.

TABLE II

Specific maneuvers typically included in a neonatal intensive care program and validated in randomized controlled trials

Maintenance of thermoneutrality
Avoidance of overexposure to oxygen
Early intravenous feeding with glucose and water
Early enteral feeding
Supplemental parenteral nutrition
Intravenous glucose and sodium bicarbonate (respiratory-distress syndrome)
Continuous distending airway pressure ± assisted ventilation (respiratory-distress syndrome)
Chest physiotherapy
Oscillating water bed (recurrent apnea)
Closure of symptomatic patent ductus arteriosus
Phototherapy (hyperbilirubinemia)
Promotion of maternal contact
Skilled assistance during neonatal transport
'Intensive-care' package

The widespread application of intensive care to the at-risk fetus and newborn infant is a relatively recent innovation. The remarkable growth of regional programs for providing neonatal intensive care has been reviewed by Butterfield [8] who estimated that between 124 and 167 such programs were in existence in North America by 1976. The aggressive treatment of extremely premature babies has pushed the limit of human viability downward to unprecedented levels. However, as smaller and more immature babies are kept alive, there is an associated increase in problems of biologic, pathophysiologic, and social complexity, and the following questions arise: Do neonatal-intensive care programs do more good than harm? What is the magnitude of their effects? What are their costs?

EVIDENCE FOR EFFICACY OF NEONATAL INTENSIVE CARE

The efficacy of neonatal intensive care has been evaluated by randomized controlled clinical trials of a number of specific elements of neonatal care. Table II lists some preventive or therapeutic interventions or services that have been found through randomized, controlled trials to be beneficial in the care of high-risk babies. The list does not include trials of antenatal treatment of the mother for the prevention of neonatal disease (e.g., Rh-immune gamma globulin for the prevention of Rh erythroblastosis, glucocorticoids for the prevention of hyaline-membrane disease, or tocolytic drugs for the prevention of premature delivery). Although the list in Table II is not exhaustive, it at least indicates that there is experimental evidence in support of practices involving the respiratory, nutritional and environmental management of sickness in infants. In most of the clinical trials cited, the outcome measures are neonatal mortality or short-term morbidity. Few trials have tested the efficacy of neonatal intensive care as measured by long-term morbidity.

EVIDENCE FOR EFFECTIVENESS OF NEONATAL INTENSIVE CARE

The effectiveness of neonatal intensive care programs in large populations has not been tested experimentally in studies using a randomized controlled design. Evaluation of effectiveness of neonatal intensive care has been based on non-experimental research, chiefly descriptive and analytic surveys.

Effect on Mortality

During the pre-intensive care era, survival was less than 10 percent among babies weighing under 1000g at birth, and only about 50 percent among those weighing 1000 to 1500g. Since the introduction of neonatal intensive care, reported survival rates have increased substantially. For example, among babies weighing under 1000g at birth, survival rates of 45 percent or higher have been reported and among babies weighing 1000 to 1500g at birth, reported survival rates have been 80 percent or higher. However, these recent reports are based on the experience of centers treating infants who have been referred for care, and they leave unanswered the question of whether neonatal mortality has changed similarly in the entire population.

There have been several recent attempts to evaluate the impact of neonatal intensive care programs on the total populations they serve. These population studies seek to avoid patient selection bias by recording clinical outcomes on all patients within a defined region to whom the program is directed. Some of these area-based studies are summarized in Table III.

TABLE III

Area-based studies of neonatal mortality of very low birth-weight infants

Author and area	Year of birth	Mortality (%)		
		Type of rate *	Birth weight category	
			501–1000 g	1001–1500 g	501–1500 g

Author and area	Year of birth	Type of rate *	501–1000 g	1001–1500 g	501–1500 g
Pakter and Nelson, New York	1962	NN	87.5	45.0	
City [28]	1971	NN	79.0	33.8	
Steiner et al., Mansfield and					
district, England [39]	1963–1971	NN			52.6
Usher, Quebec [45]	1968	NN	92.0	53.5	
	1974	NN	88.0	36.4	
Kleinman et al., 5 states [24]	1960	ENN	90.7	54.1	71.1
	1973	ENN	83.3	32.1	55.8
Kleinman et al., North Carolina	1960	ENN	92.1	54.6	71.2
white [24]	1973–1974	ENN	84.0	40.1	59.5
Hein, Iowa [20]	1972	NN			68.0
	1978	NN			47.0
Horwood et al., Hamilton	1964–1969	NN	88.1	36.6	58.7
Canada [21]	1973–1977	NN	69.4	21.6	39.2

* Abbreviations used are: NN, neonatal (0–27 days); ENN, early neonatal (0–6 days).

Paneth et al. [29] analyzed neonatal mortality rates of 501–2250g infants born between 1976 and 1978 in New York City, classified according to hospital of birth: those with newborn intensive care units (Level 3), those with capabilities for the care of most premature infants (Level 2), and those without any special facilities for premature newborns (Level 1). The distribution of maternal characteristics conferring higher risk of neonatal mortality was quite even across the three kinds of hospitals. Among 13,560 singleton low birth-weight infants, the risk-adjusted neonatal mortality rate for Level 3 hospitals was significantly lower than the rates for both Level 2 and Level 1 units. The association of mortality with level of care held across a broad range of conditions. The authors concluded that birth at a Level 3 hospital can lower neonatal mortality in low birth-weight infants.

Over the past twenty years there has been a substantial decline in neonatal mortality, especially in birth-weight groups over 1000g. It is simplistic, however, to attribute this decline to perinatal and neonatal intensive care alone. Other changes that have occurred (e.g., in maternal age and fertility, birth control, prenatal screening, and selective abortion) are known to affect mortality in newborns. Nonetheless, Kleinman, *et al*. stated, "The most likely explanation for at least part of the recent decline in mortality levels among low birth-weight infants is the development of the medical technology for successful management of premature infants and the consequent proliferation of this technology" ([24] p. 466). Similarly, Lee *et al*. noted a substantial decline in birth-weight-specific neonatal mortality in the United States from 1950 to 1975; they stated (and I agree with them) that "although the evidence is indirect, and although it is impossible to rule out the contribution of factors as yet unspecified, the most plausible explanation for the demographic trends we have noted is the steady improvement in perinatal medical care . . ."([25], p. 24).

Effect on Morbidity

It is often claimed that not only mortality rates but also long-term morbidity rates are reduced by neonatal intensive care. Selected follow-up studies of very low birth-weight infants born over the past twenty-five years show that among babies weighing less than 1500g who were born in the 1940s and 1950s, one-third of the survivors were handicapped. However, among children in the same birth-weight group born in the 1960s and early 1970s only about 10 percent had handicaps. Once again, however, these are hospital-based studies; therefore, they cannot be used to indicate the effect of neonatal intensive care on the population served.

Table IV lists some recent area-based studies of long-term morbidity among very low birth-weight infants. These studies do not show a reduction in the incidence of handicap among surviving very low birth-weight infants born between 1963 and 1977, a period when neonatal intensive care was being introduced. In fact, these studies suggest that the handicap rate has remained fairly constant: about 15 percent of survivors of very low birth-weight have serious handicaps.

Cerebral palsy is of particular interest in relation to neonatal intensive care because there are reasonably strict criteria for its diagnosis and classification and because the incidence (particularly that of spastic diplegia) is known to vary inversely with birth weight and to be strongly

TABLE IV

Area-based morbidity follow-up studies of very low birth-weight infants live-born between 1963–1977

Author and area	Year of birth	No. live-born/ No. of neonatal survivors/No. followed up	Age at follow-up	% of those followed who were free of serious handicap
Steiner et al., Mansfield and district, England [39]	1963–1971	293/139/133	6½–16 yr	87
Shapiro et al., 8 regions in USA [34]	1976	–* / –* /209	1 yr	86
Horwood et al., Hamilton, Canada [21]	1964–1969	373/154/121	9–14 yr	83
Horwood et al., Hamilton, Canada [21]	1973–1977	265/161/134	1½–6 yr	84

* Data not available.

influenced by perinatal events. In several counties in Sweden, the total incidence of cerebral palsy decreased from 2.2 per thousand live births in the period 1954–1958 to 1.3 per thousand live births by 1967–1970 [18, 19]. This overall decline was due almost entirely to a decrease in the incidence of spastic diplegia among low birth-weight infants, and it coincided with the introduction of new methods of perinatal and neo-natal intensive care in Sweden. However, more recent reports on rates of cerebral palsy in Sweden [16, 17] and Western Australia [12, 37] have failed to confirm a continuing decline in the incidence of cerebral palsy despite the increasing dissemination of perinatal and neonatal intensive care.

Retinopathy of prematurity is another outcome of considerable rel-evance to neonatal intensive care, and in this case the available evidence suggests that such care may in fact increase morbidity. Both the inci-dence and the severity of this condition are inversely related to birth weight. As survival rates increase among babies weighing less than 1500g (and particularly less than 1000g), the number of infants at risk for blindness from retinopathy of prematurity also increases. Skill-ful avoidance of excessive use of oxygen may reduce the occur-rence of retinopathy of prematurity; however, present technical skills in administering oxygen do not appear to be sufficient to prevent the disorder in the most immature infants. Indeed, Phelps [30] has used current estimates of survival and blindness among survivors to estimate the annual number of cases of blindness among very-low-birth-weight infants in the United States. Alarmingly, her calculations suggest that this number could be approaching the level during the 'epidemic' of retinopathy of prematurity in the pre-intensive care years from 1942 to 1953.

To summarize the evidence of efficacy and effectiveness of neonatal intensive care, we can be confident that intensive care interventions in the neonatal period are efficacious in reducing neonatal mortality. Neonatal mortality rate in the population is declining and it is likely that this is due in large part to the effectiveness of perinatal/neonatal intensive care. However, it is doubtful that the rate of handicap in surviving very low birth-weight infants has been much affected. The substantially increased survival rate of very low birth-weight infants of whom 10 to 15 percent may be handicapped may result (in absolute terms) in an increased number of handicapped individuals being introduced into society as a consequence of intensive care of tiny infants.

EFFICIENCY OF NEONATAL INTENSIVE CARE

There is a third perspective from which neonatal intensive care is being evaluated – the economic perspective. An economic evaluation seeks to investigate the relative costs and benefits of alternative strategies in health care – that is, to value the resources used and to weigh them against the values of the outcomes. Thus, an economic evaluation seeks to answer the question: "Is it worth doing?"

Why undertake an economic evaluation of a health program? The answer is grounded in utilitarian ethics. Resources are finite, and there are always choices to be made with respect to how best to use them. Thus, the concept of the value of resources that is applied in an economic evaluation is that of opportunity cost: since resources are finite, deploying them in one way means that a benefit is foregone in not having them available to pursue the best alternative. Neonatal intensive care is expensive [26, 31, 32], and whether we relish the question or not, it must be faced: are finite resources better spent on expanding society's capacity for providing neonatal intensive care rather than in launching or expanding other health programs? To address this question, the techniques of economic evaluation have been applied to neonatal intensive care.

TECHNIQUES OF ECONOMIC EVALUATION OF HEALTH PROGRAMS

Economic evaluation may employ one or more of the following techniques: cost-benefit analysis [2, 23] in which outcomes are converted to dollars; cost-effectiveness analysis [35, 49] in which outcomes are measured in units of health (e.g., mortality or disability days); and cost-utility analysis [33, 41] in which health outcomes are adjusted on the basis of values or utilities assigned to them by patients or members of society at large. However, regardless of the technique used, the general nature of an economic evaluation is the same: it consists of a comparative analysis of alternative courses of action in terms of their costs and consequences.

The impact of effective health care programs is felt in terms of both decreased mortality and decreased morbidity. In order for health care programs to be compared with each other, patients are assessed using a comprehensive measure of health that considers both mortality and morbidity. The morbidity component is captured by using standardized scales and measured preferences in order to adjust for lost 'quality' of survival due to disease or disability. In measuring preferences for health states on a 'utility' scale, it has become customary to arbitrarily assign the values 0 and 1 to the reference states 'dead' and 'healthy', respectively. Thus, a life year in a health state judged to be 0.75 on a utility scale would represent 0.75 quality-adjusted life years.

Economic analysis can be performed from a variety of viewpoints (e.g., those of the patient and family, the care-giving institution, the third-party payer, society as a whole). The viewpoint of the analysis should be appropriate for the decision to which the work is addressed. Two categories of decision must be distinguished: planning (or programmatic) decisions made on behalf of the community as a whole, and clinical decisions made on behalf of the individual patient. Economic evaluation is most relevant to planning decisions, which set priorities for the allocation of scarce resources. In this context, the costs and consequences of the program should be evaluated from the viewpoint of society; all costs and consequences to all parties should be considered.

ECONOMIC EVALUATION OF NEONATAL INTENSIVE CARE OF VERY LOW BIRTH-WEIGHT INFANTS

At McMaster University, we carried out an economic evaluation of neonatal intensive care of very low birth-weight infants using outcomes and costs of care before and after the introduction of a regional neonatal intensive-care program. We used the techniques of cost-effectiveness analysis, in which outcomes are measured in units of health, and cost-utility analysis, in which health outcomes are quality-adjusted on the basis of values assigned by members of society.

The methods used in our study have been published in detail [3, 4, 21, 40]. Only the main points will be summarized here. We adopted the societal perspective; i.e., we took into consideration all the costs and benefits of providing neonatal intensive-care, regardless of who pays or who benefits. We determined costs and outcomes on all very low birth-weight infants born to residents in a defined region. Before the introduction of intensive care (1964–69), such infants were treated in community hospitals by general pediatricians and the staff of a 'premature' nursery; after the introduction of intensive care (1973–77) such infants were born in or could be transferred to the regional perinatal center. In fact, 68 percent of the 1973–77 cohort actually received care in the regional neonatal intensive-care unit.

Health outcomes that were ascertained included survival to the point of discharge from newborn hospitalization and follow-up health status. The latter required the development of a health status index. The various states of health were valued by parents in order to provide a basis for quality-adjusting the observed health states [40]. Parents rated some chronic dysfunctional states in children as worse than death; thus, our empirically determined range of utility values extended below zero on the utility scale.

Costs, expressed in 1978 Canadian dollars, were measured for neonatal care [3] and for health care costs and other costs occurring after discharge from the hospital. Forecasts of lifetime costs and outcomes were made on the basis of each child's health history.

A neonatal intensive care program requires the early expenditure of large sums of money in order to achieve later gains (e.g., in numbers of life-years). Therefore, a discount rate of 5 percent per annum was applied to future costs, earnings, and health effects in order to convert the future values to their equivalent present value.[1] Sensitivity analyses

TABLE V

Health outcomes for very low birth-weight infants born before and after the introduction of neonatal intensive care, according to the birth-weight class (undiscounted)

Period	Birth weight 1000–1499 g		Birth weight 500–999 g	
	Before intensive care (1964–69) $n = 213$	Intensive care (1973–77) $n = 167$	Before intensive care (1964–69) $n = 160$	Intensive care (1973–77) $n = 98$
To hospital discharge				
Survivors (%)	62.4	77.2	10.6	22.4
To age 15 (projected)				
Life-years/live birth	9.0	11.1	1.46	3.37
QALYs */live birth	6.4	8.1	1.22	1.80
To death (projected)				
Life-years/live birth	38.8	47.7	6.6	13.0
QALYs */live birth	27.4	36.0	5.5	9.1

* QALY denotes quality-adjusted life years. Data of Boyle et al. [4].

were performed to determine the robustness of the findings to changes in discount rate, life expectancy, loss to follow-up, and utility values.

Neonatal intensive care increased survival rates and life years (Table V) and costs (Table VI). For newborns weighing 1000 to 1499g, the incremental cost (in 1978 Canadian dollars) was $59,500 per additional survivor, $2900 per life-year gained, and $3200 per quality-adjusted life-year gained over the projected lifetime. For infants weighing 500 to 999g, the corresponding costs were $102,000 per additional survivor, $9300 per life-year gained, and $22,400 per quality-adjusted life-year gained. When the increased future earnings were netted against costs as a "cost recovery", the net economic cost per life-year gained (or per quality-adjusted life-year gained) was appreciably lower. These results are summarized in Table VII.

Analyses by 250-gram birth-weight groups showed that the largest gain in survival rate for any subgroup was obtained for the 750–999 group (survival to hospital discharge increased from 19 to 43 percent). However, in this subgroup, the gain in life-years was not matched by an equal gain in quality-adjusted life-years. As a result, not only hospital costs but also postdischarge costs were very high in this weight group.

TABLE VI

Economic outcomes according to birth-weight class (undiscounted)

Period	Birth weight 1000–1499 g		Birth weight 500–999 g	
	Before intensive care (1964–69)	Intensive care (1973–77)	Before intensive care (1964–69)	Intensive care (1973–77)
Costs/live birth				
To hospital discharge				
Health care	5,400	14,200	1,500	13,600
To age 15 (projected)				
Health care	8,100	18,700	1,800	18,000
Other	4,000	2,000	200	1,900
Total cost	12,100	20,700	2,000	19,900
To death (projected)				
Health care	45,000	61,500	9,500	28,600
Other	47,100	38,600	1,500	15,000
Total cost	92,500	100,100	11,000	43,600
Earnings/live birth				
To death (projected)	122,200	154,500	19,200	48,100

* Values are expressed in 1978 Canadian dollars. Multiply by 0.877 to calculate equivalent 1978 U.S. dollars. Data of Boyle *et al.* [4].

By every measure of economic evaluation, the impact of neonatal intensive care was more favourable among infants weighing 1000 to 1499g than among those weighing 500 to 999g.

How does neonatal intensive care compare with other health care programs with regard to economic viability? Direct comparisons should be made with caution because of methodologic differences between studies. For example, other studies have not always measured costs comprehensively and from the viewpoint of society as a whole; quality-adjustment factors, determined experimentally in our study, have often been assigned arbitrarily. Nevertheless, rough comparisons are possible, and these are shown in Table VIII. Clearly, neonatal intensive care of infants 1000–1499g is already placed very favorably in relation to the cost-utility of other health programs; under 1000g, the cost-utility of intensive care is not yet as encouraging.

TABLE VII

Cost-effectiveness and cost-utility of neonatal intensive care by birth-weight class (5% discount rate)*

| | Birth-weight class | |
	1000–1499 g	500–999 g
	$	
To hospital discharge[a]		
Cost/additional survivor at hospital discharge	59,500	102,500
To age 15 (projected)		
Cost/life-year gained	6,100	12,200
Cost/QALY[b] gained	7,700	40,100
To death (projected)		
Cost/life-year gained	2,900	9,300
Cost/QALY[b] gained	3,200	22,400
Net economic cost/life-year gained	900	7,300
Net economic cost/QALY gained	1,000	17,500

* Values are expressed in 1978 Canadian dollars. Multiply by 0.877 to calculate equivalent 1978 U.S. dollars.
[a] All costs and effects occurred in year one.
[b] QALY denotes quality-adjusted life-year.
Data of Boyle et al., [4].

TABLE VIII

Comparative cost-utility results for selected programs[a]

Program [reference]	Reported cost/QALY[b] gained in U.S. dollars (year)	Adjusted[c] cost/QALY[b] gained in U.S. dollars 1983
PKU screening [6]	< 0 (1970)	< 0
Post-partum anti-D [42]	< 0 (1977)	< 0
Ante-partum anti-D [43]	1220 (1983)	1220
Coronary artery bypass surgery for left main coronary artery disease [47]	3500 (1981)	4200

continued on page 182

TABLE VIII *continued*

Program [reference]	Reported cost/QALY[b] gained in U.S. dollars (year)	Adjusted[a] cost/QALY[b] gained in U.S. dollars 1983
Neonatal intensive care, 1000–1499g [4]	2800 (1978)	4500
T4 (thyroid) screening [13]	3600 (1977)	6300
Treatment of severe hypertension (diastolic ≥ 105 mm Hg) at age 40 [38]	4850 (1976)	9400
Treatment of mild hypertension (diastolic 95–104 mm Hg) at age 40 [38]	9880 (1976)	19,100
Estrogen therapy for postmenopausal symptoms in women without prior hysterectomy [48]	18,160 (1979)	27,000
Neonatal intensive care, 500–999g [4]	19,600 (1978)	31,800
Coronary artery bypass surgery for single vessel disease with moderately severe angina [47]	30,000 (1981)	36,300
School tuberculin testing program [7]	13,000 (1968)	43,700
Continuous ambulatory peritoneal dialysis [9]	35,100 (1980)	47,100
Hospital hemodialysis [9]	40,200 (1980)	54,000

Table adapted from Torrance, G. W. and Zipursky, A. [43].

[a] These studies use similar, but not identical, methods. Generally, costs are net health care costs; however, discount rates and preference weights are not completely consistent. Differences in methods (in particular, the assumption on patient compliance) should be considered when comparing the relative cost-utility. For details, see original sources.

[b] QALY denotes quality-adjusted life-year.

[c] Adjusted to 1983 dollars according to the US Consumer Price Index for Medical Care for all urban consumers. Source: US Bureau of Labor Statistics. *Monthly Labor Review.*

MORAL AND PHILOSOPHICAL ISSUES

Toulmin [44] has noted that medicine over the last twenty years has "saved the life of ethics" in the sense that medical progress has provided difficult topics raised by concrete cases, which have challenged the dormant practical reasoning skills of philosophers. The particular case of neonatal intensive care of the tiny premature infant raises a number of moral and philosophical issues that have been touched on and will be expanded here.

Probably few would quarrel with the premise that people's preferences should count in reaching decisions that will affect them. But whose preferences should count? In the field of health, preferences for health states have been used in the field of clinical decision analysis and in the field of health program evaluation. Clinical decision analysis is concerned with decisions that must be made regarding the investigation and/or treatment for an individual patient. It is obviously appropriate in this application to attempt to measure the preferences of the particular patient for the various possible outcomes and to use them in the decision analysis. On the other hand, health program evaluation is concerned with decisions that must be made regarding alternative health care programs directed to groups of patients. Whose preferences for health states should be measured? Should it be a random sample of the general public on the grounds that it is society's resources that are being allocated to the various health care programs and so it is society's preferences that should count? Should it be the actual patient groups to whom the programs are directed (or in the case of newborns, their parents) on the grounds that who better can appreciate the true implications of a particular health state than patients or parents who have first-hand knowledge? Or should it be health professionals on the grounds that they are the most knowledgeable and/or they are the proxies of the public in the health field?

The findings of our study of the economic aspects of neonatal intensive care have potential implications for the planning of health care programs. Societies with insufficient capacity to provide intensive care for all very low birth-weight infants may choose to give priority to infants weighing over 1000g because economic analysis indicates that the impact of intensive care is more favorable in this group than in infants weighing under 1000g at birth. Societies with insufficient resources to meet all the health care needs of their citizens may choose to direct increased resources to neonatal intensive care and curtail other health care programs that are less cost-effective. Thus, analysis of the relative costs and effects of health care programs inevitably leads to questions concerning not only the planning but also the 'rationing' of health care.

Even when health care resources are limited, can rationing of medical care at a programmatic level be morally justified? Physicians have been reluctant to consider medical decisions within economic constraints, traditionally arguing that to do so violates the values of the profession as well as of patients. However, Culyer argues that "efficiency is as much a moral pursuit as justice since inefficiency means you could accomplish the same end with fewer resources and hence have some over to pursue other (moral) objectives. Similarly, an apparently just distribution of health resources is not really just if it wastefully uses resources that could be put to use in the service of other just ends" ([11], p. 7). In a similar vein, Fuchs believes that cost-benefit and cost-effectiveness analyses offer "the most rational, humane basis for effective, efficient allocation" of health care resources. "It is in the best interests of patients and professionals for these constraints to be derived from careful study of costs and benefits rather than from capricious budget ceilings and regulatory roulette. When constraints on health care are imposed without regard to costs and benefits, the nation's health suffers more than is necessary" ([14], p. xi).

Can rationing decisions be equitable? Economic appraisal of health services leads to conclusions that, while they can be valid and applicable, may not in fact be equitable. Inequity may result from the viewpoint of the analysis. When the viewpoint of the analysis is that of society, there is no assurance that the conclusions of the analysis will fairly represent the interests of patients within that society who harbor a specified condition or specified values. For example, if from the perspective of society renal transplant is judged to be more cost-effective than hemodialysis in the treatment of end-stage renal disease and dialysis programs are therefore curtailed, this will deal an inequity to patients in whom renal transplant is contraindicated or who value the possibility of long-term survival less than freedom from risk of early operative mortality.

Other types of potential inequity can also be identified. The technique of discounting future costs and outcomes adjusts for time preference, which it is meant to do; however, it may also invoke an age preference, which it is not necessarily meant to do. For example, intensive care programs have high initial costs in order to achieve later gains in outcomes such as life years and productivity. Discounting affects the later gains more than the initial costs and adversely affects the cost-benefit appraisal of intensive care programs to a degree that depends on the age of the patients in the program. The age preference will be for young adults first (because future earnings lie shortly ahead and are discounted least), infants and children next, and geriatric patients last.

Inequity may arise from the choice of comparison. Only when different treatments for the same condition are compared may patients with that condition be treated equitably (and even then not necessarily so, see end-stage renal disease, above). For example, consider the cost-effectiveness of contrasting ways of managing threatened pre-term delivery. This condition could be handled by an intensive care program initiated either before birth (aimed at postponing birth) or launched after birth (intensive care of the pre-term infant). The interests of the fetal patient would be equitably represented in such a comparison. This would not be the case, however, if neonatal intensive care were compared with coronary intensive care, or with compulsory seat-belt legislation.[2]

Inequity may arise in choosing between effectiveness and efficiency when they are in conflict. For example, in our study of neonatal intensive care of very low birth-weight infants, neonatal intensive care was *most effective* in infants weighing 750 to 999g at birth (survival rate increased from 19 to 43 percent); however, it was *least efficient* in this same group (net economic loss was $25,000 per live birth). If neonatal intensive care of very low birth-weight infants were to be rationed, which infants should preferentially receive intensive care – those that are most likely to benefit (750 to 999g) or those from whom society is most likely to benefit (1250 to 1499g)?

How should rationing decisions be applied? Fuchs recommends that when the results of economic evaluation are applied it will be important to "insulate the individual practitioner from explicit involvement on a day-to-day basis because of potential conflict with the commitment to do what is best for each patient" ([14], p. xii). Thus, the appropriate time for trade-offs is when decisions are made about construction of facilities, authorization of new techniques, training of personnel, and setting standards and procedures. The general approach suggested by Mechanic is similar: "Constraints can be provided in a general way by

putting limits on total expenditures but allowing physicians and patients
to negotiate the detailed priorities and decisions required" ([27], p. 730)
(*cf.* hospital 'global' budget, Medical Research Council annual budget,
etc.). "Alternatively, government or other planning bodies could develop detailed guidelines and regulations that mandate priorities, that
spell out contingencies and that limit professional discretion. Such rules
might prescribe what equipment can be acquired, what procedures can
be used under various circumstances, and ranges of permissible treatments for specified disorders" ([27], p. 730). A current example of
implementation of this approach is the specification of a maternal age
range for amniocentesis for fetal chromosome examination.

CONCLUSION

The aggressive medical treatment of extremely premature babies has
pushed the limit of human viability downward to unprecedented levels.
Although neonatal intensive care is effective in reducing the mortality
rate, it is doubtful that the rate of handicap among survivors has been
much affected. Thus, it is probable that in absolute terms an increased
number of handicapped individuals is being introduced into society as a
consequence of the intensive care of babies born at the threshold of
viability.

Neonatal intensive care is expensive and long-term costs for the care
of handicapped survivors are very great also. An economic evaluation
investigates the relative costs and benefits of strategies in health care by
valuing the resources used and weighing them against the value of the
outcomes. The techniques of economic evaluation have been applied to
intensive care of very low birth-weight infants. By every measure of
economic evaluation, the impact of neonatal intensive care has been
more favorable among infants weighing 1000 to 1499g than among those
weighing 500 to 999g at birth. In comparison to other health care
programs whose cost-utility ratio has been evaluated, neonatal intensive
care of infants 1000 to 1499g is already very favorably placed; under
1000g birth-weight, the cost-utility of intensive care is not yet as encouraging.

A number of unresolved moral and philosophical questions resulting
from these observations are raised for discussion. In evaluating health
care programs, whose health-state preferences should count? In applying the results of such evaluation to decisions about the spending of

scarce resources, can rationing of health care be morally justified? Can rationing decisions be equitable? Who should make them, and when is the appropriate time to apply them?

McMaster University
Hamilton, Ontario, Canada

NOTES

[1] For a discussion of the concept and rationale of discounting, see [46].
[2] This is not to say that neonatal care would lose out when compared with intensive care of adults. In fact, the reverse is probably true: cost-effectiveness of neonatal intensive care appears to be much more favorable than intensive care of critically ill adults [10].

BIBLIOGRAPHY

1. Advisory Committee on Reproductive Medical Care to the Minister of Health for Ontario: 1979, *A Regionalized System for Reproductive Medical Care in Ontario*, Ontario Ministry of Health, Toronto.
2. Akehurst, R. L. and Holtermann, S.: 1979, 'Application of Cost-benefit Analysis to Programmes for the Prevention of Mental Handicap', *Excerpta Medica* (Ciba Foundation Symposium 59 (new series)), 173–191.
3. Boyle, M. H. *et al.*: 1982, 'A Cost Analysis of Providing Neonatal Intensive Care to 500–1499 Gram Birth-weight Infants', *Research Report No. 51*, Program for Quantitative Studies in Economics and Population, Faculty of Social Sciences, McMaster University, Hamilton, Ontario.
4. Boyle, M. H. *et al.*: 1983, 'Economic Evaluation of Neonatal Intensive Care of Very-low-birth-weight Infants', *New England Journal of Medicine* **308**, 1330–1337.
5. Budin, P.: 1907, *The Nursling*, Caxton Publishing Co., New York.
6. Bush, J. W., Chen, M., and Patrick, D. L.: 1973, 'Cost-effectiveness Using a Health Status Index: Analysis of the New York State PKU Screening Program', in R. Berg (ed.), *Health Status Indexes*, Hospital Research and Educational Trust, Chicago, pp. 172–208.
7. Bush, J. W., Fanshel, S., and Chen, M.: 1972, 'Analysis of a Tuberculin Testing Program Using a Health Status Index', *Socio-Economic Planning Sciences* **6**, 49–69.
8. Butterfield, L. J.: 1977, 'Organization of Regional Perinatal Programs', *Seminar in Perinatology* **1**, 217–233.
9. Churchill, D. N., Lemon, B., and Torrance, G. W.: 1983, 'Cost-effectiveness Analysis Comparing Continuous Ambulatory Peritoneal Dialysis to Hospital Hemodialysis' (abstract), *Medical Decison Making* **3**, 355.
10. Cullen, D. J. *et al.*: 1984, 'Results, Charges and Benefits of Intensive Care For Critically Ill Patients: Update 1983', *Critical Care Medicine* **12**, 102–106.
11. Culyer, A. J.: 1983, 'Effectiveness and Efficiency of Health Services', *Effective Health Care* **1**, 7–9.
12. Dale, A. and Stanley, F. J.: 1980, 'An Epidemiological Study of Cerebral Palsy in

Western Australia, 1956–75. II. Spastic Cerebral Palsy and Perinatal Factors', *Developmental Medicine and Child Neurology* **22**, 13–25.

13. Epstein, K. A. *et al.*: 1981, 'The "Abnormal" Screening of Serum Thyroxine (T_4): Analysis of Physician Response, Outcome, Cost and Health Effectiveness', *Journal of Chronic Diseases* **134**, 175–190.

14. Fuchs, V. R.: 1982, 'Foreword', in K. E. Warner and B. R. Luce, *Cost-Benefit and Cost-Effectiveness Analysis in Health Care*, Health Administration Press, Ann Arbor, Michigan, pp. x–xii.

15. Hack, M., Fanaroff, A. A., and Merkatz, I. R.: 1979, 'The Low-Birth-Weight-Infant – Evolution of a Changing Outlook', *New England Journal of Medicine* **301**, 1162–1165.

16. Hagberg, B.: 1979, 'Epidemiological and Preventive Aspects of Cerebral Palsy and Severe Mental Retardation in Sweden', *European Journal of Pediatrics* **130**, 71–78.

17. Hagberg, B., Hagberg, G., and Olow, I.: 1975, 'The Changing Panorama of Cerebral Palsy in Sweden 1954–1970. I. Analysis of the General Changes', *Acta Paediatrica Scandinavica* **64**, 187–192.

18. Hagberg, B., Haberg, G., and Olow, I.: 1982, 'Gains and Hazards of Intensive Neonatal Care: An Analysis From Swedish Cerebral Palsy Epidemiology', *Developmental Medicine and Child Neurology* **24**, 13–19.

19. Hagberg, B., Olow, I., and Hagberg, G.: 1973, 'Decreasing Incidence of Low Birth Weight Diplegia – An Achievement of Modern Neonatal Care?' *Acta Paediatrica Scandinavica* **61**, 199–200.

20. Hein. H.: 1980, 'Evaluation of a Rural Perinatal Care System', *Pediatrics* **66**, 540–546.

21. Horwood, S. P. *et al.*: 1982, 'Mortality and Morbidity of 500 to 1499 Gram Birth Weight Infants Live-born to Residents of a Defined Geographic Region Before and After Neonatal Intensive Care', *Pediatrics* **69**, 613–620.

22. Kinsey, V.: 1956, 'Retrolental Fibroplasia: Cooperative Study of Retrolental Fibroplasia and the Use of Oxygen', *Archives of Ophthalmology* **56**, 481–543.

23. Klarman, H. E.: 1974, 'Application of Cost-benefit Analysis to the Health Services and the Special Care of Technologic Innovation', *International Journal of Health Services* **4**, 325–352.

24. Kleinman, J. C. *et al.*: 1978, 'A Comparison of 1960 and 1973–1974 Early Neonatal Mortality in Selected States', *American Journal of Epidemiology* **108**, 454–469.

25. Lee, K-S. *et al.*: 1980, 'Neonatal Mortality: An Analysis of the Recent Improvement in the United States', *American Journal of Public Health* **70**, 15–21.

26. McCarthy, J. T. *et al.*: 1981, 'Who Pays the Bill for Neonatal Intensive Care?', *Journal of Pediatrics* **95**, 755–762.

27. Mechanic, D.: 1982, 'Curing, Caring and Economics: Dilemmas of Progress', *Perspectives in Biology and Medicine* **25**, 722–735.

28. Pakter, J. and Nelson, F.: 1974, 'Factors in the Unprecedented Decline in Infant Mortality in New York City', *Bulletin of the New York Academy of Medicine* **50**, 839–868.

29. Paneth, N. *et al.*: 1982, 'Newborn Intensive Care and Neonatal Mortality in Low-Birth-Weight Infants', *New England Journal of Medicine* **307**, 149–155.

30. Phelps, D. L.: 1981, 'Retinopathy of Prematurity: An Estimate of Vision Loss in the United States – 1979', *Pediatrics* **67**, 924–926.

31. Phibbs, C. S., Williams, R. L., and Phibbs, R. H.: 1981, 'Newborn Risk Factors and Costs of Neonatal Intensive Care', *Pediatrics* **68**, 313–321.

32. Pomerance, J. J. *et al.*: 1978, 'Cost of Living for Infants Weighing 1000 Grams or Less at Birth', *Pediatrics* **61**, 908–910.

33. Sackett, D. L. and Torrance, G. W.: 1978, 'The Utility of Different Health States as Perceived by the General Public', *Journal of Chronic Diseases* **31**, 697–704.

34. Shapiro, S. *et al.*: 1980, 'Relevance of Correlates of Infant Deaths for Significant Morbidity at 1 Year of Age', *American Journal of Obstetrics and Gynecology* **136**, 363–373.

35. Shepard, D. S. and Thompson, M. S.: 1979, 'First Principles of Cost-Effectiveness Analysis in Health', *Public Health Report* **94**, 535–543.

36. Silverman, W. A., Fertig, J. W., and Berger, A. P.: 1958, 'The Influence of the Thermal Environment on the Survival of Newly Born Infants', *Pediatrics* **22**, 876–886.

37. Stanley, F. J.: 1979, 'An Epidemiological Study of Cerebral Palsy in Western Australia, 1956–75. I. Changes in Total Incidence of Cerebral Palsy and Associated Factors', *Developmental Medicine and Child Neurology* **21**, 701–713.

38. Stason, W. B. and Weinstein, M. C.: 1977, 'Allocation of Resources to Manage Hypertension', *New England Journal of Medicine* **296**, 732–739.

39. Steiner, E. S., Sanders, E. M., and Phillips, E. C. K.: 1980, 'Very Low Birth Weight Children at School Age: Comparison of Neonatal Management Methods', *British Medical Journal* **281**, 1237–1240.

40. Torrance, G. W., Boyle, M. H., and Horwood, S. P.: 1982, 'Application of Multi-attribute Utility Theory to Measure Social Preferences for Health States', *Operations Research* **30**, 1043–1069.

41. Torrance, G. W., Thomas, W. H., and Sackett, D. L.: 1972, 'A Utility Maximization Model for Evaluation of Health Care Programs', *Health Service Research* **7**, 118–133.

42. Torrance, G. W. and Zipursky, A.: 1977, 'Cost-effectiveness Analysis of Treatment with Anti-D', Working paper presented at the Rh prevention conference, McMaster University, Hamilton, Ontario, Sept. 28–30.

43. Torrance, G. W. and Zipursky, A.: 1984, 'Cost-effectiveness of Antepartum Prevention of Rh Immunization', *Clinics in Perinatology* **12** (2), 267–281.

44. Toulmin, S.: 1982, 'How Medicine Saved the Life of Ethics', *Perspectives in Biology and Medicine* **25**, 736–750.

45. Usher, R.: 1977, 'Changing Mortality Rates with Perinatal Intensive Care and Regionalization', *Seminar in Perinatology* **1**, 309–319.

46. Warner, K. E. and Luce, B. R.: 1982, *Cost-benefit and Cost-effectiveness Analysis in Health Care: Principle, Practice, and Potential*, Health Adminsitration Press, Ann Arbor, Michigan, p. 93 ff.

47. Weinstein, M. C.: 1980, 'Estrogen Use in Post-menopausal Women – Costs, Risks and Benefits', *New England Journal of Medicine* **303**, 308–316.

48. Weinstein, M. C.: 1981, 'Economic Assessments of Medical Practices and Technologies', *Medical Decision Making* **1**, 309–330.

49. Weinstein, M. C. and Stason, W. B.: 1977, 'Foundations of Cost-effectiveness Analysis for Health and Medical Practices', *New England Journal of Medicine* **296**, 716–21.

RICHARD B. BRANDT

PUBLIC POLICY AND LIFE AND DEATH DECISIONS
REGARDING DEFECTIVE NEWBORNS

Decisions about the use of surgery and/or life-support systems for prolonging or improving the lives of defective newborns are normally made by the parents in consultation with the attending physicians, sometimes after consultation with a hospital ethics committee. Decisions, however, are subject to certain legal restrictions, partly embodied in criminal law, partly by court power to appoint a guardian *ad litem* to make a decision in the place of the parents, and partly by regulations of the Department of Health and Human Services laying down requirements for hospitals receiving federal funds. Juvenile courts and child protection agencies directly or indirectly play a role. In what follows I wish to consider what, from a moral point of view, such laws and policies should be.

When I say I wish to consider what these policies should be, from a moral point of view, you will at once want to know on which general moral principles I am going to rely and why. I shall respond to this query at once, but shall not attempt to defend my answer here, except for brief remarks near the end of this paper. First, then, I affirm that a policy is justified from a moral point of view if and only if it is one which factually informed, rational, and otherwise normal persons would *want* for a society in which they expected to live a lifetime. This statement does not tell us anything about which policies such persons might want, however. So I shall affirm, second, that the policies such persons would want are those which, when adopted by the appropriate agencies of society, would be most beneficial for society in the long run. This second statement is somewhat vague as formulated. For instance, what counts as being 'beneficial'? I shall spell this concept out more fully as we go along.

First of all, I want to state what is a legal fact, at least in most states, which bears on the issue we are concerned with, and I shall explain why I think it is right that this legal fact exists. This legal fact is that in many

R. C. McMillan, H. T. Engelhardt, Jr., and S. F. Spicker (eds.),
Euthanasia and the Newborn, 191–208.
© 1987 *by D. Reidel Publishing Company.*

191

states, certainly in the states of Michigan, Wisconsin, and Minnesota, parents, at the time they would normally take their infant home from the hospital, *or later*, can go into juvenile court and sign papers waiving their parental rights, turning the child over to the state. Child protection agencies are then given custody of the child, and arrange for adoption or placement in a foster or group home, or institution. In some states parents are liable for the costs of their infant unless or until an adoption is arranged for, or unless the court finds them incapable of financial support. But in Michigan and Minnesota, for example, in practice no attempt is made to collect costs from the parents. Parents, at least in Michigan, are not required to give a *reason* for the state to take over if the parents declare that they do not want their child.

Is it good to have this legal 'out' for the parent? I believe it is. The state can mandate provision of food, shelter, and medical care, or the cost thereof, but it cannot mandate love or psychological support. The state cannot even manage to collect for support in many cases – for example, if the mother is an unwed teenager. So, from the point of view of the welfare of children, it seems best for the state to stand ready to take over and it ought to do so.

This conclusion may be questioned. The immediate response of many to the question whether parents must be responsible for (and also have decision rights over) the care of their child is: "Of course, the parents have the responsibility for the infant. It's theirs, isn't it? Didn't they produce it?"[1]

This response may reflect the influence of traditional tort law on our thinking. In tort law, the cost of an accident falls on the victim. If I fall downstairs and am confined to a wheelchair thereafter, that is my problem (unless I have accident insurance). Certainly it is not anyone else's problem, unless the loss was caused by the negligence of someone else. The same with the defective baby: the loss is on the parents, unless the defect was a result of, say, the fault of the manufacturer of some food or medicine. So we tend to think. But there is another way of looking at the matter. Workmen's compensation laws call for payment for injury on the job, irrespective of fault. The same is true for no-fault automobile insurance. In New Zealand there is social insurance for all accidents. So, in view of the fact that a defective child may result from an activity of which society approves – that of having a family and rearing the next generation – and in view of the fact that there was no negligence on the parents' part, it would be in accord with present trends that the *state* provide for the care of a defective infant. This would certainly be true if it *mandated* that the infant be given aggressive hospital treatment so that its life be saved.

AN APPRAISAL OF REGULATIONS ON LIFE-SUSTAINING TREATMENT

Let us now consider the main question: What should public policy mandate about life-sustaining treatment for defective newborns, in which types of cases should there be discretion about treatment, and in whom should the discretion be vested? We are, of course, not interested in what the present public policy is, but what it should be, from the point of view of morality.

Some think the issue is settled by the alleged fact that every infant has a *right* to life. Some may think there is a legal right to life, which requires life-sustaining treatment in all cases. And, of course, there is if legislatures mandate it. There is, however, no such *constitutional* right; the Fourteenth Amendment says that a state may not deny equal protection of the laws. Hence you might say the Constitution demands that states that prohibit killing adults must also prohibit killing defective infants. True, but the Constitution does not demand the provision of all possible medical technology for saving anybody's life. In any case, we are concerned with whether infants have a *moral* right to life. Do all infants, defective to whatever degree, have a *moral* right to life-sustaining treatment? One writer answers by saying, "Simply because of his or her humanity, every human being is a person possessing rights. The right to life is the most basic and paramount of all" ([13], p. 248). But here we should be careful not to make what I think is a philosophical mistake. For when someone says that something should be done for an infant because the infant has a moral right, he seems to overlook the fact that what it *means* to say that someone has a certain moral right is to say, no more and no less, that some or all people have certain moral obligations with respect to the person said to have the right. In other words, to say that a person has a certain right is the same thing as to say that it is wrong to treat him, or fail to treat him, in certain ways. So, if there is doubt whether a person can morally be treated in a certain way, it is no answer to say that he has a certain corresponding right; for insofar as there is doubt whether he ought to be treated in a certain way, there is equal doubt about whether he has a right, or what is the scope of the right. So an attempt to resolve the question how infants or fetuses should be treated by discussing the question whether infants and fetuses have a right to life is essentially confused.

Some philosophers say that a fetus has a moral right to life if it is a *human being*, others that it has such a right only if it is a *person*, and give explanations of what it is to be a person: a person must have a self-consciousness, a sense of past and future, a capacity for making plans and having desires, and so on. All of this discussion is irrelevant. The basic question is whether it is wrong to kill or withhold life-supporting treatment from a fetus or newborn whose mental state, or prospective mental state, is such and such, and all the discussion about who has rights and what exactly they are is only a detour which brings us around to the very same questions with which we started, none the wiser for the detour.

So let us directly approach the question whether, from a moral point of view, regulations should mandate life-sustaining treatment for defective newborns. It will be helpful to approach the question by examining the recent conclusions of the President's Commission. Three points are made: First, the decision must ignore "negative effects of an impaired child's life on other persons, including parents, siblings, and society" ([14], p. 218); Second, prospective handicaps should lead to a negative decision

only when they are so severe that continued existence would not be a net benefit to the infant. . . . Net benefit is absent only if the burdens imposed on the patient by the disability or its treatment would lead a competent decision maker to choose to forego the treatment . . . . For many adults, life with severe physical or mental handicap would seem so burdensome as to offer no benefits . . . . From the perspective of an infant, who can be helped to develop realistic goals and satisfactions, such frustrations need not occur ([14], pp. 218–219).

Third, within these restrictions a decision about life-sustaining supports is to be made by the parents and physicians if they agree, and by a hospital board or court if they do not.

Let us begin with the first proposal: that the prospective costs, however great, to the family and society should be *altogether* ignored. Taken literally, this proposal cannot be right. We do not use such standards elsewhere. One estimate of U.S. Army Policy in saving lives by providing artillery and other support concludes that the policy implies that the Army regards the life of an average private to be worth about $250,000. In a suit for negligent killing, courts gauge the worth of a life in terms of the lifetime earning power of the decedent. Extra wages demanded by workers in high-risk occupations work out to a much smaller estimate of the value of a life. Moreover, we could build ships that are virtually unsinkable in a storm, but it would be uneconomical to do so. We could build only homes that provide some protection in case of a tornado, but we do not do so because of the added expense. So we normally do take into account the impact on others in deciding whether to take steps to save lives. Why should the President's Commission think not in the treatment of defective newborns? It offers no argument.

People who agree with the Commission may think of human life as being something different from what, in fact, it is. As far as I can see, human life, or what is worthwhile about human life, is a succession of *experiences* (associated with the body), many of which can be remembered later, and some of which are anticipated, planned and desired in advance. Let us say, then, that life is essentially a connected stream of experiences. When we sustain a life, we prolong that stream of experiences. When we fail to sustain it, the result is an earlier termination of the stream. It is not as if we destroy an immortal soul; if we have an immortal soul it cannot be destroyed. Some writers speak of human life as being 'sacred'. But we ourselves – and we cannot be accused of selfishness in our own case – set a *finite value* on the worth of continuing *our own* stream of experiences; we would not want to prolong our own experiences at the cost of bankrupting our children, especially if we thought the stream would not be very good (for instance, if we anticipated having to spend the final year of life in bed, unable to do any creative work).

But, if the President's Commission is wrong in thinking the unfavorable impact on others should be ignored, what kind of trade-off should we acknowledge? The utilitarian would want a plan maximizing the welfare of human beings whoever they are, and at whatever stage of life. So he would say that if the lifelong care of a defective newborn would cost $1,000,000, we should proceed to spend the money that way, if we had to choose, only if the money could not be spent to produce a better life stream of experiences elsewhere (for example, by providing better education for children who could benefit). We must be careful here, for one of the values we do not want to lose is that of general caring for others, and especially for children; we want to avoid thinking of their lives in monetary terms. Perhaps it is therefore better, if we are thinking how to compare the benefits of life-sustaining treatment for defective newborns with costs elsewhere, to think of the impact on the infant's family. What are these? If the family is not well insured, the costs of surgery and continuing care may mean that the life of the family is lived at a spartan level for many years. The siblings of the defective child may have to be deprived of a college education. There are, moreover, serious disruptions in the family. The life of the parents may come to revolve in a small circle around the child. The family may feel unable to have a social life because it is uncomfortable to have guests to a meal, given the unpredictable behavior of the defective family member. One could go on, but surely the continued presence of the child may well reduce dramatically the quality of life of the family. Of course, sometimes the opposite will be the case: the needs of the defective child may serve to unify the family. What I propose is that a satisfactory policy will take into account *both* the total prospective benefit to the infant and the total loss to the family, and will maximize net benefit, doubtless giving the benefit of aggressive treatment to the child if the divergence is not large.

There is another way of thinking of matters, which I owe to Derek Parfit (which he presented at a lecture at Oxford), which highlights the fact that if the life of a defective infant is not sustained, the parents may feel able to replace it by a normal child. The reasoning follows.

Suppose a woman wants a child, but is told that if she conceives a child now it will be defective, whereas if she waits three months she will produce a normal child. Obviously we think she should delay. Of course, if she delays, she will not have the *same* child as the one she would have had if she had not delayed; but we do not think we need worry about any rights of the child she might have had.

Suppose, however, a woman conceives but discovers, five months later after amniocentesis, that the fetus will develop into a defective child. Furthermore, the probability is good that she can have a normal child later if she has an abortion and tries again. Now this time there is still the same reason for having the abortion that there was formerly for the delay: that she will produce another child with a better life. Ought she not have the abortion? If the quality of the child's life is poor, he could well complain that he was injured by being brought to term, and in fact, some court suits along this line have actually been filed. I believe that the vast majority of persons would think this woman should have an abortion. The reason amniocentesis is becoming so frequent is that many women fear there may be congenital defects.

Now suppose a woman cannot discover until after birth that her child is seriously defective. She learns then that, were she to conceive again, it is highly probable that she would have a normal child. Are things really different from the previous cases during the first few days? One might think that a rational person would want, in each of these cases, the substitution of a normal child for a defective one, of a better life for a worse one.

So, it seems, in deciding what should be done about sustaining the life of a defective newborn, we have to compare not only the good of its life with the possible harm done to other family members (and society), but also with the better life that could be lived by a child which might be born to take its place. Why is not all of this relevant?

So much for the Commission's first contention that costs be wholly ignored. That brings us to the second one: that a life should be sustained if there will (probably) be net benefit to the infant over its lifetime, taking the point of view of the aspirations, etc., of the infant.

How is one to decide whether a life is worthwhile from the individual's point of view? The Commission mentions pain and frustration as negative weights; if a life were nothing but these, with no countervailing benefits, it would overall be bad. How might we decide whether it is good or bad *for* the infant? One way of deciding is this (and possibly this is what the Commission had in mind): Suppose we draw a curve corresponding to a person's lifetime, points below the curve representing experiences *disliked* at the time, the distance below the x-axis being fixed by how strongly the person disliked the experience at the time.[2] (Positions on the x-axis represent successive moments of experience during the individual's life.) Then we could also draw points above the line, representing how strongly the individual liked the experience he was having at the moment, the distance from the x-axis representing how strongly the individual liked his experience at the time. Now we can draw a curve connecting these sets of points and ideally compute the area between the curves and the x-axis. If the area above the line exceeds that below the line, then life has a net benefit for that person, the amount corresponding to the size of the area.

There is another way of estimating whether a life is good or bad for a person overall. We might say that a person's life is good overall if the individual, toward the end of it, could recall all of it vividly, and be glad that he had lived that life. *How* glad he is would presumably determine how worthwhile his life has been to him. One trouble with this proposal is that it seems impossible to recall a whole life vividly at one moment (not to mention the practical problem of predicting in advance how a person then would feel). And, even if a person does recall it to some extent, whether the picture attracts or repels may very well be subject to the mood of the moment: if he is happy the picture looks rosy, whereas if he is depressed the picture looks grey. Still, you might prefer this criterion for whether a life is worthwhile for a person since it is less hedonistic; it does not rate a life just by noting how enjoyable its successive moments were to the individual at the time.

Now if one of the foregoing is accepted as the criterion for a life better for a person than not, how do we apply it to the case of defective newborns? How do we decide whether a given newborn should be given treatment, in view of the prospective value of his life to him? If Dr. John Lorber's statistics [7, 8, 9] about spina bifida are right, we have some useful information to consider.[3] For then we know that probably, if the newborn has some observable symptoms, which Lorber enumerates, even if treated aggressively, it has a 60 percent chance of being dead within seven years and will probably have gross paralysis, some leg deformity, frequent bone fractures, incontinence of urine and feces, a marginally normal intelligence, and be repeatedly subject to further surgery if a shunt is required to relieve hydrocephaly. On this basis Lorber recommends selective treatment only for those infants without the symptoms he enumerates.

But the objective physical results likely for the infant are only part of what we should know to make decisions about treatment. What do they tell us about the worth of an individual's future life to him? Fractures, incontinence, and operations are misfortunes to which nearly everyone is subject at one time or another, and they are not devastating. If there is relatively continuous severe pain or frequent worry about early death, that is another matter. We must remember, however, what writers often seem to overlook: that we are talking of a whole life, during part of which a person will likely not have the psychological support of parents.

What strikes me as a very serious problem for the value of a life is the possibility of long stretches of unrelieved boredom or tedium when, during the day, one looks forward to nothing but going to sleep. It is true that low I.Q. and handicaps do not necessarily mean poor quality of life in adult years, at least not directly. But they do limit opportunities, and these opportunities may be important for making life worthwhile. What is needed in life to prevent unrelieved tedium? A. H. Maslow [10] has devised a list of human 'needs', which we might look at to assess a

defective newborn's prospects for a good life. Among the needs a
defective child will likely have difficulty with are activity, sex, love and
belongingness, esteem by others and self-esteem, understanding, and
what Maslow calls 'self-actualization' (development of one's own special
abilities). (It is interesting to note that apparently an animal does not
need much of some of these in order to feel cheerful.) J. Griffin, in a
forthcoming volume tentatively titled *Wellbeing*, lists the making of
autonomous choices, a sense of accomplishment, enjoyments, and deep
personal relations as important to a good quality of life. For a relatively
satisfying life, a human being seems to require, on the basis of my own
experience, interpersonal relations including friendly conversations,
projects of interest such as collecting stamps or solving complex problems, responsibilities with social pressure to discharge them, probably
some love relationships, and the ability to look forward to a few exciting
activities and experiences involving others. A report of the University of
Michigan Institute for Social Research roughly supports the foregoing
judgments. It concludes that

> Those people whose feelings of well-being are distinctly negative are all deprived of some
> critical element of their lives – social support, good health, employment, or status. . . .
> There are obviously many things people learn to do without, but for most people
> marriage, health, and work . . . are major contributors to a positive outlook on life ([3],
> p. 232).

Dr. Lorber tells us that among the total group of spina bifida patients
aggressively treated, only 10 percent can hold a job. (I do not know if
'sheltered shops' are available in England. Many Down's syndrome
children in this country are able to find life-long employment there.)
Most mentally defective children can watch television with enjoyment,
but it seems doubtful that a person can make much of a life out of this.
So for many defective newborns – we must remember that Lorber is
talking only of spina bifida children, not Down's syndrome, or any of
the myriad children who have suffered severe brain damage before or
after birth or had seriously premature births – there will probably be no
interesting job available to them, and hence no pressure to perform
tasks responsibly (but Down's children do seem intent on performing
simple manual tasks), very little activity, no sexual relations, relatively
low esteem by others and little basis for self-esteem, little prospect for
'understanding' if the person has a low level of intelligence, and little
that can be called 'self-actualization'. A seriously defective newborn

may enjoy plenty of love and support in his family during his early years, but as he and his parents grow older (and particularly after the death of his parents), he is apt to have little of this. It seems he will be able to have his physical needs satisfied, but will miss the major distinctively human goods.

There are qualifications to be added to this somewhat gloomy prognosis. First, there have been improvements in treatment and many of the children Lorber classified as hopeless would probably do much better at the present time. Second, many children who would have been regarded as hopeless cases now can be given training – say, with behavior-learning techniques – and learn to perform socially useful tasks and live in groups where there is some peer support. Third, the elimination of institutional care in favor of small foster or group homes is psychologically stimulating and provides social interaction. (Indeed, this may be much better than life in the child's own family where, despite professions of love and seeming concern, the child may be resented or even hated, and live an essentially isolated life.)

It seems to me that, as matters stand today, defective newborns fall into three main classes. First, some are so seriously defective that at best they will have a short and unpleasant life, despite anything medicine can do for them. It is a favor for them to allow an early death. Second, there are some whose lives will be only marginally beneficial to them, but at a high economic and/or psychological cost to others. The family should not be expected to bear the burden of providing this marginally valuable existence at great cost, and the infant should be aggressively treated only if society is prepared to pay what is necessary to provide a life that is reasonably worthwhile, given the child's potentialities. Third, there are those who have the capacity to survive and over the long term make a reasonably decent life for themselves, or even a normal life. These should, of course, be aggressively treated, and someone – family or society – should provide the necessities for them to develop their capacities and live good lives. Such children will presumably be acceptable for adoption if their parents do not wish to undertake care for them. There is, of course, a fourth class, that of children whose lives will be only marginally beneficial to them, but whose parents are willing to accept them as part of the family and whose condition is such that their presence will not be a significant burden to the family. Then, of course, aggressive treatment is indicated.

Unfortunately, while there will be many infants that clearly, on the day of birth, can be identified as belonging squarely in one of these classes, there will be many borderline cases. Of course, a decision need not be made on the day of birth; it can be delayed for months until the diagnosis and prognosis become clear (so long as it is not so delayed that the infant becomes aware of the situation and can begin to suffer from anxiety about what is going to happen, or that attachments with parents form, which are painful to break). It is manifest that it is psychologically important for all concerned that a decision whether to continue aggressive treatment be made as early as possible.

This brings us to our third problem: *Who* is to make the decision about continuation of aggressive treatment? What is needed is an individual or group acquainted with the exact symptoms of the child and prognosis for the child's future, indeed long-term future if the prognosis does not rule out the possibility of this. The chooser should also know the circumstances of the family, whether the presence of the infant will be a severe burden to them. The chooser should also know what kind of life the individual will have if he becomes a ward of the state – what kinds of care and education are available, whether all assistance will cease at age 26, and so on. Some writers have urged that society has a *duty* to provide care good enough to make life worthwhile for wards of the state, but unless and until that is done the chooser should bear in mind what kind of care will actually be furnished and what life will probably be like in that situation. The decision will be an especially difficult one if the infant can count on a marginally acceptable life if he is cared for in a family, where such care would be a heavy burden for the family, but a life on the whole not acceptable if he has to be a ward of the state.

Traditionally, the parents of the child have been recognized as having a decisive voice in such decisions, but unless the parents stand ready to accept the child into their family, it is far from obvious why they should have this traditional prerogative. On the other hand, it may be said that the parents, at least in consultation with the attending physician, are in a position to make the best decision from the point of view of the child; they may know more of the facts and will have the interest necessary for giving careful thought to the issue. But it is clear that the scope of their right to decide should be limited. On the one hand, they should not be free to sentence an infant to further suffering if the medical prognosis is such that further treatment would only prolong life briefly and be painful for the patient. On the other hand, they should not be free to mandate no aggressive treatment for a child whose defects are relatively minor and who, in the judgment of child care agencies, can be adopted.

Even with these restrictions, however, there is a question whether the parents and the physician are very well qualified to make decisions about continuing aggressive treatment. The physician may be a very busy person who has given relatively little thought to the issues involved – he may never have visited the state-provided foster homes or schools, and have no idea what is in store for a defective child who becomes a ward of the state. And, unless the parents are intelligent and well-educated, they will not be able to think through clearly what prolonged life would be like for their child, or what their own life would be like with such a child in their midst. Nor will they, normally, be familiar with the quality of state-provided facilities. They may be emotionally un-settled, subject to social pressures from friends or self-appointed ad-visers, and all too ready to rely on the advice of their physician.

What should be available for the decider to use is systematic statistical information along the lines Dr. Lorber provides, but brought up to date, improved and expanded to cover a wider range of defects. Ideally, the physician ought to be able to refer to the results of such statistical studies and say, "The medical profession, in view of the statistics about past cases, would recommend in this case that such-and-such be done." However, this kind of ideal situation does not yet obtain. Of course, if the child does not clearly fall in the first class identified above – of infants that in effect are already destined to an early death – and the parents wish to take the responsibility for the child themselves, there appears to be no real problem; the parents may decide they want to opt out later, but that seems to be a risk worth taking, everything con-sidered.

But if this is not the case, it appears we shall have to look to a hospital ethics committee for the decision for problematic cases. Such a com-mittee would presumably include the attending pediatrician and perhaps a second pediatrician, a neurologist, preferably a psychoneurologist, at least one social worker (who will be familiar with what is in store for the child if it becomes a ward of the state), a specialist in ethical decisions – preferably a philosopher attached to the medical staff, but possibly a specially trained clergyman provided his theological views do not com-mit him to advocating aggressive treatment for absolutely all infants because they are God's property, etc. – and perhaps a sensible layman. The members of such a committee must be sufficiently public-spirited to be willing to give thought to the problems. Such a committee seems to be the best solution for the decision problem at present and, incidentally, would provide a legal shield for the physician. It is not easy to see how it can be helpful to involve the courts; a judge would seem to be far worse qualified than a hospital ethics committee to make such decisions. If there is no standing ethics committee in a hospital, presumably it will always be possible to assemble an ad hoc committee that is willing to listen to the details of a single case.

How do the foregoing remarks differ from the recommendations of the President's Commission? (1) Most important, they permit taking into account not only the future 'net benefit' for the child, but also the total impact on everyone affected, including the family and society, bearing in mind the possibility of the parents' having a normal child in the future, if treatment of the present child is discontinued or the child is made a ward of the state. (2) They attempt to make a start at filling in the concept of 'net benefit' for the infant, conceived as stretching over a lifetime (consistently, I think, with what the Commission says), but developed along lines of widespread (but far from universal) thinking among moral philosophers. (3) They are somewhat more restrictive than the Commission about leaving decisions about treatment in the hands of the parents in consultation with the physician. The parents are not free to mandate continued aggressive treatment where this is medically contraindicated, or to forbid such treatment when the defects of an infant are relatively minor, and their authority lapses unless they are prepared to accept their infant at the end of the aggressive treatment. In problematic cases, unless the parents want aggressive treatment and are prepared to accept the child when it is ready to leave the hospital, the decision should be made by the hospital's ethics committee – ideally supported by generally accepted professional standards, somewhat along the lines of Dr. Lorber, but expanded to other types of problems and based on up-to-date statistics representing modern modes of treatment. The ethics committee would be free to mandate no further treatment in light of its judgment about the benefits to everyone concerned.

THE MORAL STATUS OF THE PROPOSAL

Since the foregoing proposal implies non-treatment for some infants, and is therefore a virtual sentence of death for them, it is sure to be

questioned by some. Not, perhaps, for those infants whose prognosis is
so poor that they are in effect already irremediably dying, or whose
future contains so much pain and is in any case almost certainly so short
that it would clearly be doing them no favor to prolong their existence.
But there will be a sizable group that parents and physician, or hospital
committee, will assign to the non-treatment group, either because of a
somewhat negative prospect for an acceptable life from the infant's own
point of view over the long term, or else a somewhat positive prospect
for the longer term conjoined with the near certainty of very heavy costs
to family or society.

This problem naturally leads us to look at general theories in normative ethics to see if there is any one with plausibility and that would
forbid this conclusion I have suggested. The conclusion suggested has
been selected to conform to what has historically been the most influential theory: a variant of a utilitarian test of public policies.[4] According to
the utilitarian thesis, a policy is morally justified if the total net benefit
of its adoption, direct or indirect, is greater than the total net benefit of
adoption of any other possible policy. The theory thus affirms that the
moral test of a policy is its maximizing the net long-term benefit over
everyone involved. Thus the theory directs that criminals should be
treated in a way not necessarily best just for *their* welfare, but in a way
best for the long-range benefit of everyone, criminals included. In our
case, the test is the maximal benefit of the whole society, not necessarily
the maximum benefit of the infant, although in most cases a policy
mandating the maximal net benefit for the infant will not diverge from
one aiming at the maximal net benefit of society.

Now suppose that my recommendation of a policy for not treating
some defective newborns is implied by this utilitarian theory. Would
that count as a serious recommendation? The present is not the place for
discussing the merits of the currently much-maligned utilitarian theory,
but I think this view is the one rational informed people would prefer to
support as a morality for their society, as contrasted with other normative theories or with no theory at all. If so, the fact that utilitarianism
calls for this policy is no mean point in its favor.

At the present time the chief *systematic* normative theory contrasting
with utilitarianism is that of John Rawls. This is not in respect of his
background theory – that an act is right if the principle involved is one
that would be chosen by rational persons behind a veil of ignorance – for
a defendant of utilitarianism might say that his principles, too, would be

so chosen.[5] But it is in respect of his positive normative principles, especially the so-called Difference Principle, that economic institutions should be arranged so as to favor the worst-off group (say by tax or welfare benefits) up to the point where further favoring would result, in the long run, in making them still worse off than they would otherwise be. This principle might seem to apply to our problem, since a handicapped child is very badly off. Should such children be given favored treatment up to the point where more benefits to them would in the long run be self-defeating? About this suggestion one can say that Rawls' theory is addressed to a very important but somewhat narrower range of problems having to do with the social and economical system and with people who are more or less normal and expected to live a full life. We can be sure that Rawls himself did not have this application in mind, and the difference between our problem and the problems he addresses is likely so great that difficulties would arise in an attempt to transpose his arguments, used to support his view for its intended domain, in support of some view for the problem we are considering.

Some critics of Kantian inclinations might assert that failing to treat defective newborns because of great psychological or economic costs to others is failing to treat them as ends in themselves. And it is true that the utilitarian proposes, if he advocates non-treatment in this situation, to make a newborn worse off than he otherwise could have been because of costs to others. But there is another side to matters. A newborn's family also consists of people, and if society imposes severe burdens on them for the sake of the newborn, is it not using *them* as means to *his* ends? It is not very clear to me what the Kantian principle implies to be done when the interests of parties are conflicting.

There are various philosophers who think we know that no one ought to kill innocent human beings, no matter what their life prospects are or what the cost to others will be, without their consent. This view derives mostly from the Christian tradition, but, when shaken loose from speculative theological underpinnings, its logical status appears to be no more than a basic intuition. It would take us far afield to inquire to what degree such intuitions should be taken seriously, but at least we can say they do not enjoy the status of being implicates of a well-worked-out system of metaethical and normative theory.

NON-TREATMENT VERSUS ACTIVE TERMINATION

Suppose it has been decided that the condition of a given newborn is such that it ought not to be treated, either for its own sake in that the quality of its life will be negative, or on account of the very great cost, psychological or economic, to others, with only a very marginally desirable existence for the infant. There is then a troubling problem: the infant may survive for a long time, gradually deteriorating to death, and its condition while alive will be worse if it is not aggressively treated, rather than if it is. Some, on this account, favor aggressive treatment of virtually all infants, even though they think it would be better if they would die quickly.

There is of course an alternative: what has been done with severely defective infants from earliest times – that they not be allowed to survive at all. The infant could be given a terminating anesthetic. Call it 'delayed abortion' or 'legal miscarriage' if you will. Such an idea seems hardhearted, but it is surely kinder than allowing slow deterioration until death arrives, with or without medications. It could be no worse for the infant than undergoing a general anesthetic, and it is better than a late abortion, which can be painful to the fetus. I concede that the idea of actively giving an infant a lethal anesthetic is somewhat horrifying, although, strangely, the idea of just letting it die miserably does not seem to bother people so much. What is done quietly and *sub rosa* we find easy to accept; it is a 'medical' decision.

Active termination by anesthetic is currently contrary to law. But the law about neonates, when compared with the law about abortions, seems very strange. For example, if a woman learns during the sixth month of pregnancy that the fetus will probably be born with defects, she is free to have an abortion. (Indeed, she is free to have an abortion for no reason at all.) Consider a woman who is a carrier of hemophilia. If she discovers by amniocentesis that her child will be male, then, although there is a 50 percent chance a male child will be normal, and given the fact that hemophiliacs sometimes have good lives anyway, she is not only free to have an abortion, but many people think it is her moral obligation to do so. As Peter Singer points out [12], it would be more rational to wait until after birth, when it can be definitely determined whether the infant is a hemophiliac, and then permit non-treatment or termination at that point. The mere timing of the termination of a life seems morally trivial, unless there were serious reasons to think that delayed decisions would undermine our social moral fabric and lead to the erection of gaschambers, as obviously it would not. There is nothing sacrosanct about birth as the time at which a child's legal right to life begins. The Supreme Court decided that 'state interest' in a child begins at the point at which it is viable – a decision that was largely arbitrary. There is no reason why the Court might not decide that the date of one month after birth is the time at which seriously defective infants acquire a legal right to life. This would be a more coherent policy than one vesting decision about abortion in the hands of the parents up until nearly the end of pregnancy, and vesting no power in the hands of parents, or parents in consultation with physicians and a hospital ethics board, to make the same terminating decision soon after birth, when there is much better evidence on which to base a decision.

Fortunately, there is hope that these problems may be partially resolved within the next few years, when better methods of prognosis through prenatal testing will enable physicians to identify fetuses with prospectively serious defects so that they can be aborted during early pregnancy. Such abortions, barring changes in the views of the Supreme Court, will be legal and accepted by the general public.

University of Michigan
Ann Arbor, Michigan, U.S.A.

NOTES

[1] This seems to be the view of Professor J. M. Gustafson [5].

[2] Identifying where these points should go is not theoretically easy, and involves the traditional philosophical problem of the measurement and interpersonal comparison of utilities. For recent discussions of this problem see [1], [2], [6], and [15].

[3] For some criticism, see [4].

[4] The utilitarian theory is accepted in the Report by a Working Party [11].

[5] John Harsanyi does, for example, see [6].

BIBLIOGRAPHY

1. Bergstrom, L.: 1982, 'Interpersonal Utility Comparisons', read at a conference in Vienna and available from the Department of Philosophy, University of Uppsala, Uppsala, Sweden.
2. Brandt, R. B.: 1979, *A Theory of the Good and the Right*, Clarendon Press, Oxford, United Kingdom, Ch. 13.

3. Campbell, A.: 1981, *The Sense of Well-Being in America,* McGraw-Hill, New York.
4. Freeman, J. M.: 1974, The Shortsighted Treatment of Myelomeningocele: A Long-Term Case Report', *Pediatrics* **53**, 311–313.
5. Gustafson, J. M.: 1973, 'Mongolism, Parental Desires, and the Right to Life', *Perspectives in Biology and Medicine* **16**, 529–557.
6. Harsanyi, J.: 1977, 'Morality and the Theory of Rational Behavior', *Social Research* **44**, 623–656.
7. Lorber, J.: 1971, 'Results of Treatment of Myelomeningocele', *Developmental Medicine and Child Neurology* **13**, 279–303.
8. Lorber, J.: 1973, 'Early Results of Selective Treatment of Spina Bifida Cystica', *British Medical Journal* **4**, 201–204.
9. Lorber, J.: 1974, 'Selective Treatment of Myelomeningocele', *Pediatrics* **53**, 307–308.
10. Maslow, A. H.: 1970, *Motivation and Personality,* 2nd ed., Harper & Row, New York.
11. Report by a Working Party: 1975, vol. I, 'Ethics of Selective Treatment of Spina Bifida', *The Lancet,* January 11, 1975, 85–88.
12. Singer, P.: 1979, *Practical Ethics,* Cambridge University Press, New York, pp. 136–138.
13. Trinkaus, W. R.: 1982, 'Decision Making for Newborns', in A. E. Doudera and J. D. Peters (eds.), *Legal and Ethical Aspects of Treating Critically and Terminally Ill Patients,* AUPHA Press, Ann Arbor, Michigan. (AUPHA Press now Health Administration Press, Washington, D.C.)
14. U.S. President's Commission for the Study of Ethical Problems in Medicine and Biomedical and Behavioral Research: 1983, *Deciding to Forego Life-Sustaining Treatment,* U.S. Government Printing Office, Washington, D.C.
15. Waldner, J.: 1972, 'The Empirical Meaningfulness of Interpersonal Utility Comparisons', *Journal of Philosophy* **69**, 87–103.

SECTION IV

RELIGIOUS AND MORAL ADMONITIONS IN THE CARE OF DEFECTIVE NEWBORNS

CHOOSING AMONG EVILS

The prospect of choosing among evils in any context is not attractive. The forbidding character of such choices seems especially acute in those situations in which the evils faced bear directly on the life of a wanted infant, born to parents benevolently disposed to it. Even anticipating the necessity of such choices tends to generate anxiety for the parents or others responsible to make this type of decision. Our moral training has directed us toward the good and away from evil. By instruction, example, and experience, we fashion concepts of good and evil. Normative judgments of right and wrong are similarly reached. The accent of our moral education points us toward the good and the right. The prospect of embodying the lesser evil in our moral character is discomforting at best ([22], p. 230).

With experience and maturity we discover that preferred goals and means of attaining them are not always available, that some situations force upon us choices that are not fully redeeming in the ways that we would prefer. Our deficiencies in moral training with regard to choices among evils are likely to leave us paralyzed in the face of the need to decide or act. Then, in a crisis of conscience, a choice is made, an action follows, and we may be morally apprehensive both about the intended end and the means by which it is sought. Rightly or wrongly we may feel guilty. But the encounter with guilt ought not to be dismissed lightly. For there are potential dangers in a too ready embrace of lesser evil. The temptation is to describe the lesser evil simply as a good. Doing so may enable us to avoid guilt but risks initiating a practice of self-deception with ominous, immoral potential ([22], p. 242, cf. [6]).

Some cases in neonatal medicine are of the variety in which seemingly only greater or lesser evils are within reach. The good that we wish is beyond our technico-medical grasp. The President's Commission for the Study of Ethical Problems in Medicine and Biomedical and Behavioral Research characterized these situations as 'ambiguous cases' (cf. [34]).

R. C. McMillan, H. T. Engelhardt, Jr., and S. F. Spicker (eds.),
Euthanasia and the Newborn, 211–231.
© *1987 by D. Reidel Publishing Company.*

Clearly beneficial therapies, to use the language of the Commission, are not available and an imminent death is not sure if certain interventions take place. In short, there is a factual uncertainty regarding prognosis, given the current state of therapeutics. The factual uncertainty can occasion a moral uncertainty with regard to the requirement of any or all supportive measures. Our hesitancy in the face of the unknown can turn into an inability to make the hard decision that is necessary. This sort of decisional inertia can compound the pain and suffering for the newborn and others committed to care.

Ethicists seem more troubled than physicians or parents by the necessity to select among evils. For example, John Lorber writes, "We must decide our priorities to ensure that, with all the intensive effort and good will, we shall not do more harm than good" ([28], p. 300). Similarly, Raymond S. Duff admits that in these sorts of cases there may be no single right choice, that dilemmas should be fully explored, and that the "least detrimental alternative" should be chosen ([9], p. 218). Lay people tend to be anguished about their choices but settle on what they think is 'best'. The justification, more often than not, is intuition or common sense. Ethicists tend to engage in an elaborate casuistry, defending a justifying exception to a strict rule or proposing a principle, like the principle of double effect, that absolves the agent of responsibility for the evil that results. The perfection or absoluteness sought by ethicists seems to be of less concern to others who may be more aware of the imperfection, waste, and disorder that nature can produce in reproduction. Compromise and balance, in these circumstances, are not vices.

Two cases will illustrate how choices among evils are, in fact, made in the routine practice of neonatology in a Level III intensive care nursery. However, prior to reviewing these cases, we should discuss briefly the concept of evil and the principle of beneficence. Unfortunately, a comprehensive review and analysis of the moral concepts and reasons invoked in justifying choices among evils are beyond the scope of the present assignment. Some of these concepts and arguments will be mentioned but not explicated or evaluated. In addition, I shall resist disclosing my bias about these matters until the concluding sections of the essay in which we shall consider if it can be morally licit to effect the deaths of certain infants in order to achieve the lesser evil.

EVIL AND BENEFICENCE

The concept of evil in philosophy and theology is heterogeneous and complex in character. Theology seems more concerned with evil since the integrity of certain doctrines of God is at stake. Theologians attempt to explain or reconcile claims of God's goodness and power with the experience of evil in creation. Not only are God's *attributes* of goodness and power called into question by the so-called 'problem of evil', but the *reality* of God, insofar as God is described in orthodox theology, is challenged.[1] Secular philosophical interest in evil is not prompted by a concern to explain or defend God's being or character. Rather, secular philosophy endeavors to give a 'natural' account of evil in terms of disvalue ([33], p. 420).

Evil is not easy to define satisfactorily. However, let us use the definition of evil by G. H. von Wright as our common understanding. Evil, according to von Wright, is "anything – be it institution, an act, a state of affairs or of character – which is harmful in that sense of 'harmful', which is the opposite of beneficial, *i.e.*, for that which is bad for the good of a being" ([45], p. 46). In other words, evil is a subcategory of harmful, and harmful is anything that affects the good of a being unfavorably or adversely. The 'good of a being' will not be specified here. Rather, let us assume that the good for humans is subject to diverse, reasonable understandings, none of which is so compelling as to establish it to the exclusion of other competing visions of the good. In short, the environment is that of a moral pluralism, and evil is that which unfavorably or adversely affects the good of a being as justifiably defined by that being, or, in the case of infants, as defined by that being's surrogate.

The forms of evil are usually classified in terms of the agency of their actualization. One form of evil is moral evil. Moral evil involves human agency. It is understood in relation to notions of human freedom and responsibility. It can refer to an evil intention with a bad effect, or it can refer to a bad intention alone without regard to consequences. Examples of moral evil include first degree murder, theft, and fraud. Another form is non-moral evil, evil that does not involve human agency. Some commentators refer to it as natural evil, but non-moral will be the preferred designation here. Examples of non-moral evil include pain and suffering in and of themselves, apart from considerations of their source. These harms, however, can proceed from human action or from nature. A person may be harmed in an assault by another person or by a disease. Or, said differently, non-moral evil may be the result of personal agency (moral evil) or non-personal agency (non-moral evil). Evil can be distinguished further in terms of genuine and *prima facie* evil, and intrinsic and instrumental evil. These additional distinctions contribute to a more robust understanding of evil but, for our purposes, they can be ignored.[2]

A final distinction regarding moral evil is, however, directly relevant to the present inquiry, for moral evil is of two types. One type of moral evil is that which is against autonomy (e.g., unjust imprisonment). A second type of moral evil is a harm to another that is intended by the agent without a violation of the autonomy of the injured. An example here would be the torturing of non-human animals. Whereas the first type of moral evil is against autonomy, the second type of moral evil comes in the course of acting on the principle of beneficence, the moral principle directly relevant to our topic.

The principle of beneficence contains two parts. The first part refers to the "duty to *confer* benefits and actively to prevent and remove harms" ([2], p. 148). The second part "requires balancing of benefits and harms" ([2], p. 149). The first part is a principle of positive beneficence. The second part is a version of the principle of utility. The second part of the general principle of beneficence, the warrant for balancing benefits and harms, takes recognition of the fact that the "moral life does not permit us simply to produce benefits and avoid harms, and thus a balancing principle is essential" for both consequentialist and deontological moral theories ([2], p. 159). Accordingly, benefits are balanced against harms, benefits are balanced against alternative benefits, and harms are balanced against alternative harms. Utility as a part of beneficence is concerned with the interest or good of the individual at issue. It does not warrant the sacrifice of the interests and rights of an individual in order to serve the interests of society as a whole because beneficence is only one of several principles (e.g., autonomy, justice) that guide moral conduct.

As might be expected, both parts of the principle of beneficence are subject to debate.[3] Several questions suggest the nature of this dispute: What counts as a benefit and harm? Whose values will determine the identification and ordering of benefits and harms? What are the limits to the duty of beneficence?[4] The unsettled answers to these and other questions regarding the principle of beneficence suggest the potential for conflicting judgments in situations in which beneficence is the operative moral action guide. The debate about paternalism in adult medicine illustrates the directions that these interpretive disagreements may follow. In neonatology, the prospect for dissent may be even more pronounced. One cannot, as in adult medicine, begin with a determination of the competency of the patient. If competent, the adult patient's wishes are followed. If incompetent, an appropriate surrogate is appointed who speaks on behalf of the patient until competency is regained. With newborn infants, however, conflict usually turns on disparate judgments of the child's best interests held by the infant's parents, physicians, or others. Parents and the infant's physicians bear role responsibilities for the infant. Their respective performances of their duties toward an infant under the warrant of the principle of beneficence can lead to differing interpretations and evaluations of the present and prospective evils for this infant and family. These are unfortunate, and tragic, confrontations, not because they are between people benevolently disposed to an infant, but because the choices open to them are among natural and/or moral evils ([30], p. 208). However, without a clear and compelling conception of the good that provides a basis upon which to select among evils, it is not easy to know better and worse choices or ways to choose. The best face that can be put upon these choices of a lesser evil is one that presents the choice as one of a greater good, realizing that 'good' is given an unusual meaning (cf. [32]).

Painful examples of such choices confront parents of infants born with serious physical and/or mental handicaps. The non-moral evils of pain and suffering for the infant[5] and the family and of costs to the family and society constrain one to choose among evils.

TWO CASES

Two possible cases will illustrate the tragic nature of these situations. An infant was born and placed for adoption. The adoption was anticipated, and an agency had arranged in advance to place the child with a couple who already had one child. Soon after taking the infant home a rash developed on its back. The rash was diagnosed as a common childhood infection that would resolve within a few days. Several days later the parents decided that the infant was too sleepy and lethargic for something more serious not to be involved. The next day the infant became cyanotic, was admitted to the hospital, placed on antibiotics, and monitored. A diagnosis of herpes encephalitis of unknown source was made. Seizures developed, the baby became apnic, bradycardic, and was electively intubated. The herpes infection spread to the central nervous system. No other organ systems became involved.

The adoptive parents were conscientious people who had become attached to this infant even though they had been with it for only a few days. They had planned for this infant, and considered themselves morally responsible for the infant even though the adoption had not become final.

The physicians advised the parents that the single anti-viral agent that could be used in treatment would decrease the chance of mortality but would not decrease the possible morbidity. The consensus judgment of the physicians was that with treatment the infant had a 50 percent chance of survival. Unfortunately, the infant also would have a reasonably certain prognosis of severe mental retardation with a possible I.Q. of less than 50. Institutionalization of the infant was considered probable because of anticipated continued seizures, spasticity, chronic pulmonary infections, and other complications. In short, nursing care of the infant, if it survived, probably would be beyond the capacities of the adoptive parents. The child that they had wanted might live but would not be a part of their family in the way that they had imagined.

These were warm, caring, attractive parents. They quickly won the admiration and sympathy of the physicians and nurses who cared for their infant. They were seen as kind and generous people who were being dealt with unfairly by a situation for which they were not responsible. The parents were faithful members of a Protestant church. Their pastor visited the baby. His counsel was sought by the parents with regard to the extent of treatment for their newly adopted child. The medical staff communicated to the parents a willingness to be less aggressive in their treatment of the infant. They were open to orchestrating their care in a way that would permit the infant's disease or some complication to cause its death. Doing so would spare the child a troubled life and spare the parents and sibling the burden of care. Of course, the intention behind this option was not explicitly stated to the parents but the other-regarding motive was clear to all concerned.

While the parents considered their options, full treatment was undertaken. With respect to the infant, the parents did not consider its continued life to have an absolute value. They did not accept the proposition that life in any condition is better than death. Neither did they accept the view that this infant had a justifiable claim upon their unlimited sacrifice. And, they were unable to see any of their options as good. In other words, the evils they faced clustered under the headings of morbidity and death. They had to decide whether a likely early death was more in the best interests of their infant than a longer, medically complicated life ending in a later death. Which would be the lesser evil, death or a life of limited capacity and pleasure?

The parents also considered the effect the life or death of this infant would have on their marriage and family. They were as committed to their natural child as they were to this adopted child. They were concerned about the possible emotional and financial costs associated with the infant's survival, and gradually came to realize their probable losses if the child lived or died. These were not wealthy people. Only the husband worked. He earned a liveable wage. They lived modestly but comfortably. Their lives were ordered, goal-oriented, religiously grounded, and committed to doing their best for their children. Making a rash judgment about the care of this baby was not in their character. They were conscientious people, consulting with the physicians and their pastor in order to decide what was best for the infant primarily and for themselves secondarily. For them, continued treatment of the baby was equivalent to the lesser evil. Their dreams for this newborn and their collective future were in conflict with the reality of the baby's problems.

The parents decided that treatment should proceed without reservation. All things considered, they decided that parenting carried no guarantees for good or evil. Their decision to adopt, in their judgment, carried a family commitment to not abandon an infant who had been abandoned once already. The possible burdens associated with the baby's survival were not unappreciated. To the contrary, they asked many questions of themselves and others. And, to their credit, they endeavored to consider the prospects, positive and negative, in as honest a fashion as they were able. In short, they took the duties of parenting seriously and accepted the risks associated with it. Thus, the decision was made to shoulder the burdens at present because, in their judgment, the desired continued life of this infant was a lesser evil than its immediate death. This assessment was linked to a pledge to do what they could to make the life of this infant as comfortable and pleasurable as they could, if it survived. If complications developed that were life-threatening at a later time they would have another opportunity to assess the evils. At that time death might be judged the lesser harm.

Let me add a footnote to this case study. The family was insured for hospital and physician expenses through the husband's employer. Unfortunately, however, the insurance would not cover the expenses of this baby because the adoption was not final. The hospital was sympathetic to their dilemma but maintained the demand that the parents were liable for the bills. The couple never refused the obligation, which grew rapidly in the intensive care unit. But despite their financial exposure they agreed that the lesser evil was treatment.

The second case is unlike the first with regard to the medical problems of the infant. It is like the first in that the parents exhibited an admirable conscientiousness in a distressing situation. The mother was in her early thirties. They had a daughter three years earlier. The current pregnancy was planned. They considered themselves faithful Roman Catholics, even though they did not conform to the official teaching of the church regarding the practice of contraception. Both parents were college educated, articulate, family- and career-oriented.

Their second pregnancy resulted in the birth of an infant with multiple anomalies. The urinary bladder was not enclosed within the body, the genitalia was ambiguous. There was a mild hydrocephalus, a missing sacrum, no anus, agenesis of the large bowel, and a meningocele at the base of the spine. The meningocele was large and growing larger. The baby's urine and stools were being excreted onto the exposed urinary bladder. There were no known defects of other organs.

This infant was extensively evaluated by the relevant specialists. The baby was found to be chromosomally male. The genitals were judged non-functional, however, and it was recommended that the infant be raised as a female, if it survived. Surgical responses to the anomalies were contemplated. A diverting colostomy to prevent the bowel from emptying onto the exposed bladder and efforts to enclose the bladder within the body could have been performed. The meningocele was unsightly. However, any surgery on the sack was considered more cosmetic than therapeutic. In addition, surgery on the meningocele was not expected to restore function to the baby's legs which had atrophied in utero. A shunt to relieve the mild hydrocephalus was not immediately needed.

The infant was placed on prophylactic antibiotics, given intravenous nutrition (feeding was difficult due to the abnormalities of the colon and excretion increased the risk of infection), and kept warm while the parents decided for or against the initiation of the possible surgeries. The parents were told that ostomy bags for urine and stools would decrease the risk of infection and would facilitate the nursing care of the baby. But, these procedures were not expected to affect the infant's quality of life. The physicians told the parents that the baby could be reasonably expected to experience mild to severe mental retardation, if it survived. Efforts to redirect the draining hydrocephalus would require shunts approximately every three months initially. Again these procedures were not anticipated to affect the ultimate prognosis for the infant other than to contribute to a decrease in the expansion of the meningocele. The baby was expected to be wheelchair-bound, develop severe scoliosis, and ultimately bed-bound if it survived. Almost by any measure, the prospects for this child were not attractive.

As before, the evils at issue are those that relate specifically to the infant primarily and family secondarily. It is difficult to define an infant's interests apart from or independently of its primary care providers. Nevertheless, such efforts to isolate the child for decision purposes are undertaken by parents and physicians. However, I am skeptical of the ability or wisdom of doing so. The relative evils for the child in this case are reasonably clear: the evil of death or the evil of a life with severe handicaps. The severity of the evil of a life with handicaps would be influenced significantly by the level and character of support available from the parents. Hence their attitudes, capabilities, and resources bear in an important way on the assessment of evils for the infant with respect to its continued life in their custody.

The treatment of infants with meningoceles has been debated in the medical literature, both on medical and moral grounds.[6] One of the several specialists consulting on this case considered the possible surgeries a legitimate option, but the strength of his commitment to this course was limited. The number, type, and severity of the anomalies were sufficient to cause the physicians not to recommend anything other than nursing care if they were asked for a recommendation.

Being Roman Catholic, it was presumed (more accurately, feared) that the parents would require that the surgeries be initiated. It was believed that the family's religious beliefs would commit them to a sanctity-of-life ethic that would consider the evil of a life with handicaps as less than the evil of death. This presumption was heightened when it was discovered that the infant's uncle was a priest in a local parish. After being presented with the diagnosis, options for intervention, and prognosis, the parents asked for time to consult with the uncle.

The parents were very concerned about the present and future pain and suffering of this child. They had planned for this to be their last pregnancy. The duties of parents to mantain and nurture their children were seen as duties under God. They did not wish to be unfaithful to their religious commitments. Neither did they wish to lessen whatever opportunity their baby might have. The burden of care and the likely effect this child would have on the family was not underestimated. Nevertheless, they reasoned that they would cope with the emotional and financial burden without limiting the opportunity of their first child. The focus was on the interests of the newborn alone, to the extent this was possible. Like the parents in the first case, this couple, in consultation with their ordained relative, were concerned about the best interests of this child insofar as those interests were defined in terms of the lesser evil.

To the surprise of the medical staff, the parents refused all surgery. They authorized nursing care only. Nutrition and warming were continued; antibiotics were stopped. Within a few days the infant died of electrolyte imbalance, even though efforts were made to correct it. The parents accepted the view that the multiple procedures offered to them would not be therapeutic. Rather, they would contribute to a prolonged pain and suffering for the infant not believed warranted. They used the language of Roman Catholic moral theology in their decision. They judged all interventions other than nursing care 'extraordinary'.[7] The possible manipulations were seen to impose a 'grave burden' upon their baby. As such the interventions were not obligatory. The baby was expected to die quickly, and this loss was already being mourned. They simply could not bear to impose on the baby the pain and suffering necessary to the purchase of a continued life. Thus, not only were the interventions judged extraordinary, there was not a proportionate reason to embark on such a course. They did not desire or intend the infant's death directly, though they understood death as the probable consequence of their decision. They intended to avoid for the infant the evil of compounded pain and suffering. Invoking a form of the principle of double effect, the parents reasoned that the evil of death was justifiable for proportionate reasons.[8] In short, their decision was believed to be, in the words of Richard McCormick, "the best possible service of all of the values in the tragic and difficult conflict" ([31], p. 46).

In these two cases the parents, in a deliberate manner, approached a decision with unavoidable non-moral evil consequences. Both sets of parents focused primarily on the best interests of their baby. To the extent possible, they tried to avoid a choice between their interests and the newborn's interests, or between the interests of another son or daughter and the interests of the infant in immediate peril. No interested party was valued higher than another. It could be claimed, however, that the critically ill infants, in fact, were of equal value with other family members only in some abstract sense of the term 'equal value'. The distinctions of value, it could be argued, are not desired or made by the parents. They are forced on the parents by the range of defects brought by nature. It is not unfair to choose the interests of one over the interests of another. To ignore the burden on others that the care of these sorts of infants brings is to diminish unfairly the value of the lives of others if their interests are sacrificed in the process. Parents who carefully weigh the well-being of other family members in making decisions regarding the care of defective newborns, so the argument would go, are as worthy of respect as those parents who withdraw from this sort of calculus.

In each case the parents weighed the evils of pain, suffering, and a life of handicap against the evil of death. The parents of the baby with herpes encephalitis judged death a greater evil. The parents of the baby with multiple anomalies judged treatment a greater evil. Their respective decisions were based on the particular circumstances of their child and the values, moral and non-moral, they held as a family. Some form of evil was inevitable, no matter how they chose. They sought actively to remove and prevent harms, and doing so required them to balance harm against harm or evil against evil. In short, they applied the principle of beneficence in their own ways.

Who can say that the choice of either set of parents involved the best choice among moral evils? These are the borders, gray zones, or margins, call them what you like, of the moral life where certainty is replaced by reasonableness. If these parents chose incorrectly, they have only committed a prima facie wrong, they chose an evil other than the lesser one. Their good-faith effort to choose the lesser evil, and in that sense to do the right thing, properly can be analyzed but, in my opinion, not blamed. If they did an evil, it was an evil incurred in the pursuit of a good and innocent of the more onerous evil of violating a person's autonomy. The moral path is not always clear. And, in a context of moral pluralism, one ordering of evils may be no more compelling than a rival ordering. The parents of the child with multiple anomalies did not wish death for their child. Neither did they wish the life that was projected. But in order to avoid or prevent the evil to the child of continued existence, the parents did not seek actively or directly to terminate the infant's life. They were content to let the baby die from its diseases, to let 'nature take its course'. The question that we consider next is whether parents or someone else can effect the death of a similarly situated newborn infant as a licit choice among evils.[9]

SELECTIVE INFANTICIDE: A LESSER EVIL?

As suggested, the controversy regarding a choice among evils is not limited to concerns for the identification, ordering, and balancing of evils as these affect decisions to intervene or not to intervene. The so-called 'Baby Doe Rules' are visible evidence of this form of the controversy [34]. A second form of the controversy related to the management of defective newborns concerns the practice of 'beneficent euthanasia' (cf. [24, 25]). Can death by human hand be a lesser evil than a prolonged, painful dying in nature's time?

Hints of the connection of this question to the whole issue of selective treatment is found in the literature on the care of newborns with spina bifida. Clearly John Freeman, an advocate of full treatment, sees the link. Freeman writes,

Is it moral to encourage the survival of a child who will be a paraplegic, incontinent, and will require multiple surgical procedures for hydrocephalus, orthopedic deformity, and bladder dysfunction? . . . If we elect *not* to treat a child, what becomes of him? Is he to be fed and watered while the physician waits for him to develop meningitis? Is he to be sedated and fed inadequately so that he dies slowly of starvation without making too much noise? Or are we to kill him overtly? Or covertly? Actively rather than passively? ([18], p. 14)

Later in the same article Freeman admits "active euthanasia might be the most humane course for the *most severely* affected infants, but it is illegal. 'Passive euthanasia' is legal, but is hardly humane." He continues in conclusion that, "until active euthanasia for the most severely affected children becomes acceptable to society, we must opt for vigorous treatment, to make these children and their families as intact as we are able" ([18], p. 21).

John Lorber, an advocate of selective treatment, similarly sees the relation. Lorber writes, "The main object of selection is not to avoid treating those who would die early in spite of treatment, but to avoid treating those who would survive with severe handicaps" [27]. He considers selective treatment not a 'good solution', merely a 'least bad solution' to what he characterizes as a 'desperate, insoluble problem'. With regard to euthanasia, Lorber says, "I wholly disagree with euthanasia. Though it is fully logical, and in expert and conscientious hands it could be the most humane way of dealing with such a situation, legalizing euthanasia would be a most dangerous weapon in the hands of the state or ignorant or unscrupulous individuals" ([26], p. 204).

Another approach to the issue of killing severely defective newborns is by extension of the logic in favor of abortion. Here the concern is to establish the moral significance of the birth canal. Why is the abortion of a defective fetus licit and killing a similarly affected newborn not? In short, what is the status of a fetus and newborn? Michael Tooley has considered this question at length. His general conclusion is that

new-born humans [even normal ones] are neither persons nor even quasi-persons, and their destruction is in no way instrinsically wrong. At about the age of three months, however, they probably acquire properties that are morally significant, and that make it to some extent intrinsically wrong to destroy them. As they develop further, their destruction becomes more and more seriously wrong, until eventually it is comparable in seriousness to the destruction of a normal adult human being ([43], pp. 411–412).

Further, and perhaps equally challenging, Tooley dismisses species membership as a morally significant factor in judgments about killing. He· sees the morality of abortion, infanticide, and killing nonhuman animals as interrelated.

Steering a course through the debate about the morality of killing severely defective newborns would require an extensive examination of relevant moral concepts as they are understood by proponents on both sides. Concepts like person, right to life, sanctity of life, quality of life, acting and refraining, and potentiality are debated vigorously. Though important to the question of choosing among evils, such an exposition is far beyond the limits of this paper.[10] Let us turn away from the valued discipline of metaethics to the front line of moral decision-making in neonatology.

Raymond Duff and A. G. M. Campbell confessed to the world that there are cases in which parents in agreement with physicians choose an earlier death for a defective newborn infant. They went on to express their belief that physicians 'deep down' believe that there are cases in which "death may be a prudent choice and achieving death (in fact, killing) a sorrowful and painful obligation." As if this admission and perception were not enough to send shock waves through medical and lay circles, they advocated a change in the law to permit selective euthanasia ([13], pp. 118–120). They criticized the prevalent disease-oriented philosophy to patient care that will not permit a patient to die if it can be prevented. Duff claims that the vested professional interest in disease or its care ought not to prevail. If it does, he fears that "a policy of coercive living through the application of medical technology may result" ([9], p. 218). In its stead, Duff and Campbell favor a person-oriented philosophy that intends the relief and freedom of the patient from pointless, dehumanizing treatment ([13], p. 120). Speaking alone, Duff allows that such an approach would permit death by active or passive means to escape an excessive and cruel disease or an oppressive, dehumanizing therapy. He observes that there may be no single right choice in these situations. Nevertheless, the dilemmas should be fully explored and the 'least detrimental alternative' should be chosen in each case ([9], p. 218). To our loss, we are not told how to know the 'least detrimental alternative'.

Duff and Campbell are not overly fearful of abuse if the law permitted selective euthanasia. The natural affection of parents and the supervision of physicians are believed competent safeguards. They believe that parents are responsible for wrestling with these choices. The agony and suffering associated with the decision should help to protect against abuse, especially when the decision is made and implemented openly. In their judgment society should intervene only if (1) harm is being done to someone, (2) a better alternative is available, and (3) if society will support those on whom it imposes an unwelcome choice. The people who are most involved with the infant – parents and physicians – should decide according to what they 'feel' is correct. They conclude: "In view of the complexities of human experience and human tragedy and the difficulties and conflicts in deciding the proper use of medical technology, this approach to the problem of life and death control seems to make sense" ([13], p. 121; cf. [10, 11, 12]).

The provocative suggestions of Duff and Campbell require greater scrutiny and elaboration before they can be judged adequate to warrant the changes in policy that they propose. Neither have they provided a sufficient moral justification for their various practices and proposals. Their views have not been mentioned as a model of moral argument.

Rather, they are meant to illustrate that lay people and medical professionals, as well as philosophers, take seriously the notion that hastening the deaths of certain infants is morally permissible. Reason, intuition, and common sense variously are called upon to advance the claim that selective killing can be a morally licit choice among evils.

Consider another type of case, that of a newborn with a severe dermatological disorder. A female infant was born to a woman in her early twenties. At delivery the baby did not require resuscitation but was taken to the intensive care unit immediately because of extensive excoriation of the skin over the forearms, hands, legs, and feet. Large blisters and additional excoriation were found on the buttocks. Other than the obvious skin disease the baby was found to be normal.

A diagnosis of epidermolysis bullosa dystrophica was made after seven days (the skin biopsy takes this long). The immediate problems were several: (1) continued excoriation and blister formation with bleeding accompanied any type of handling of the baby, (2) protein loss, blood loss, and fluid loss from the lesions were similar to that of a third degree burn, (3) infection, (4) lesions in the mouth prohibited oral feeding so nutrition also was a significant problem. Chronic problems associated with this diagnosis also are significant: (1) there is a constant need for careful handling of the baby, (2) bandages need to be changed several times each day, (3) medicated baths and special ointments are required, (4) constant abrasion and breakdown of the skin cause scar formation with fusion of the toes, fingers, and scaring deformities that result in loss of mobility.

The infant was placed in isolation and into an incubator to provide warmth. Intravenous fluids were begun. This was difficult since any kind of phlebotomy of IV insertion required more handling of the infant, therefore, more excoriation of the skin. The infant was given multiple transfusions of fresh frozen plasma and packed red blood cells.

The dermatology consultants recommended local skin care, analgesics, no vigorous resuscitative efforts, and no ventilatory support since this illness is so debilitating to the patient and his or her care-providers. The infant's skin condition progressed, spreading over previously unaffected portions of the body. Massive fluid losses and electrolyte losses continued. Infection became a problem. Antibiotics were given. The baby became anuric, developed hyperkalemia, renal failure, and died on the fifteenth day of life.

What should have been done? The considered judgment of all of the physicians was that there was nothing they can do to save the life of this baby. The nursing staff and family suffered during the course of treatment. They believed that the medical management of the baby was prolonging its life only to increase its pain. The parents had planned this pregnancy. They were not eager to see the baby die. At the same time they did not want it to continue in pain and suffering unnecessarily. Given these circumstances would 'selective euthanasia' have been morally permissible? Would it have been morally allowable to effect this infant's death by human agency without appeal to the concept of 'extraordinary care' or the principle of double effect? Does the principle of beneficence permit killing in this type of situation as a means to choose among evils?

There is a growing body of moral literature addressing these questions. Much of it is emotionally charged but some of it is cool, rational, and analytic.[11] Efforts are being made to refine the meaning of person, our understanding of the status of newborns (normal and/or defective), and the basis of our duties toward infants. One purpose of these inquiries is to sort out what we are obliged to do, what we are obliged not to do, and what is purely elective (i.e., not subject to strict prescription or proscription).

There is a tendency in these discussions to move away from species membership as a sufficient condition for moral standing and for being the subject of rights. Peter Singer comments:

The biological facts upon which the boundary of our species is drawn do not have moral significance. To give preference to the life of a being simply because it is a member of our [human] species would put us in the same position as racists who give preference to those who are members of their race. . . . [The life of a newborn is of] no greater value than the life of a nonhuman animal at a similar level of rationality, self-consciousness, awareness, capacity to feel, etc., . . . A week-old baby is not a rational and self-conscious being, and there are many nonhuman animals whose rationality, self-consciousness, awareness, capacity to feel, and so on, exceed that of a human baby a week, a month, or even a year old. If the fetus does not have the same claim to life as a person, it appears that the newborn baby does not either, and the life of a newborn baby is of less value than the life of a pig, a dog, or a chimpanzee ([41], pp. 76, 122–123).[12]

Engelhardt agrees that newborns are not persons, at least, in a 'strict sense' (self-conscious, rational, and self-determining) ([15], p. 184). They are persons in a 'social sense'. He writes:

others must act on their behalf and bear responsibility for them. They are, as it were, entities defined by their place in social roles (for example, mother-child, family-child) rather than beings that define themselves as persons, that is, in and through themselves. Young children live as persons in and through the care of those who are responsible for them, and those responsible for them exercise the children's rights on their behalf ([14], p. 183).

Accordingly, infants have a different value than comparable animals in Engelhardt's theory because they have a different "moral role within particular communities of persons". Imputing personhood to infants serves to establish general practices that "secure important goods and interests, including the development of kindly parental attitudes to children, concern and sympathy for the weak, and protection for persons in the strict sense when it is not clear that they are still alive" ([15], p. 190).

These views would seem to shed some light on what is morally permissible to do in cases relevantly similar to the newborn with epidermolysis bullosa dystrophica. Recall that no cure was available, that management of the infant was difficult and painful to the baby, and that its life expectancy was believed to be days. Would it not have been reasonable, merciful, and justifiable to have shortened the baby's dying by a direct action? Would not such an action be consistent with the principle of beneficence? Could not such an action represent a choice for a lesser evil? Is it morally justifiable to treat non-humans in pain more compassionately than we treat our own kind? If killing infants in this sort of condition is wrong, a moral evil, then is it justifiable or excusable?

In my judgment a choice among non-moral evils (pain, suffering, and death) is *not* a moral evil. This position deviates from the classic Roman Catholic doctrine of double effect. In the case of double effect, Roman Catholic moral theologians offer a way to choose among non-moral evils such that if properly made does not involve a moral evil. They hold that it is morally evil to intend, rather than simply foresee, the death of an individual. This is not my view. In cases like the one of epidermolysis bullosa dystrophica, one would not simply foresee that stopping treatment would lead to death, but that in addition it would be morally proper to hope that a quick death would ensue. And if death is judged the lesser evil that can be attained, then it would be morally proper to insure its actualization. I realize that this view is controversial, but the facts of certain conditions and the burden of moral decision making requires that this alternative be conscientiously considered.

CONCLUSION

No one disputes that treatment decisions for severely defective new-borns are hot-beds of medical, moral, and legal debate. Often the choice available to those individuals responsible for the care of these infants is limited to a choice among evils. No one is happy that only evil options are, at times, available. However, not to decide for or act in a manner that pursues the least evil results unnecessarily in a greater evil. Choosing among evils requires wisdom and courage.[13] We need wisdom properly to select among means and ends. We need courage to act on wise choices. When faced with situations that demand "sound and serene judgment regarding the conduct of life" ([3], p. 322), may we have the courage to 'sin boldly', if in fact we 'sin' at all.[14]

Institute of Religion and Baylor College of Medicine
Houston, Texas, U.S.A.

NOTES

[1] There are a great number of volumes and articles analyzing the nature of good and evil. Among the better scholarly analyses are works by John Hick [23], who employs a more traditional methodology, and David Griffin [19], who develops a theodicy methodologically based in process theology.

[2] See [19], p. 22f, for a more complete statement of these distinctions. In short, genuine evil is "anything, all things considered, without which the universe would have been better." *Prima facie* evil is "anything that may be judged evil at first glance, superficially, i.e., when considered from a partial perspective, and/or within a limited context". Intrinsic evil is that which is bad in itself, "apart from considerations of utility to some other being, or to a later moment in the life of the being in question." Something can be "instrumentally evil insofar as it is destructive of the potential intrinsic good of something else".

[3] For an extensive analysis of the principle of beneficence and its application to problems in bioethics, see [37].

[4] These and other questions are discussed in [37] and [2].

[5] It may be that infants do feel pain but are not developed enough to suffer. A judgment depends on how suffering is interpreted, see [4] and [36].

[6] See, for example, [17, 18, 26, 27, 28, and 29].

[7] See, [5], pp. 270–271.

[8] The principle of double effect is an effort to preserve the 'absolute' nature of moral rules by distinguishing evils that are intended from those that are not prevented or intended though foreseen. See, [5], pp. 272–274; [31] and accompanying chapters; [8], pp. 157–164; and [16]. The principle has four conditions: (1) The act itself must be good or morally indifferent. (2) Only the good effect can be intended. The evil effect is foreseen and allowed, not intended or sought. (3) The evil effect cannot be a means to the good end.

Put differently, the same action must lead to both effects. (4) There must be a proportionately grave reason for allowing the evil to occur.
[9] In addition to a consideration of the act itself, a comprehensive examination of this issue would include an analysis of the arguments regarding who might properly 'do the deed'. We cannot decide that question here.
[10] Many of the relevant concepts are discussed in [1, 14, 15, 21, 35, 38, 41, 42, 43, and 44].
[11] Among the more considered work is that by Michael Tooley [42, 43, 44], Peter Singer [41], H. Tristram Engelhardt, Jr. [14, 15], and Warren Reich and David Ost [35].
[12] Charles Hartshorne and Michael Tooley share this view. Cf. [20, 43].
[13] For discussions of courage and medicine, see [39] and [40].
[14] I address a broad range of moral questions in neonatology in a forthcoming volume [38].

BIBLIOGRAPHY

1. Bayles, M. D.: 1984, *Reproductive Ethics*, Prentice-Hall Inc., Englewood Cliffs, New Jersey.
2. Beauchamp, T. L. and Childress, J. F.: 1983, *Principles of Biomedical Ethics*, 2nd ed., Oxford University Press, New York.
3. Blanshard, B.: 1972, 'Wisdom', *Encyclopedia of Philosophy*, vol. 7, Macmillan Publishing Co., New York, pp. 322–324.
4. Boeyink, D. E.: 1974, 'Pain and Suffering', *Journal of Religious Ethics* **2**, 85–98.
5. Bok, S.: 1978, 'Death and Dying: Euthanasia and 'Sustaining Life: II. Ethical Views', *Encyclopedia of Bioethics*, Free Press, New York, pp. 268–278.
6. Burrell, D. and Hauerwas, S.: 1974, 'Self-Deception and Autobiography: Theological and Ethical Reflections on Speer's *Inside the Third Reich*', *Journal of Religious Ethics* **2**, 99–117.
7. Department of Health and Human Services: 1984, 'Nondiscrimination on the Basis of Handicap; Procedures and Guidelines Relating to Health Care for Handicapped Infants; Final Rule', *Federal Register* 49 (8), January 12, pp. 1622–1654.
8. Donagan, A.: 1977, *The Theory of Morality*, University of Chicago Press, Chicago, Illinois.
9. Duff, R. S.: 1978, 'A Physician's Role in the Decision-Making Process: A Physician's Experience' in C. A. Swinyard (ed.), *Decision Making and the Defective Newborn*, Charles C. Thomas, Springfield, Massachusetts, pp. 194–219.
10. Duff, R. S.: 1981, 'Counseling Families and Deciding Care of Severely Defective Children', *Pediatrics* **67**, 315–320.
11. Duff, R. S.: 1979, 'Guidelines for Deciding Care of Critically Ill or Dying Patients', *Pediatrics* **64**, 17–23.
12. Duff, R. S. and Campbell, A. G. M.: 1973, 'Moral and Ethical Dilemmas in the Special-Care Nursery', *New England Journal of Medicine* **289**, 890–894.
13. Duff, R. S. and Campbell, A. G. M.: 1979, 'On Deciding the Care of Severely Handicapped or Dying Persons', in R. Munsen (ed.), *Intervention and Reflection*, Wadsworth Publishing Co., Inc., Belmont, California, pp. 116–123.
14. Engelhardt, H. T., Jr.: 1975, 'Ethical Issues in Aiding the Death of Young Children', in M. Kohl (ed.), *Beneficent Euthanasia*, Prometheus Books, Buffalo, New York, pp. 180–192.

15. Engelhardt, H. T., Jr.: 1983, 'Viability and the Use of the Fetus', in W. B. Bondeson
    et al. (eds.), Abortion and the Status of the Fetus, D. Reidel, Dordrecht, Holland,
    pp. 183–203.
16. Foote, P.: 1978, 'The Problem of Abortion and the Doctrine of the Double Effect', in
    Virtue and Vice, University of California Press, Berkeley, California, pp. 19–32.
17. Freeman, J. M.: 1974, 'The Shortsighted Treatment of Myelomeningocele', Pediatrics
    53, 311–313.
18. Freeman, J. M.: 1974, 'To Treat or Not to Treat', in J. Freeman (ed.), Practical
    Management of Meningomyelocele, University Park Press, Baltimore, Maryland, pp.
    13–22.
19. Griffin, D. R.: 1976, God, Power, and Evil, Westminster Press, Philadelphia, Penn-
    sylvania.
20. Hartshorne, C.: 1985, 'Scientific and Religious Aspects of Bioethics; in E. E. Shelp
    (ed.), Theology and Bioethics, D. Reidel, Dordrecht, Holland, pp. 27–44.
21. Hauerwas, S.: 1977, 'The Demands and Limits of Care: On the Moral Dilemma of
    Neonatal Intensive Care', in S. Hauerwas, R. Bondi, and D. B. Burrell, Truthfulness
    and Tragedy, University of Notre Dame Press, Notre Dame, Indiana, pp. 169–183.
22. Hauerwas, S.: 1980, 'Selecting Children to Live or Die', in D. J. Horan and D. Mall
    (eds.), Death, Dying, and Euthanasia, University Publishers of America, Inc., Frede-
    rick, Maryland, pp. 228–249.
23. Hick, J.: 1978, Evil and the God of Love, revised edition, Harper and Row, San
    Francisco, California.
24. Kohl, M. (ed.): 1975, Beneficent Euthanasia, Prometheus Books, Buffalo, New York.
25. Kohl, M. (ed.): 1978, Infanticide and the Value of Life, Prometheus Books, Buffalo,
    New York.
26. Lorber, J.: 1973, 'Early Results of Selective Treatment of Spina Bifida Cystica', British
    Medical Journal 4, 201–204.
27. Lorber, J.: 1976, 'Ethical Problems in the Management of Myelomeningocele and
    Hydrocephalus', Nursing Times 72, p. 5–8.
28. Lorber, J.: 1971, 'Result of Treatment of Myelomeningocele', Developmental Medicine
    and Child Neurology 13, 297–303.
29. Lorber, J.: 1974, 'Selective Treatment of Myelomeningocele: To Treat or Not to
    Treat?', Pediatrics 53, 307–308.
30. MacIntyre, A.: 1981, After Virtue, University of Notre Dame Press, Notre Dame,
    Indiana.
31. McCormick, R. A.: 1978, 'Ambiguity in Moral Choice', in R. McCormick and P.
    Ramsey (eds.), Doing Evil to Achieve Good, Loyola University Press, Chicago,
    Illinois, pp. 7–53.
32. Nielsen, K.: 1985, 'Critique of Pure Virtue', in E. E. Shelp (ed.), Virtue and Medicine,
    D. Reidel, Dordrecht, Holland, pp. 133–150.
33. Nozick, R.: 1981, Philosophical Explanations, Harvard University Press, Cambridge,
    Massachusetts.
34. President's Commission for the Study of Ethical Problems in Medicine and Biomedi-
    cal and Behavioral Research: 1983, Deciding to Forego Life-Sustaining Treatment, U.S.
    Government Printing Office, Washington, D.C., pp. 197–229.
35. Reich, W. T. and Ost, D. E.: 1978, 'Infants: Ethical Perspectives on the Care of
    Infants', Encyclopedia of Bioethics, Free Press, New York, pp. 724–735.

36. Robinson, D. N., Shaffer, J. A., and Bowker, J. W.: 1978, 'Pain and Suffering', *Encyclopedia of Bioethics*, Free Press, New York, pp. 1177–1189.
37. Shelp, E. E. (ed.): 1982, *Beneficence and Health Care*, D. Reidel, Dordrecht, Holland.
38. Shelp, E. E.: Forthcoming, *Born to Die?*, Free Press, New York.
39. Shelp, E. E.: 1984, 'Courage: A Neglected Virtue in the Patient-Physician Relationship', *Social Science and Medicine* **18** (4), pp. 351–360.
40. Shelp, E. E.: 1983, 'Courage and Tragedy in Clinical Medicine', *Journal of Medicine and Philosophy* **8**, pp. 417–429.
41. Singer, P.: 1979, *Practical Ethics*, Cambridge University Press, Cambridge, Massachusetts.
42. Tooley, M.: 1972, 'Abortion and Infanticide', *Philosophy and Public Affairs* **2**, 37–65.
43. Tooley, M.: 1983, *Abortion and Infanticide*, Clarendon Press, Oxford, United Kingdom.
44. Tooley, M.: 1978, 'Infants: Infanticide: A Philosophical Perspective', *Encyclopedia of Bioethics*, Free Press, New York, pp. 742–751.
45. von Wright, G. H.: 1963, *The Varieties of Goodness*, Routledge and Kegan Paul, London, United Kingdom.

MARVIN KOHL

MORAL ARGUMENTS FOR AND AGAINST MAXIMALLY TREATING THE DEFECTIVE NEWBORN

I

This paper explores the issue of whether and in what circumstances active euthanasia of newborns could be justified. Allegations that active infanticide of severely deformed children under the age of approximately one month does not have the same potential for undermining moral practice as infanticide under other circumstances, in that a full bonding with an infant and an acceptance of the infant into society has not occurred, will as well be assessed. This paper does not purport to examine all the moral arguments, a task clearly beyond the scope of a single paper. It only examines some of the more salient ones, and only does so from a particular moral point of view. Nor does it pretend to address the theoretical and practical difficulties generated when one moves from a relatively clear-cut paradigm case of a seriously defective child under one month of age known to be hydranencephalic, a condition where both cerebral hemispheres are absent and are replaced by cerebral spinal fluid, to other cases where the child is less seriously defective or defective in a significantly different way. Expressed another way: this paper focuses upon a small part of the problem of whether it is morally right or wrong to maximally treat known hydranencephalic infants from birth to the age of about a month, and considers only those interpretations of right and wrong that are grounded upon a neo-Hobbesian[1] moral point of view. It considers the case of Paul Doe, a three-week-old known hydranencephalic, and claims that the death of this infant is not a harm to it because mere physical process, life in and of itself, is not always a good. To be more specific, it claims that the loss of an objectively meaningless life is not the loss of a primary good.

Let us first consider the question of social bonding, forgetting, for the moment, what Paul Doe may or may not experience in terms of having ties with others. Some writers, like Ashley Montagu, argue that at birth

R. C. McMillan, H. T. Engelhardt, Jr., and S. F. Spicker (eds.),
Euthanasia and the Newborn, 233–252.
© 1987 *by D. Reidel Publishing Company.*

the human infant has to complete its gestation outside the womb and that persons, socialized individuals, come into being only through a long process of social interaction and education. Others argue that some bonding occurs as early as the prenatal period. Still others maintain that the issue is not one of bonding but a question of when intense bonding occurs, and that intense bonding, the kind of tie where the death of the child results in deep grief and an intense sense of loss, does not typically occur until after the first year.

Now it is tempting to argue that bonding is typically developmental and that separation or death is easier the earlier it occurs. After all, are we to assume that if ending the life of a seriously defective infant is not a harm to that infant, it is generally *not* better (in terms of possible harm to others) to do so as soon as one reasonably can?

Notice that the difficulty is not with the developmental thesis. Bonding is typically developmental and separation *is* generally easier the earlier it occurs. The trouble, I suspect, is with the words 'typically' and 'generally'. For they suggest that in some cases the general thesis will not be true.

What, in light of this, ought we to do? Should we make the exception to the rule? Or should we be content to recognize that bonding can be idiosyncratic? I urge the latter. We should neither try to make fit what does not truly fit nor be overly pessimistic and assume that nothing ever can fit. Hence, a means ought to be provided by which exceptions, the problematic cases, can be taken care of. We should recognize that bonding can be idiosyncratic; that in some situations a close tie is established early, while in other situations fairly late, if ever.

Having admitted this, let us return to the case of Paul Doe. Born essentially without the complete brain structure of a human being, Paul possesses only a brain stem, which serves primarily to control respiratory function ([1], p. 480). It seems reasonable to hold, therefore, that where there is no capacity for cognition, there is no opportunity for the child to be aware of ties, aware in the sense of having more than rough prehensions. So that, even if it be granted that there is far greater physical dependency with such an infant, it nonetheless seems to be true that infants who lack even minimum cognitive power are infants who also lack a necessary condition for social bonding or, perhaps more accurately, they lack the necessary condition for an awareness of that bonding.

But the problem is not as simple as all this. For even if the infant cannot have this tie, other cognizant human beings can, including health care workers and parents. Indeed, the attachment of other parties may be, and often is, greater because of the infant's defects and great dependency. People, even in an intensive care infant nursery, do get attached to defective children, often in a relatively short period of time, and simply to dismiss this possibility without reason or explanation will not do.

On the other hand, the exception does not make the rule. Significant positive bonding is rare in cases of hydranencephalic infants.[2] The reasons for this are fairly clear – the shortness of time, the professionalism of the health care staff, and the typically limited contact between the child and its parents. In this sense, the case before us, the case of Paul Doe, is a typical one. It is a case where no significant bonding has occurred. Moreover, it is a case where the parents with reasonably full information view their child's existence as wrongful and, therefore, give their consent to withdraw maximal treatment, knowing that that withdrawal will probably result in the death of their child.

In so limiting our paradigm, I do not wish to suggest that atypical cases are unimportant. Quite the contrary. They raise a host of important questions concerning the rights of parents. The only suggestions I wish to make at this point are, first, that since it may make a moral difference if parents are bonded to and wish their hydranencephalic infant to live as long as it can, we should distinguish these cases from cases where that bonding has not occurred; and, second, that a discussion of the complexities generated by the former are beyond the scope of the present paper.

II

Thomas Hobbes is perhaps the most neglected of the great ethical theorists. And with this neglect an understanding of ethics, one based upon a realistic understanding of human nature, largely came to an end. For Hobbes, above all other thinkers, understood that ethics must have the power of coercion. This does not mean that we must accept his materialism, egoism, or the conclusion that monarchy is the best form of government; for, like all bold and explosive thinkers, Hobbes made some grand mistakes. But when we consider his mistakes, we see that they are largely derivative and, in the main, due to moving too quickly from the ethical to the political realm. The great strength of Hobbes lies elsewhere. It lies in his fundamental doctrine that human nature is dominated by fear of loss, and that the primary function of ethics is the protection of the primary good, namely, life. When strained of its non-essentials, the doctrine is that humans are dominated by fear of loss of life and that the major function of ethics is objectively to allay this fear.

But it is not enough to enumerate these claims without saying how they are related to each other, and without more carefully refining them in order to arrive at what we have called a neo-Hobbesian moral point of view. It would not be adequate to merely say that, according to Hobbes, "the cause which moveth a man to become subject to another is the fear of not otherwise preserving himself". For we do not understand how it is that the wills of most men are governed by fear. Similarly, we do not understand why the primary function of ethics is to protect the primary rather than the highest good or to protect all the goods necessary for a full life.

Hobbes explicitly says that fear of death and the desire for power are the two basic notions that move most men, if and when they would have the choice, to construct a form of governance. But he does not say that fear of death and the desire for power are the only human motives. Nor does he say that only corporeal substances have the ability to effect human behavior. What has power is that which has the ability to change things. So the question of which things have power is an empirical one, and Hobbes readily admits that things such as the imagination have power. Critics tend to confuse these points. In their attempt to vilify and refute Hobbes, an activity that unfortunately has become philosophic ritual, they tend to confuse canalizations of motives for the motives that more generally move men. In doing so they neglect Hobbes' own introduction to the *Leviathan* ([4], p. 20) where he distinguishes the passions, which are the same in all men – desire, fear, hope, etc. – from the objects of the passion, which do not have this similitude.

There is a restless desire of power in all men, "a perpetual and restless desire of power after power, that ceaseth only in death" ([4], p. 80). This desire leads to the state of nature where the life of man is "solitary, poor, nasty, brutish, and short". The reason being that there can be no legitimate peace and security without a central and dominant power that protects the weak from the strong, and the strong from the weak; for even a weak man may have the power to take the life of an otherwise stronger man.

Aversion is the turning away from an object. Fear is a strong aversion coupled with the conscious or unconscious opinion that the object is harmful. Fear of death is, at root, an elliptical way of saying that there is a strong aversion to the loss of life because one is of the opinion that that loss is a harm. Thus it is not death per se that is feared but rather the loss of life, and this is feared because that loss is viewed as being a great harm. Another way of saying this, that is Hobbesian in spirit, if not in letter, is to say that life is the primary good, thus the loss of life is the primary evil. The primary function of the policy is to protect that primary good, and that the goodness of this good is determined by the fact that it is generally desired by mankind, and the badness of death determined by the fact that it is generally abhorred by mankind.

Few moral philosophers have stressed the importance of protecting life as did Hobbes. The heart of his doctrine is to be found in Chapter 14 of the *Leviathan*. Here Hobbes discusses the right to the defense of one's own life, the right the correct understanding of which is vital to our moral understanding of the Paul Doe case. Hobbes suggests that a right may be transferred or renounced. The nature and limits of how we may give up a right or grant it to others is perhaps not sufficiently clear. What is clear is that rights are not absolute in the important sense that some are alienable. However, not all rights are alienable; not all rights can be surrendered. And the first of these inalienable rights is the right to the defense of one's own life. Hobbes' explanation of this entitlement is as follows:

Whensoever a man transferreth his right, or renounceth it; it is either in consideration of some right reciprocally transferred to himself; or for some other good he hopeth for thereby. For it is a voluntary act; and of the voluntary acts of every man, the object is some *good to himself*. And therefore there be some rights which no man can be understood by any words, or other signs, to have abandoned, or transferred. As first a man cannot lay down the right of resisting them, that assault him by force, to take away his life; because he cannot be understood to aim thereby at any good to himself ([4], p. 104).

What are we to say about this doctrine of Hobbes? It is quite certain that there is empirical warrant for the claim that human beings generally hold life to be a good, and since they generally do not give up a good except in exchange for another good for themselves, it follows that, when assaulted, they typically neither transfer nor renounce their right to life. I think very likely that the objections raised against Hobbes' egoism fail to touch this doctrine. Contrary to advocates of psychological altruism, exceptions do not make the rule. Even if some men are

willing to renounce or transfer this right on the basis of complete
self-disinterest, most men are not. Hobbes' basic point is that the
purpose of social morality is not to regulate the lives of a few saints or
their like, but to regulate and protect the lives of ordinary men and
women. This much, I think, we must grant to Hobbes.

Yet there remains much that needs be added to the theory. We must
not assume that, because life is generally a good, it is always a good.
From a Hobbesian perspective – since what makes something a good is
the fact that what is deemed to be of value is something that has or is
capable of standing the test of mankind, that it has been desired by most
men over the span of their existence or that it is capable of being freely
desired by most men over some comparable and reasonable span of time
– it follows that if some forms of life have almost never been desired and
have been typically avoided, then these forms of life cannot properly be
called good. We have already suggested that the loss of an objectively
meaningless life is not the loss of a primary good. It is not the loss of a
good because, once the notion of an objectively meaningless life is
properly understood, it becomes clear that mankind, with sufficient
reason, has not generally held such life forms to be a good but rather an
evil.

The distinction between an objectively meaningless and an objectively meaningful life is not an easy one to draw. There are two reasons
for this. The first is historical or perhaps evolutionary in nature. Prior to
the significant changes in medical technology that have taken place in
our lifetime, human progeny who, because of nature or accident, were
physiologically so low functioning as not to be able to possess or achieve
any goals minimally healthy human beings typically have or choose to
pursue, would have died at birth or succumbed to the general exigencies
of life. In other words, the physiological condition of those who are here
being described as having objectively meaningless lives was such that
they typically died at birth or shortly thereafter. This is a vitally important point because it explains, in no small way, why Hobbes and most
men of good sense prior to our time held that life and objectively
meaningful life were identical. The reasoning was straightforward.
Observe those who live and those who die. Those who live, even if they
be close to subsistence, can give their lives purpose and worth by
choosing goals. Of course these goals may not involve the pursuit of the
highest or the higher goods, but a life that is not fully meaningful may,
nonetheless, be meaningful.[3] Similarly, observe those who are about to

die. If the death is not preventable, then, aside from posthumous interests, the problem of having goals is largely futile; a problem that will, so to speak, resolve itself shortly. This is no longer true or as true as it once was. Natural selection no longer always takes care of those who would have heretofore died. Therefore it is a mistake, given the accomplishments of modern science and technology, to assume that biological existence equals meaningful existence.

The second difficulty involves that formidable task of showing how what is true can be shown to be true. How can we show that statements of the form "Paul Doe has an objectively meaningless life" are true or false? The first point to notice is that, whether we be successful or not in verbally characterizing the notion of an objectively meaningless existence, there are biologically living beings who possess the characteristics in question. That is why we have insisted upon focusing upon the hydranencephalic. Hydranencephalics may be rare, but they do exist. Of course, a critic may be inclined to say that, in the phrase 'objectively meaningless existence', we have a denotation without adequate connotation. This is very well. Half a cake is better than none. For the more serious charge would be to have a reasonably clear signification, say like the signification of the word 'unicorn', and not to have any objective referent.

What, then, are we to say about the signification of the term 'objectively meaningless life'?

By life is here meant the genetic capacity to initiate, build up, replicate, or destroy protoplasm, a capacity that permanently ends with death. Subjectively, judgments as to meaningfulness are correct when the individual being described earnestly believes his or her life is not vain. Objectively, such judgments are correct when the claim that the life in question is not vain corresponds to relevant external conditions. If this admittedly rough and preliminary analysis is correct, it means that meaninglessness wears the semantic pants, that our understanding of the concept of meaningful life derives primarily from our understanding of meaningless life and not vice versa. It is therefore closer to the mark to say that meaningless existence is one thing; irrevocably meaningless existence another. A life is irrevocably meaningless when an individual cannot possess, can no longer possess, or cannot achieve any goals *and* when one or more of these conditions are irreversible. Perhaps better put: subjectively meaningless existence is one thing; objectively meaningless existence another. A life is subjectively meaningless when an individual earnestly believes he or she cannot possess, can no longer possess, or cannot achieve any goals. A life is objectively meaningless when any of the forementioned intersensual and intersubjective conditions exists and is known, or is capable of being known, to be irreversible. Certain cases of irreparable brain damage, monolithic or anhedonic personality, permanent coma, and impending inevitable death are some examples.

In other words, some judgments about the meaninglessness of life are correct. Subjectively, they are correct if the individual who is being described earnestly believes his or her life is vain. Objectively they are correct if, given the individual's dominant goals or his very capacity to have goals, the judgment that his life is vain corresponds to relevant external conditions.

Why, it will naturally be asked, is having an objectively meaningless life such an evil? Why not be content with organic life, even if it be objectively meaningless? And why not just admit that nothing is good unless life itself is good?

To assume that life is a good because it comes first is to confuse primacy with goodness. For it does not follow that every condition of a good is a good. Suppose we consider a cure for cancer to be a good (albeit a concrete one). Suppose further that the condition of having cancer is also a necessary condition for its cure. Now it may follow that the having of cancer is primary, but it does not follow that, because it comes first, it must be a good. The "nothing is good unless life itself is good" argument is fallacious. It is fallacious because it rests, as Richard Robinson observes, on the false principle that every condition of a good is a good.·

Not every condition of a good is a good. Suffering is an evil although it is a condition of pity and pity is a good. Life does not have to be itself good because it is a condition of there being any good. It is consistent to say that something is good and yet life is not a good ([10], p. 54).

As to the question of why having an objectively meaningless life is such an evil, we can only refer back to our Hobbesian perspective. What makes something a good or an evil is that it has been or is capable of so being judged by mankind, in that it is held desirable or undesirable by mankind on the grounds of sufficient reason. Hence to say that an objectively meaningless life is an evil is to say that, where it has existed, it has been averted by most men and with sufficient reason. Omitting the grossly ignorant, the superstitious, and the fearful, ordinary men and women strongly prefer not to live objectively meaningless lives.

The theoretical basis of our ethical theory, at least in motivational terms, is the principle of meaningful life, – viz., that it is necessary for the minimal well-being of each individual to have goals and the capacity of attaining some of them. The fact that mankind has generally recognized this principle means that they do not desire mere organic life, but desire meaningful life. And it is mankind – neither individuals nor societies – who is the irrefutable and ultimate arbiter of the good.

It is of course plain that this leaves undiscussed many questions with which any complete treatise on ethics ought to deal. A great deal obviously remains to be said in order to make meaningful life and other principles of Hobbism clearer. But enough, I hope, has been said by way of preliminary to explain why we claim that the loss of an objectively meaningless life is not the loss of a good.

III

Let us now turn our attention to a very able and contrary point of view. Philip Devine's *The Ethics of Homicide* [3] seems to be on the right track in several regards. First, in maintaining that an ethics of homicide should be developed as a branch of morality in its own right rather than merely as a derivative part of a theory of justice or as a set of corollaries to another more comprehensive moral theory. Second, that the ethics of homicide directly relate to whether or not human beings have an interest in continuing to live, for if it can be shown that there never is an interest in direct or indirect voluntary death, then, whether one knows it or not, one has made the essential case for absolute pacifism. Third, that the essential opposition to what appears to be morally permissible killing is due to the belief that, when a homicide is wrong, it is considered wrong in itself, apart from the bad side effects it is also likely to have.

Devine never very clearly states the 'in-house' alternatives to his own nominal moral interest theory. He seems to believe that if one holds an interest theory one must hold one essentially like his own or that the alternatives to his own theory are not worth considering. Since on either alternative he is mistaken, I think it will be wise to briefly consider alternative interest theories before considering in detail the arguments for his own position.

Let us grant, for the sake of argument, that the judgment "X is a good homicide" would never have been made by an advocate of a moral interest theory unless the homicide was considered valuable because of some interest taken in X. Let us also grant, for the moment, that the interest to live itself and all our other interests are at root conditional on continued living.[4] Now there are several different ways of analyzing these claims. We can say that interest may be defined as "anything that is the object of desire". We can say, as Perry does, that an interest is a favorable attitude somewhat broader and less subjective than what is usually called desire and that moral good is "the fulfilment of an organization of interests" ([8], p. 14). Or we can say that an object of an interest is what is truly good for a person whether he desires it or not, because what counts morally is not individual desire but whether or not genuine harm occurs. Now let us, for simplicity's sake, label these alternative approaches (1), (2), and (3). According to (1), to say that an infant has an interest in continuing to live is to say that that infant desires to live. According to (2), an infant has a moral interest in living only if living fulfills a minimum of other, presumably 'higher', interests. According to (3), an infant has an interest in continuing to live, whether he desires it or not, depending on the quality and quantity of harm that is involved. The initial oddity is that, although Devine uses the language of the moral interest theoretician, his logic is such as to avoid the assets and liabilities of the aforementioned approaches. Of course, this may merely indicate an oversight on our part, and may mean that Devine has managed to avoid the perils of the more typical approaches. Or it may mean that we have before us a closet moral theist, as his opening remarks seem to suggest ([3], p. 10), and that most of the talk about interests derives from an unexamined 'classical moral theology'.

We are now in a position to consider Devine's argument. The difference between his own theory and other theorists he tells us is that these other theorists [11] think that:

an interest must be grounded in a desire, albeit in some cases the desire may only be a possible or future desire of an existing individual. That is to say, if an act is to be a violation of someone's rights, it must be contrary to desires he could experience *now*, or desires he *will* experience in the future. I am maintaining, to the contrary, that at least some desires are expressions of pre-existing interests, and that it is unnecessarily strained, when someone entertains clearly self-destructive desires, to refer to his potential desires to explain how his desires and interests are in conflict. (I do not suppose that someone could have an interest in having something he could never view except with aversion.) Accordingly, an infant can have an interest in continuing to live, although he can possess no articulate desires of any sort, and if we kill him he will never develop any. His existence, as a self-maintaining system of a complex sort is sufficient to ground the claim that he has an interest in continuing to live, and hence also (if our common moral notions are not in error) a right to do so ([3], p. 69).

The key passage here is that every infant has an interest in continuing to live and that its existence (as a self-maintaining system of a complex sort) is sufficient to justify that claim. Be not deceived, seduced, and mistaken concerning the nature of homicide, says Devine. All infant death is evil. All infant life is good. For we have received from nature standards and rules for the knowledge of truth, and nature's lesson is devastatingly simple: the death of an infant is always a harm to that infant, because since life (mere existence as a self-maintaining system) is always a good, the loss of life is always a harm.

It is tempting to say that, whatever may be the merits of this approach, it is not an interest theory – or it begs the question. After all, how can an interest in continuing to live be identical with the fact that one is alive? How can one's existence as a mere organic being be sufficient to ground the claim that one has an interest in continuing to live, and hence also a right to do so? In short, how can a state of being stand as its own justification?

One possible explanation is that death seems to be viewed, not neutrally as the ending of life, but as the loss of life. But even this move will not do. For Devine is then faced with the problem of explaining that the loss of something is necessarily a harm. Admittedly, the loss of life is a loss; for it seems certain that the loss of X is indeed the failure to keep X. But if I should lose a cold or an enemy, where is the harm? To assume that everything one loses incurs a harm to the loser, as Devine seems to do, assumes that each and every loss is a loss of a good, a move that decidedly begs the question at issue.

A related argument concerns the evil of death and the correlate claim that death is an evil incommensurable with other evils. The argument is as follows:

. . . there is something uncanny about death, especially one's own . . . I do not want to deny that a suicide can be calmly and deliberately, and in that sense rationally, carried out. But then someone might calmly and deliberately do something blatantly foolish or even pointless, and it is sometimes rational to act quickly with passionate fervor. But if, as seems plausible, a precondition of rational choice is that one knows *what* one is choosing, either by experience or by the testimony of others who have experienced it or something very much like it, then it is not possible to choose death rationally. Nor is any degree of knowledge of what one desires to escape by death helpful, since rational choice between two alternatives requires knowledge of both. . . . the opaqueness of death is a logical opaqueness. . . . [for] such a choice presents itself inevitably as a leap in the dark. . . . The difference between these choices [undergoing a sex-change operation, taking LSD, and so on] and that of death is a logical one. While it is logically possible . . . to get an idea of what it is like to have taken LSD from someone who has done so, death is of necessity that from which no one returns to give tidings ([3], pp. 24–28).

Now, as regards this statement, all that I can say is this. It does not seem to me to express any evidence to show that death is an evil. In fact, if we accept the logic of the statement, what follows is that death is incommensurable and, therefore, cannot be known to be either good or evil.

Devine largely confines his attention to arguing that death is logically opaque, that it is not logically possible to get an idea of what death is really like. But it seems clear that, if death is that epistemically dense, then it is strictly speaking not opaque, but connotatively almost empty. And if it is connotatively almost empty, then all the talk about choosing death as if one were choosing something – as opposed to merely leaving life – is cognitively misleading.

In so far as *the notion of death is a negative notion, only denoting the lack of life*, there is no leap into something. Strictly speaking, there is no 'something'. There is no thing to fear. To the extent fear is rational, we may fear dying or the loss of life if and when it is a good, but to fear death believing that it is actually something is like believing that, when there is nothing in one's pocket, that nothing somehow exists. Without being bound by superstition or theistic sentiment, death signifies the lack of life and nothing more. Contrary to Devine and the tradition he represents, death is not a leap into the unknown but, so to speak, a leap into nothingness. Unless we adore intellectual mystification, nothingness is nothingness, and not ontological 'somethingness'.

This point seems fatal to Devine's supporting argument. For he would have us believe that, when we choose death, we are actually choosing something, something that is logically opaque. Since we know what life is like, and cannot possibly know what death is like, the choice of death is at best a blind choice, if not outrightly irrational. But if the aforementioned explanation is correct, then the reason why death is an opaque notion is because there is nothing 'behind it' in that it simply and solely denotes the end of the life of a being who once lived. The choice between life and death is not like the choice between leaving London and going to Cimmeria. It is more like the choice between staying in London and leaving London to go nowhere forever. We are inclined to believe that the rationality of the latter choice turns upon the reasons for leaving, and not upon knowing something about nowhere. Similarly, the choice between leaving life to 'go to death' is like leaving a place we know something about to go nowhere forever, and the rationality of this choice depends upon the reasons for leaving, and nothing else. In fact, there is something absurd about claiming that there is a choice between the knowable and the logically unknowable, and then insisting that we cannot leave the former unless we know what the latter is like.

Expressed differently: Devine would have us believe that the death of Paul Doe is an evil because death per se is an evil. But what we have shown is that that case has not been made. We have urged that the notion of death is logically dense because it is, in a vital sense, denotatively empty, and that because of this, whatever rational judgments may be made must be directed solely to the question of whether or not ending the life of Paul Doe is an evil, in the limited but important sense of being a harm to Paul Doe. If the loss of an objectively meaningless life is not the loss of a good, and if Paul Doe has an objectively meaningless life, then it follows, contrary to what Devine and others may feel, that the death of Paul Doe is not a loss of a good to him.

Before enlarging upon the explanation of why the loss of an objectively meaningless life is not the loss of a good, we should perhaps address that part of Devine's argument that has thus far been neglected. It is the argument which, for want of a better label, may be called the argument for moral vitalism. The argument is as follows: The aim of every living being – plant, animal, or human – is to persist as a living being. To thwart this aim is an evil. Hence the death of any living being is an evil to that being. Or in Devine's own words:

Loss of life . . . is the central harm inflicted by an act of homicide. This is a harm that can be inflicted on any organism; plants, nonhuman animals, and human organisms of every state of development including the embryonic can all suffer loss of life. A consequence is that plants (and consequently animals and all members of the human species without exception) have interests . . . ([3], pp. 20–21). For all living beings have an interest in continuing to live . . . ([3], p. 32).

In a parallel vein, he writes that we can talk about and should take seriously the interests of species. For both individuals and species have interests:

It will not do to refuse to admit the existence of such interests [self-preservation] on the grounds that "a whole collection, as such, cannot have beliefs, expectations, wants, or desire," since such conditions are not necessary to the existence of interests. We can easily view the perpetration of a species through its characteristic mode of reproduction as an act, not only of the individual organisms that engage in pre-productive activity but also of the species itself, acting through its members. It is thus possible to attribute *an aim of preserving itself* to species as a whole and to see *this aim* as frustrated when the species becomes extinct (emphasis added) ([3], p. 111).

The point of quoting this passage at length is not to lose the thread of the underlying argument in the difficult question of whether or not species can have interests but, rather, to show that Devine uses the term 'aims' and 'interests' interchangeably. Thus he seems to believe that if a living being has some sort of teleological aim, then this is tantamount to that being always having an interest in staying alive, because staying alive is always in the interest, presumably the best interest, of that organism.

In order to exhibit adequately the importance of the distinction between having an interest in a teleological sense and having an interest in the sense of an act being in one's own best interest, I must ask the reader to travel with me and briefly visit the metaphysical realms of teleological naturalism and supernaturalism, the two great strongholds of moral vitalism. Before, our primary concern was with determining impartially whether loss of life was a loss of a good in the sense of being contrary to the best interests of the infant; now we have to ask whether the loss of life is contrary to the natural or supernatural aim of an individual organism.

If we begin by accepting the tenets of naturalistic vitalism – the belief that the functions of a living organism are due to some power or force that preserves its life – we may seem to have before us a self-evident claim. For being appears to necessarily mean aiming at self-preservation. And it is evident that if every organism must aim at self-preservation, then they must aim at self-preservation. Equally undeniable is the immediate inference from the claim of those super-naturalists who hold that, because God makes each living being aim at preserving itself, each living being so aims. In short, metaphysical vitalism is irrefutable. But it is irrefutable because it largely assumes what it seeks to prove and typically protects these assumptions under a cloak of intellectual obscurantism.

But if metaphysical vitalism guarantees that each living being aims at preserving itself – that is, grounds the claim that each has an aim, in this sense therefore, each has an interest – then I cannot see how one can leap from this to the claim that his interest is a good, unless there is another, hidden premise that logically helps us make this leap. Is it premise (1) that "whatever living beings naturally aim at is good"; (2) that "continued living, no matter what be the condition of that life, is always an actual good"; or (3) that "the aim of continued living is a good because God gave us the aim and God, by definition, is all-good"? It is difficult to say. Premise (3) plunges us into the problems of theism which Devine purports to avoid. Premise (2) has the dual fault of not being self-evident and of clearly begging the question. Premise (1) is plausible but requires an independent criterion for what is good or else it lapses into (2). It is not necessary here to know what Devine's hidden premise is: it suffices to say that without such a premise his metaphysical vitalism does not provide adequate grounds for his moral vitalism. In other words, the residuum of understanding we have so far obtained is that, even if we admit that metaphysical vitalism is irrefutable, that in itself does not necessarily make the case for moral vitalism. Whatever may be the merits of vitalism, it is a far cry from what is typically held to be a moral interest theory; for to have an aim is one thing, to have a morally good one, another.

IV

Let us now pass to a fuller explanation of why the loss of an objectively meaningless life is not the loss of a good. In the first place we have explained why it is a mistake to be content with the language of 17th century thinkers or to tacitly assume that by the right to life they meant the right to mere organic life. It was admitted that human life is generally meaningful. What this means is that most surviving human progeny live meaningful lives. But most is not all. We have suggested that the gap between having a meaningful and a meaningless life may be proportional to our ability and willingness to protect and sustain objectively meaningful forms of human existence. With our new abilities there come new and, as in the paradigm before us, heart-rending problems.

The greatest danger perhaps is that, because many of us are unfamiliar with this new concept, and because initial conceptualizations – like any new concept formation in a science – will probably be rough, perhaps imprecise, it will be dismissed out of hand. The great danger is that, because of conceptual conservatism and impatience with an admittedly new conceptualization, we may not be able to extend understanding and adequately map an area of increasing concern.

To map a new area is not to say, in itself, what one should do with that area. To say that a human life is objectively meaningless when we know or are capable of knowing that the individual cannot possess, can no longer possess, or cannot achieve any goals – is neither to say nor suggest that such individuals must necessarily die. Nor is it to suggest that it follows from this characterization alone that "the loss of an objectively meaningless life is not the loss of a good". The question of how we know the latter is true is an independent one. Although we have urged that the question is best answered by appealing to the fact that mankind, with sufficient reason, has not generally held such life forms to be a good, but rather an evil, the point we have insisted on is that the existence of something does not, in itself, make it a good.

Even if this be granted – even if one grants that some humans, including hydranencephalic infants, lead objectively meaningless lives, even if one also grants that to exist as a bare organic being is for a human not necessarily a good – one may object, and I think with good cause, that it is not sufficiently clear just *why* the loss of an objectively meaningless life is not the loss of a good.

Can we, then, better explain what it is that makes such a loss not the loss of a good? Can we more fully describe the reasons or sentiments that seem to generate judgments of this kind? It would be a mistake, perhaps only a lapse into intuitionism, to say no. At the same time it would be a greater mistake to claim more for the explanation that follows than it can actually deliver. Elsewhere I have urged that we judge certain kinds of death not to be an injury to the decedent when his life is known to be irrevocably meaningless or when irreparable meaninglessness is known to be imminent [5]. The argument, in essence, is as follows: Since, as a matter of fact, it is highly improbable that a fully informed man would choose to live an objectively and completely meaningless life, the act of ending that life is not wrongful because it is not an injury to that person. More generally, we do not injure human beings when we allow their lives to end or put them to death even if they cannot, or have failed to, state their preference if they are living an objectively meaningless life, if the state of affairs that warrants that judgment is irreparable and irreversible, and if there is no or insignificant evidence to indicate that they would not accept the judgment that their lives were meaningless ([5], p. 583).

In 'Voluntary Death and Meaningless Existence' [6], I enlarge the above argument to read that if, in addition to the aforementioned requirements, the act in question is a great kindness, then to the extent it is and *ceteris paribus*, we should end or allow that life to end. The merciful ending of life is morally permissible where it is not an injury to anyone and where, and to the degree, it rests on one or more of our moral duties, especially the duty of beneficence. An attempt is also made to distinguish between *believing* that one is leading an irrevocably meaningless life and *knowing that that is the case*, a distinction that in the present paper parallels the distinction between a *subjectively* and *objectively* meaningless life.

But I became increasingly discontented with my appeal to the 'fully informed' man. After all, what does the fully informed man know that warrants his judgment? Presumably he 'sees' that it is not an injury to the individual because that individual is living an objectively meaningless life. Does he perhaps 'see' or sense something else? Does he not somehow understand that a human being who cannot possess minimum life values and goals has a vain existence, an existence that for its possessor is pointless and worthless? Does not our ideal observer, our fully informed person, sense that the loss of a human life that is objectively meaningless is not the loss of a good because the loss of a vain existence, at least for a human, is not the loss of a good for that individual?[5]

To be quite candid, I did not realize the importance of filling in the grounds for the intuitions of the fully informed until I read Robert Coburn's excellent paper [2]. Coburn approaches the problem from a Kantian-Rawlsian perspective. Among other things, he suggests that an ideal moral legislator, a morally neutral hypothetical chooser with complete knowledge of general truths, would opt for the permissibility of infanticide where "the defects at birth are so severe that the individual's life will not be worth living and the effects on those most directly affected of either actively or passively procuring the infant's death are in the main positive and substantial" ([2], p. 347).

This rather fascinating and detailed agreement between Rawlsian constructivism and our Hobbesian morality should, no doubt, help to give us confidence in the former. But from the perspective of the latter it is difficult to see how a morally neutral theory, in itself, would generate

Coburn's conclusions. Coburn's analysis is admirable in many ways. But it has one essential defect. If the theory is morally neutral, then it cannot generate the conclusions that it does. If, on the other hand, it can generate these conclusions because it tacitly assumes a principle akin to the meaning of life principle, then it is not, strictly speaking, a Rawlsian theory. To assume, as Coburn does, that an ideal legislator would be able to recognize a life not worth living simply on the basis of non-moral general truths seems to press rational credibility. But if he is assuming that the ideal legislator recognizes the principle of meaningful life – *viz.*, that it is necessary for the minimal well-being of each individual human being to have goals and the capacity for attaining some of them – then, he is appealing to a very important moral fact. Rawls tells us that moral facts have no place in a constructivist doctrine:

The idea of approximating to moral truth . . . has no place in a constructivist doctrine . . . the parties in the original position do not recognize any principles of justice as true or correct and so as antecedently given; their aim is simply to select *the conception most rational for them*, given their circumstances. This conception is not regarded as a workable approximation to the moral facts: *there are no such moral facts* to which the principles adopted could approximate, (emphasis added) ([9], p. 564).

If it be admitted that the ideal legislator recognizes that some lives are not worth living, then this conclusion is most rational for him because he has some standard for judging worth or at least for judging vain lives. If, contra Rawls and Coburn, one is persuaded that one cannot generate conclusions concerning the worth of defective infants without an appeal to a moral fact closely akin to the principle of meaningful life, then one will naturally hold that, where Rawlsianism differs from Hobbesianism, the former is mistaken and ought to be corrected.

Consider again the case of Paul Doe, a case of a defective infant under one month of age known to be hydranencephalic, a condition in which the cerebral cortex is absent, though skull or cranial meninges, brain stem, and optic nerves are intact. Why do we know the loss of this child's life is not, for the child, a loss of a good? Because we explicitly or implicitly appeal to a moral fact. The moral fact, negatively stated, is that a human life is vain when it is objectively meaningless. When positively stated it is that it is necessary for the minimal well-being of each human to have goals and the capacity for attaining some of them. The genuine moral legislator, one who is truly informed, judges the death of Paul Doe not to be a loss of a good because, in addition to other social truths, he makes a judgment based upon the aforementioned moral fact.

V

I have now completed what I hope is a plausible explanation of why the loss of an objectively meaningless life is not the loss of a good. It only remains to guard my argument from being understood in a more sweeping sense than it has been intended or is properly able to bear. Although I have suggested that if it is morally permissible to end the life of an infant it is better, *ceteris paribus*, to do so as early as one reasonably can, nothing that I have said purports to be sufficient to make a full moral case. It is only maintained here that separation is typically easier the earlier it occurs, that death is not always an evil for the decedent, and that having an objectively meaningless existence is a good example of one such exception. Morality may demand that we should regard every act of evaluation with regard to the aggregate effect on life. But the claim that the loss of an objectively meaningless life is not the loss of a good does not necessarily lose its force because there may be more to morality.

State University of New York
Fredonia, New York, U.S.A

NOTES

[1] I shall, for reasons of style, use the terms 'neo-Hobbesian' and 'Hobbesian' interchangeably. However, the theory that follows is, strictly speaking, neo-Hobbesian. It is neo-Hobbesian because, although it resembles Hobbes in enough fundamental respects to warrant the judgment that it is far closer to his view than to other traditional moral conceptions, it is not close enough to warrant the judgment of identity or true fidelity. No doubt, Hobbes would have been comfortable with the claim that it is largely through fear that man enters into moral union with his fellows; that just as you cannot take up custard with a hook, you cannot have social morality without the power of coercion; and that the primary function of ethics is the protection of the primary good, namely, the protection of what I have called objectively meaningful human life. I am also inclined to think that he would not have been averse to a partial explanation of desirability in terms of a principle of sufficient reason or a vision of excellence involving a plurality of higher goods, provided each had sufficient empirical safeguards. The latter, however, is no more than interesting speculation.

[2] I am indebted to David Klein for this point and for much of my, albeit limited, knowledge about brain-damaged infants.

[3] For a discussion of some of the implications of confusing the having of a meaningful life with the having of a richly or fully meaningful life, see [7].

[4] I am here merely following Devine in using desires and interests as interchangeable terms. See [3], p. 29.

[5] Although my analysis takes considerable license with his point, I am indebted to F. C. White for his essential insight concerning the nature of vain activities. See [12].

BIBLIOGRAPHY

1. Bergsma, D. (ed.): 1973, *Birth Defects Compendium*, 2nd ed., Alan R. Liss, New York.
2. Coburn, C.: 1980, 'Morality and the Defective Newborn', *Journal of Medicine and Philosophy* **5**, 340–357.
3. Devine, E.: 1978, *The Ethics of Homicide*, Cornell University Press, Ithaca, New York, and London, United Kingdom.
4. Hobbes, T.: 1968, *Leviathan; Or the Matter, Forme and Power of a Commonwealth Ecclesiastical and Civil*, in M. Oakeshott (ed.), Collier Books, New York.
5. Kohl, M.: 1978, 'Karen Ann Quinlan, Human Rights and Wrongful Killing', *Connecticut Medicine* **42**, 579–583.
6. Kohl, M.: 1978, 'Voluntary Death and Meaningless Existence', in M. Kohl (ed.), *Infanticide and the Value of Life*, Prometheus, New York, pp. 206–217.
7. Kohl, M.: 1983, Is Life Itself a Value?, in P. Kurtz (ed.), *Sidney Hook: Philosopher of Democracy and Humanism*, Prometheus Books, New York, pp. 189–192.
8. Perry, R. B.: 1909, *The Moral Economy*, Charles Scribner's, New York.
9. Rawls, J.: 1980, 'Kantian Constructivism in Moral Theory', *Journal of Philosophy* **77**, 515–573.
10. Robinson, R.: 1964, *An Atheist's Values*, Clarendon Press, Oxford, United Kingdom.
11. Tooley, M.: 1973, 'A Defense of Abortion and Infanticide', in J. Feinberg (ed.), *The Problem of Abortion*, Wadsworth, Belmont, California, pp. 51–91.
12. White, F. C.: 1975, 'The Meaning of Life', *Australasian Journal of Philosophy* **53**, 148–150.

RICHARD C. McMILLAN

ANCIENT ADMONITIONS AND THE SANCTITY OF PERSONHOOD

The view that man is distinctly unique in the natural order because of his creation in the image of God has exercised a profound influence upon Western thought for centuries. Man, in this view, is affirmed to be an autonomous creature, owing his existence to God, and, therefore, ultimately responsible to deity for the way that existence is lived. Informed by this view, human thought regarding the nature of man was, until the last century, undertaken primarily by theologians and philosophers.

With the advent of experimental psychology in the last quarter of the nineteenth century, modern science turned its empirical gaze upon human nature. That study, by and large, concluded that the human being is a complex biological organism, unlike other biological organisms only in degree of complexity, particularly with respect to its neurological structures. Human behavior is determined by the reinforcement of the natural, physical environment – just as is the case with other animals – and human agency is no more than a myth bred of ignorance and superstition.

Interestingly enough, however, this modern view of human nature has not freed us to deal with the profoundly impaired newborn in the same manner in which we might deal with a severely deformed member of any other species. To decide that man is simply a complex biological organism does not, *ipso facto*, lead to the conclusion that infanticide is ethically permissible. While the scientific image of man views his behavior as determined by environmental reinforcement, his history of environmental response has created what we call 'culture' and that cultural heritage contains concepts of the 'good'. Whether or not the good is simply what man has found to be positively reinforcing, part of that tradition informs man that he should not kill his fellow man. While a 'sanctity of life' ethic resulting solely from cultural experience may not carry the force of a divine imprimatur, as does the concept of

R. C. McMillan, H. T. Engelhardt, Jr., and S. F. Spicker (eds.),
Euthanasia and the Newborn, 253–270.
© *1987 by D. Reidel Publishing Company.*

253

imago Dei, it is nevertheless a moral concept of considerable influence in our society.[1]

The admonition, "Thou shall not kill", while expressed in a variety of ways and always having exceptions according to social exigency, has been a fundamental norm for human civilization. Its status is perpetuated because it obviously protects the essential element of human community – the person. However, human community is disrupted not only when life is taken; it is equally disrupted by fear generated in the absence of respect for human life. Positive human relationships are sometimes difficult at best, but in the presence of fear that one's life is not valued, such relationships are profoundly distorted.

Then one encounters a common but nonetheless curious extension of this ancient admonition – that death is an evil. In his discussion of euthanasia, James Rachels provided an illustration of this extension:

The reason why it is considered bad to be the cause of someone's death is that death is regarded as a great evil – and so it is. However, if it has been decided that euthanasia – even passive euthanasia – is desirable in a given case, it has also been decided that in this instance death is no greater an evil than the patient's continued existence ([23], p. 80).

This extension is also presupposed in Earl Shelp's discussion in that death is one of the evils in the decision-making dilemma [26].

But, is this equation accurate? Certainly murder is an evil because one person acts so as to end the earthly existence of another *person*. In the act, not only is the personhood of another human being ended, but the potential for human community is likewise terminated. Nonetheless, is it legitimate to extend the ancient prohibition against murder to the notion that death is an evil? Murder is evil, and it is evil because of what it denies to the person whose life is taken, not because the result – death – is evil in itself.[2]

DEATH

Insofar as I can determine, death has several alternative interpretations:

(1) Death is the end of biological life, a fact of nature and a parameter common to all forms of life.

(2) Death is the end of life; beyond death there is nothing.

(3) Death is the end of a specific form of earthly existence beyond which there may or may not be some form of continued existence.

(4) Death is only one event in a continuum of existence.

(5) Death is the natural end of a mortal, finite existence which, when consciously and personally accepted, gives significant meaning and compelling opportunity to the present of existence.

The first interpretation is a statement of biological fact. Death is part of the natural scheme of things and all interpretations of death must begin with this given. Biological life is simply not unending, at least insofar as individual organisms are concerned. As a matter of fact, life for many organisms seems to be predicated upon death; one organism dies so that another might live. This statement of fact does not make the event of death less final or its contemplation less disquieting; but, viewed from this perspective, it would not seem that death can be assigned status as an evil. Death is simply a fact of natural, biological life; it represents the end of that form of life just as conception represents its beginning.

The remaining four interpretations add value judgments to this biological fact. The second, for example, states the fact, but adds the notion that there is nothing beyond death. This may or may not be the case – we simply do not know. But, if this judgment is correct, does death thereby constitute an evil? If we assume that the antithesis of good is evil, that the antithesis of life is death, and assert that life is good, are we not led to conclude that death is evil? Such an argument is of questionable logical merit because it makes a fundamental assumption that must be challenged: that life is a good. Is life an intrinsic good or is it a necessary condition for the attainment of goods? However regrettable, even tragic, experience teaches that life can *support* as much evil as it does good. Life itself appears to be a neutral but necessary condition; the experiences of life, for a rational, personal being, give life its quality and meaning.

This, of course, helps one understand why death is typically viewed as evil – it is the end of existence for persons who attribute a certain level of meaning and degree of quality to their lives. We normally do not contemplate death with joyous anticipation because death represents an end for individual growth and experience, and equally important, finally disrupts human relationships. Death represents the constant and ultimate reminder of the limited and temporary nature of human existence, of its mortality and finitude. But, is death, therefore, an evil or is it, in a strange but common sense way, a fact of life?

Perhaps the third interpretation is the most rationally honest interpretation, for, except that death is the end of biological life, we simply do not know what – if anything – lies beyond death and, as a result, have been unable to arrive at a totally satisfying understanding of the meaning of death for creatures who have attained personhood. We are reminded that it is only those organisms that have attained this status who are capable of questioning the nature and meaning of death and of assuming this, or any, interpretation.[3] Death, therefore, represents a profound and ever-present unknown, an unknown that has plagued human consciousness since the beginning of time. Moreover, while modern man knows more about the process of death than his ancestors and is, to an increasing degree, able to postpone it for a time, death remains the great mystery. As a matter of fact, death may be more mysterious for contemporary man because many of our ancestors naturally and uncritically accepted the religious interpretation of its meaning.

The fourth interpretation is a kind of summary statement of this ancestral point of view. It is the interpretation of death typically associated with religious faith and perpetuated through creed and dogma. Whether life transcends death through the return of the divine spark to divinity, through another earthly life, or through some form of existence beyond the limits of time and space, this interpretation does not divest death of its essential mystery – for one exercises faith in, but cannot prove, continued existence – but it does rob death of its finality and should reduce the anxiety commonly associated with its contemplation. While religions typically do not teach that death should be sought because life transcends it, the religious interpretation should ameliorate the fear of death and should resolve the pointlessness in life which many affirm because of the fact of death. For the most part, reflection on the resurrection of the body or the postmortem existence of the soul in the Christian tradition has not so much addressed death as it has the quality of life of the individual. Death is not to be sought because of an afterlife; rather, life is to be lived in keeping with Christian morality because of the afterlife.

The last interpretation may build on any of the preceding notions. It may affirm biological fact on the one hand, or it may evolve from religious conviction on the other. It is, however, a compellingly positive interpretation of death from a personal, existential point of view ([15], pp. 434ff). This view of death is directly related to the individual's personal affirmation of life and is part of an aggressive search for authenticity of being. Death is accepted as a fact of one's life; that death will come is certain, when and under what conditions it will come are the unknowns. Therefore, while willing one's future through self-transcendence as one 'writes' one's personal history, the individual affirms the present as the only certainly and actively intends the experience of the full potential of the present. From the existential point of view, the possessor of personhood lives in terms of two mysteries: neither life nor death can be fully explained. But, one *is* through decision – through assuming control of one's essentially mysterious existence – and the full and personal acceptance of death gives a new dimension of meaning and significance to one's decisions, to one's affirmation of the relational self in the present.

Whatever interpretation of death one elects, I would argue that death is not an intrinsic evil, no more than life is an intrinsic good. Individual human life simply has two biological parameters: conception and death. Life is the necessary but neutral condition for the attainment of goods. Death, rather than an evil, is the neutral end of biological life.

It is extremely important that the conditions of death, which we may judge to be evil, not be confused with the fact of death. Two illustrations will demonstrate our tendency to be selective. We say that a great wrong has occurred when a young child is killed by a drunken driver. This, we say, should not happen; it is evil, and some, following the principle of *Lex talionis*, advocate taking the life of the driver. But, on the other hand, we commonly hear the evaluation that an individual's death was a 'blessing in disguise' when that individual was suffering through an incurable terminal illness. The former response reflects our evaluation of irresponsibility, which brings about the untimely and unjust end of an innocent life. The latter response typically reflects several unexpressed judgments: (1) I am glad that X did not suffer any longer; (2) I am relieved that X's family does not have to continue to suffer with him; and (3) I would not want to suffer endlessly and pointlessly. We are apparently of the opinion that death can be a blessing under certain conditions; therefore, in all circumstances we do not consider death an evil. Attention to normal conversation indicates that most of us wish for peaceful, sudden death as opposed to an agonizing, protracted period of dying. Death is the fact; it is the conditions of death on which we place value judgments. Why, then, is that option viewed as inappropriate in the case of the profoundly defective neonate? Why do we feel that we must undertake aggressive intervention in order to prolong a pointless existence? If an individual, of whatever age, is incapable of attaining, sustaining, or regaining personhood, life for *that* individual does not constitute a right (as nature seems to provide no 'right' to life) or a good (as no rational person would choose to live that life).

A major difficulty, however, is that a reasonable analysis of death is impersonal and, from the point of view of 'human beingness', death is personal and its impact cannot be trivialized. We have a strong emotional reaction to death precisely because it is finally personal, and cold logic or reason fail to remove the personal quality of death. The fundamental personal anxiety associated with death is that I will die. Death is, on one level, an abstract concept; on yet another level, it is a reality of relational life when one must cope with the loss of a loved one, close friend or colleague; but on the most personal level, death is a reality I must face alone. Moreover, death threatens the 'third mode' of human beingness – the future. Because of its uncertain timing, death implies loves unfulfilled, goals unattained, relationships that never become more than superficial, experiences that never escaped the realm of dream or wish, mistakes not corrected, hurts not healed. Death is the constant reminder that human life will never be totally fulfilled.

But again the crucial point – death represents a threat to a *personal* being, a being conscious of meaning and purpose in life. It is not such a threat to the severely impaired newborn because, apart from a minimal level of 'human beingness', death is a neutral end of biological existence. It is precisely the confluence of the cognitive and the affective in the person that makes death a threat and that has led to the common identification of death as an evil. For the profoundly impaired neonate who has not attained this personal sense of the meaning of death, must we always judge the conditions of death to be evil?

Nihilism results when attention to death preempts one's attention to the full and meaningful experience of life. The fact of death, to the contrary, should intensify one's attention to the present of life. It is man's existence that is dominated by the finality of death; his being, however, is expressed in his courageous living of the present as it emerges from his past and intends his future.[4] While its conditions can be truly evil in nature, is death itself an evil against which the full armament of modern medicine and moral theory must be arrayed?

PERSONHOOD

From the point of view of personhood, a right to life is a right to a quality of life in community. It is not a right to transcend death. And this quality of life, it seems to me, has to do with the opportunity to actualize personhood. The essence of our democratic political and social structure as it impinges on quality of life is that no citizen shall be denied the opportunity to attain a full and responsible citizenship; no person will be assigned, by society, to an inferior or second-class status. If there is a 'right' to personhood, that right could be similarly stated: no individual should be arbitrarily or capriciously denied the opportunity to pursue the realization of personhood by other persons. However, non-treatment for the profoundly defective newborn does not constitute a denial of opportunity – nature has denied that opportunity. Treatment for the profoundly defective newborn, on the other hand, may assign that individual to a far worse fate than second-class social membership or limited opportunity for personhood. Treatment, in fact, may assign that individual to an existence of such negative quality that no rational person would choose to live that life or, for that matter, wish that life for another.

The concept of personhood[5] as it relates to medical practice has been widely discussed [9–12, 29, 31] and represents a fairly controversial issue ([16], pp. 35–37). Apparently a major objection is that personhood, like beauty, is seen to reside largely in the eye of the beholder.[6] The concept is, nonetheless, frequently encountered in the context of deliberations addressing abortion [4, 25] but will also be found in discussions regarding the termination of life after birth ([30], chs. 6, 7). Whatever its merit, the concept of personhood will most likely figure prominently in attempts by theologians, philosophers, ethicists, attorneys, and physicians to resolve the quality of life/sanctity of life controversy.

The temptation to defend the importance of the concept for ethical discussion in medicine will be resisted,[7] and I will devote attention to the specification of two characteristics from Joseph Fletcher's initial list [10], which may inform treatment decisions with respect to the profoundly defective newborn. While the characteristics are Fletcher's, the interpretations are mine.

1. *Minimal intelligence.* This characteristic will include Fletcher's fundamental characteristic – neo-cortical function – as that function is prerequisite for the characteristic as I will develop it. If, as Fletcher rightly pointed out, the cerebral cortex is severely damaged or absent, there can be no consciousness, no thought, or no subjective states common to human experience. As Fletcher indicated, apart from "the synthesizing function of the cerebral cortex, the *person* is non-existent. Such individuals are objects but not subjects" ([10], p. 31]). While that

statement may be a bit jolting, the presence of the cerebral cortex is fundamental for the development of personhood following any acceptable definition.

I include neo-cortical function under this characteristic because I cannot follow Fletcher's interpretation of minimal intelligence. The difficulty arises from the common definition of intelligence – the interpretation to which Fletcher ascribes – as some level of I.Q. After years of study in psychology, I remain uncertain as to just what I.Q. is – except that it is what is measured by intelligence tests. Typically this is a measure of what one knows, of the assemblage of facts one has been able to accumulate. It is fundamentally a 'storage bin' concept of human cognition.

Jean Piaget, on the other hand, developed an alternative view of intelligence. According to that view, the infant enters the world with no concept of the difference between self and other. Slowly, through interaction with the world, the infant begins to distinguish between self as object and the world as object(s). As John H. Flavell wrote, there is simultaneously a process of objectifying external reality and a process of growing awareness of self – "the self comes to be seen as an object among objects. . . . Cognition really begins at the boundary between self and object. . . " ([7], p. 16)]. According to Piaget:

Intelligence thus begins neither with knowledge of the self nor of things as such but with knowledge of their interaction, and it is by orienting itself simultaneously toward the two poles of that interaction that intelligence organizes the world by organizing itself ([21], pp. 354–355).

In this view, intelligence is the individual's ability to structure and organize the world of experience. Intelligence is a process, not an accumulation of facts; it is a dynamic, not a static, concept. The process begins with the distinction between self and other and continues as these two poles of experience interact.

Here we have an indicator of personhood that can be medically determined without waiting to assess the ability to accumulate facts. If there has been extensive neural damage, even if the cerebral cortex is present, so that the original state of egocentricism will never be overcome to any minimal degree, cognition will not take place and personhood will not develop because the individual will be unable to develop a concept of self, or of world. The individual will never be able to structure the world sufficiently as to allow even a minimal sense of relationship, and meaningful responses will be impossible.

In the absence of certain distinctly human capacities – for self-consciousness and relating to other people – the usual connection between biological life and our notion of the good is effectively severed. Just as the presence of unrelievable pain can preclude the attainment of those basic human goods that make life worth living, so the absence of fundamental human capacities can render a life valueless, both to its possessor and to others ([2], p. 32).

2. *Control of existence.* In a more complete discussion of personhood, I would have much more to say about this characteristic and would take a slightly different approach. The fundamental notion, however, remains the same: a person is that being who exercises control, to one degree or another, over the nature, quality, and direction of his or her life. Paul Tillich has written:

Personality is that being which has power over itself. . . . 'Person' in this sense . . . is a moral concept, pointing to a being which we are asked to respect as a bearer of a dignity equal to our own and which we are not permitted to use as a means for a purpose, because it is purpose in itself. This is the basis of personality, the individual human being, the person who alone among all beings has the potentiality of self-determination and, consequently, of personality ([28], p. 115).

For our purposes, self-determination is the key. Will the infant ever be capable of any degree of self-determination or will it face a life of total dependency? While I cannot document this hunch, it is my feeling that being out of control is one of the most anxiety-producing experiences. This is, I think, the basic fear associated with illness, whether it be of physical or psychological etiology.[8] This does not, however, indicate my agreement with the philosophical notion that the basic quest of man is the 'will to power'. The will to power, I think, is the wish for personal control perverted by the absence of autonomy and the recognition of human integrity. The person simply wishes to control, to a meaningful degree, the nature, quality, and direction of his personal existence. Will the profoundly defective newborn, even if capable of the wish, ever be able to actualize any degree of self-determination? For the infant to be saved through aggressive medical intervention when the prognosis is a 'life' of total and complete dependency, to live a life totally at the mercy of others, is to project no personal life at all. It is, rather, to sentence the infant to the life of a perpetual prisoner to one's profound deformity. In essence, it is a life of personal alienation, regardless of the caring response of others.[9]

If the profoundly defective newborn cannot be assisted, if assistance cannot help it achieve some degree of personhood, should treatment be undertaken? Should a life with no personal future be sustained? The potential for personhood is bequeathed by nature, nurtured by relationships, and actualized by the individual. It is, I think, the potential that provides any right that may exist. If nature does not so bequeath, relationships have nothing to nurture, and the individual nothing to actualize. In this case, no right exists.

To assess the potential for personhood requires a dual projection: (1) that the organism in question possesses certain characteristics which would lead a reasonable observer to conclude that, in the normal course of events, the organism will attain personhood; and (2) that these characteristics can be nurtured by human relationships of such quality as to lead one to expect that some degree of personhood will be achieved. Potential is, by definition, not actual, but certain indicators do allow one to make a projection of potential – indicators such as those just discussed.

We seem, however, curiously selective in our willingness to evaluate potential. A newborn, for example, cannot walk, but most physicians would not hesitate to assess that potential. While the skill itself is not present, the prerequisite characteristics are (or are not) present – the requisite musculoskeletal structures and the necessary neurological connections. On the other hand, the potential of the newborn for becoming a concert pianist would not be possible to project (other than the necessary physical structures and, possibly, some vague indication from the infant's genetic heritage). Yet, in the case of the *profoundly impaired* newborn, the judgment of potential is not like the second, but more like the first. In evaluating severe or profound impairment, the judgment of potential would not seem all that problematic; if, that is, we are not fundamentally guided by the notion that death is evil.

McCormick has argued that life itself is to be valued precisely because it is the necessary condition for other values. The problem of treatment or non-treatment then revolves about the potential for human relationships – the guideline he recommends for such decisions. While every human life is a value, will that life support the quest for those higher values for which life is the necessary condition? His conclusion appears to be that non-treatment may only be entertained as a possibility when the potential for human relationships will be lost in the mere struggle for survival and maintenance of life ([20], pp. 544–548).

Quality-of-life assessments ought to be made within an overall reverence for life, as an extension of one's respect for the sanctity of life. However, there are times when preserving the life of one with no capacity for those aspects of life that we regard as *human*, is a violation of the sanctity of life itself ([19], p. 35).

Abraham Maslow developed a simple yet profound hierarchy of human needs that illuminates this distinction ([17], ch. 5). According to Maslow, the hierarchy is one of 'relative prepotency' in which gratification becomes as important as deprivation in motivation because gratification releases the organism to higher levels of goal-setting and achievement ([17], pp. 83–84). The first level of the hierarchy Maslow called the physiological level. These needs relate to the basic survival of the organism qua organism and they must be satisfied before the organism can seek satisfaction at higher levels. If the 'life' of the profoundly impaired newborn will be solely and totally dominated by survival – by simply maintaining organismic existence – can one seriously view this as a positive life at all? In another context, Maslow argued that deficiency motivation is productive of psychological illness while growth motivation is productive of psychological health ([18], ch. 3). Do we, in good conscience, wish to will a life of deficiency motivation – a life which the severely impaired child surely faces? As Fletcher has pointed out:

It is *personal* function that counts, not biological function. Humanness is understood as primarily rational, not physiological. This 'doctrine of man' puts the *homo* and *ratio* before the *vita*. It holds that being human is more 'valuable' than being alive ([8], p. 350).

DECISION

In deliberations about treatment or non-treatment, an important point is often overlooked. If life is pointless and meaningless by any acceptable standard, if it can neither attain, sustain, or regain personhood, that form of life is incapable of decision. We speak and act as if it can or could and, with the adult, are advised to consider the 'history' of the individual, or, with the newborn, decide in terms of net gain or benefit through empathy. According to the President's Commission: "As in all surrogate decision-making, the surrogate is obligated to try to evaluate benefits and burdens from the infant's own perspective." In the view of the Commission, this standard "excludes consideration of the negative effects of an impaired child's life on other persons, including parents, siblings, and society" ([22], p. 219).

But the newborn is incapable of choosing, the precondition for setting goals. How can we decide, then, as the infant would, particularly when it suffers from a defect the magnitude of which is totally beyond our experience? I would argue that, first, unlike an elderly comatose patient whose history might provide some basis for decision for that individual, we have little if any basis for decision for or in the place of the infant, but we have a substantial and compelling basis for decisions in terms of others. Furthermore, I would argue that to act as if the infant could make the decision is to, in a fundamental and very real sense, *shift responsibility* for the decision *to the infant*. To attempt, in the role of proxy, to decide through empathy is to attempt to utilize the preferences, values, and goals of the incompetent individual. We, in a sense, make the decision as we judge they would. From the proxy standpoint, the incompetent person provides the general direction for our decision. But, the general direction of the treatment or non-treatment decision for the newborn cannot be shifted to the newborn.

Robert Weir contends that proxy or surrogate decisions for newborns are 'fatally flawed' because it is impossible for the adult proxy to empathize with the defective newborn. Instead, he argues that the 'best interest' theory provides the most positive avenue to decision-making. One should determine "whether available treatment would on balance be beneficial or harmful to the anomalous neonate. . ." ([30], p. 199). The key to his argument is that one not focus on the impact of the child's continued life on others; but that decisions be made solely on the basis of the impact of the infant's continued life on the infant. However, in the absence of chronic intractable pain, can a decision of best interest be made in a relational vacuum?

If one opts for a 'best interest' principle of treatment/non-treatment decisions for the defective newborn, care must be exercised that one consider long-term as well as short-term benefit. While the 'life' of the profoundly defective newborn may be preserved, that may not be in the child's best interest. Weir admits that "most if not all competent persons can conceive of circumstances that would present, for them, a fate worse than death" ([30], p. 206). But more than imagining fates personally worse than death, we must consider long-term relational realities. Given the rapid development of the biomedical technology that forces this problem on us and projecting a 'best world' scenario, we might be tempted to maintain all defective newborns because ideal support services would be in place and some glimmer of hope provided by medical advance. But we cannot project a best world and the best interest of the child may derive from that relational fact. Patents are not always sufficiently loving or wealthy to provide for the child's care.

Society does not seem inclined to financially support extensive research in neonatal care or the ideal institutional services frequently required by severely impaired children. And, while the Federal Government apparently wishes to be involved in such decisions, it has shown no inclination whatsoever to facilitate a best world of maximum care for the profoundly impaired newborn. Furthermore, if the parents of the child are sufficiently loving, what happens to the profoundly impaired child when these devoted parents are, for any number of reasons (e.g., the age and size of the child, the complexity and magnitude of the care required, the death of the parents), no longer able to provide love and care?[10] The long-range consequences of life for an infant cannot be ignored and they are primarily relational in nature.

In a recent article, John Arras argues that the 'reasonable person' standard cannot be applied to treatment/non-treatment decisions with the severely impaired neonate because the reasonable person will employ a concept of normalcy common to the adult decision-maker, which may place unrealistic constraints upon the infant's potential ([2], p. 30). But this projection of external standards is precisely the problem also with 'best interest' or 'net benefit' standards. It is impossible to empathize with the profoundly impaired newborn. Therefore, all our judgments for them are fundamentally projections on them. Richard Hare clearly understood the projective nature of empathy in attempting to decide for defective newborns. In his judgment, we can do no better than to "put ourselves imaginatively in the places of those affected, and judge as if it were our own future that was at stake" ([14], p. 367). With the newborn, unlike persons with a history of established relationships, I see no way to avoid the fact that decisions are made by others for others, employing the standards of others. The adult decision-maker cannot lay aside his/her accumulated experience in order to make a decision for an infant with no accumulated experience. Human compassion and the nature of the situation indicate that we cannot avoid "worries about the child's future life with a potentially abusive parent or in a hopelessly inadequate state institution. . ." ([2], p. 28). The *profoundly* impaired newborn will be inordinately dependent on others if it survives. The degree of that dependence must not be ignored and its relational implications cannot be avoided in decision-making.

Absent pain, life for the newborn is neutral; it is a condition of existence shared with all other biological organisms. That life has meaning and quality because of what it portends, because of its potential for personhood. If that neutral life has no potential for personhood, it may be viewed as of negative value because of what it portends for others – for parents who must bear the grief and suffer the emotional and financial drain; for society that will, in one way or another, contribute substantially to the care and sustenance of this meaningless life; for health care professionals who must experience the frustration of administering pointless, often painful treatment. Please be aware that these considerations result from the judgment that *personhood is not possible* for the infant. For the profoundly defective newborn, decisions cannot be made for them or on their behalf. Nature has made that decision. Decisions are made by others based on the assessment of the infant's condition. The decision is fundamentally a relational decision. In the absence of a history, apart from established relationships, and with no clear perspective of their wishes, three global assessments are required: (1) the degree of the infant's abnormality, (2) the effects(s) of this abnormality on the quality of life the child may enjoy, and (3) the burdens that will befall the family and society ([13], p. 85).

CONCLUSION

It is my judgment that two fundamental notions in this debate need closer scrutiny. On the one hand is the notion that death itself is an evil. Is death an evil or do we confuse the conditions of death – which may or may not be evil – with the fact of death itself – which I contend is no more than a fact of life. Second, is life a good in itself or is it a good "precisely because most of the other things we value cannot be realized without life?" ([5], p. 76) Life is a neutral but necessary condition to the attainment of goods by rational, personal beings.

If life and death are viewed as fundamental facts of human existence, does it not follow that our judgments are based on those values we associate with 'human beingness' or personhood? Arthur Dyck clearly understood that quality-of-life decisions rest solely upon values. According to Dyck, in quality-of-life decisions, life itself is not good, "only life of a certain kind, life with a certain degree of intelligence, potential for development, or whatever, is considered valuable" ([6], p. 16). This is no less the case with judgments seeking to employ conditions of personhood. Such decisions are not, therefore, based on *a priori* rules or considerations of the greatest good for the largest number, but on the common personhood we share and the potential of the newborn to achieve even a minimum level of that personhood.[11]

According to Ramsey, because God's creative activity has bestowed life on man (and on defective newborns), physicians, parents, clergymen – all who might entertain questions of treatment or non-treatment – are to respond in terms of what might be called the 'normal child principle'. As Ramsey wrote: "Decisions to treat or not to treat should be the same for the normal and the abnormal alike" ([24], p. 206). But if man is the creature of God, what about two of man's crowning relational attributes: compassion and responsibility? Does not compassion force us to raise questions regarding the potential for personhood? And does not our sense of mutual responsibility compel us to question the propriety of treatment regardless of our ability to administer it?

Mercer University School of Medicine
Mason, Georgia, U.S.A.

NOTES

[1] As Amundsen points out, [1] the concept of *imago Dei* altered Western thought and practice with respect to the treatment of defective newborns, and the intrinsic sanctity of human life became a benchmark for medicine. Strangely enough, as Western society has been secularized and the religious doctrine of the *imago Dei* has become but one option among many, high technology and seemingly unlimited resources have appeared to sustain, if not the intrinsic sanctity of human life, at least the notion that active euthanasia is not morally permissible (it is also, of course, not legally permissible). It seems difficult for twentieth-century man, with his technological capacity and intellectual sophistication, to conceive of any problem that cannot be solved – if not today, then tomorrow. Death, therefore, does not provide a commonly accepted solution to the problems faced by the profoundly defective neonate.

[2] I will accept, for purposes of this discussion, Earl Shelp's definition of evil ([26], p. 213).

[3] Contrary to, for example, Tooley [29] and Singer [27], I contend that species membership is critically important from a moral standpoint because it is our species that reflects on these matters. Moral dilemmas, after all, result from human relationships. Despite our flights of fancy, we are not privy to the moral reflections of other species, or forms of life.

[4] A distinction should be made between existence and being. Existence connotes qualities of 'thingness', 'itness', the occupation of time and space, a being-there. Being, on the other hand, is concept denoting the ability to intentionally transcend existence and, in some meaningful sense, control the nature, quality, and direction of one's life.

[5] I would much prefer the term 'human beingness', but as I am attempting to analyze the same structure, use of that term in this context would represent no more than a semantic game employed to avoid a controversial term.

[6] I am more concerned that the characteristics of personhood not be viewed as expressions of what man ought to be. Indicators (the word I prefer) of personhood are rather expressions of minimal capacities that allow and facilitate 'human beingness'.

[7] While the term 'personhood' is not used, one will find references to qualities constituting personhood or 'human beingness' in the writings of philosophers who reject the use of the concept (e.g. the essays of Richard Brandt and Marvin Kohl in this volume).

[8] I find some support for this notion in Jurrit Bergsma's discussion of 'dis-ease' ([3], ch. 2). In that state of illness. "Man is no longer the sole ruler of his body. he has to share this rule with something as yet undefinable. This is dis-ease in its rawest form" ([3], p. 29).

[9] In the abstract context of ethical, as opposed to clinical, discussion, specification of defects that may warrant non-treatment considerations is dangerous for a number of reasons. First, there is always the problem of the severity of the condition (e.g., spina bifida cystica or hydrocephalus). Second is the fact that abnormalities are often multiple as is typically the case with Trisomy 21 (Down's syndrome). Some neonatal conditions seem hopeless even with aggressive treatment (e.g., Trisomy 18) while others present complicated management strategies requiring multiple surgeries and extensive long-term rehabilitation processes, assuring no more than a very uncertain outcome for the infant (e.g., exstrophy of the cloaca). And, despite the sophistication of modern medical science, some conditions simply seem to defy treatment (e.g., De Lange syndrome). Furthermore, add to this the fact that many readers will disagree with the examples given. Whether we like it or not, the fundamental fact is that treatment/non-treatment decisions remain, at this point, largely situational.

[10] Appeals to love are not often as satisfactory in the resolution of dilemmas in this context as some assume. All too often, there is an underlying equation of love with self-sacrifice. It is argued that parents should 'love' their child regardless. I fear that this, however, ignores a number of other equally important aspects of love: the love of oneself, which is an integral part of relational love; the willing of the best for the loved one regardless of standards or oughts imposed from external sources; the love one has established with others. Human love is not well served or understood when it is equated with masochism or martyrdom.

[11] Utilitarianism is a noble and honored (at least by some) ethical theory (or set of theories). But my argument would be misunderstood if it were viewed as purely utilitarian in nature or intent. I am not suggesting that we assess ends or outcomes in a utilitarian sense, but that we evaluate a continuum of relational experiences based upon a commonly shared nature – our 'human beingness'. 'Human beingness' (or personhood) is not understood as a guarantee of any value, meaning, or good; it is simply a quality, realized on the basis of biological life, which makes such attainments possible. The values, meanings, or goods of "human beingness" will be realized, to one degree or another, in subsequent relationships.

BIBLIOGRAPHY

1. Amundsen, D. W.: 1987, 'Medicine and the Birth of Defective Children: Approaches of the Ancient World', in this volume, pp. 3–22.
2. Arras, J. D.: 1984, 'Toward an Ethic of Ambiguity', *The Hastings Center Report* **14**, 25–33.

3. Bergsma, J. and Thomasma, D. C.: 1982, *Health Care: Its Psychosocial Dimensions*, Duquesne University Press, Pittsburgh, Pennsylvania.

4. Bondeson, W.B. *et al.* (eds.): 1983, *Abortion and the Status of the Fetus*, D. Reidel, Dordrecht, Holland.

5. Brody, H.: 1981, *Ethical Decisions in Medicine*, Little, Brown, and Co., Boston, Massachusetts.

6. Dyck, A. J.: 1977, 'Ethics and Medicine', in S. J. Reiser *et al.* (eds.), *Ethics in Medicine*, MIT Press, Cambridge, Massachusetts, pp. 114–122.

7. Flavell, J. H.: 1963, *The Developmental Psychology of Jean Piaget*, D. Van Nostrand, Princeton, New Jersey.

8. Fletcher, J: 1977, 'Ethics and Euthanasia', in R. F. Weir (ed.), *Ethical Issues in Death and Dying*, Columbia University Press, New York, pp. 348–359.

9. Fletcher, J: 1974, 'Four Indicators of Humanhood – The Enquiry Matures', *The Hastings Center Report* **4**, 4–7.

10. Fletcher, J: 1972, 'Indicators of Humanhood: A Tentative Profile of Man', *The Hastings Center Report* **2**, 1–4.

11. Fox, R. C. and Willis, D. P.: 1983, 'Personhood, Medicine, and American Society', *Milbank Memorial Fund Quarterly* **61**, 127–147.

12. Grobstein, C.: 1983, 'A Biological Perspective on the Origin of Human Life and Personhood', in M. W. Shaw and A. E. Doudera (eds.), *Defining Human Life: Medical, Legal, and Ethical Implications*, AUPHA Press, Ann Arbor, Michigan, pp. 3–11.

13. Habgood, J. S. *et al.*: 1975, 'Ethics of Selective Treatment of Spina Bifida', *The Lancet* **I**, 85–88.

14. Hare, R. M.: 1976, 'Survival of the Weakest', in S. Gorovitz *et al.* (eds.), *Moral Problems in Medicine*, Prentice-Hall, Englewood Cliffs, New Jersey, pp. 364–369.

15. Heidegger, M: 1962, *Being and Time*, J. Macquarrie and E. Robinson (trans.), Harper, New York.

16. Macklin, R.: 1983, 'Personhood in the Bioethics Literature', *Milbank Memorial Fund Quarterly* **61**, 35–57.

17. Maslow, A. H.: 1954, *Motivation and Personality*, Harper, New York.

18. Maslow, A. H.: 1962, *Toward a Psychology of Being*, D. Van Nostrand, Princeton, New Jersey.

19. McCormick, R. A.: 1978, 'The Quality of Life, The Sanctity of Life', *The Hastings Center Report* **8**, 30–36.

20. McCormick, R. A.: 1977, 'To Save or Let Die: The Dilemma of Modern Medicine', in S. J. Reiser *et al.* (eds.), *Ethics in Medicine*, MIT Press, Cambridge, Massachusetts, pp. 544–548.

21. Piaget, J.: 1954, *The Construction of Reality in the Child*, M. Cook (trans.), D. Van Nostrand, Princeton, New Jersey.

22. President's Commission for the Study of Ethical Problems in Medicine and Biomedical and Behavioral Research: 1983, *Deciding to Forego Life-Sustaining Treatment*, U.S. Government Printing Office, Washington, D.C.

23. Rachels, J: 1975, 'Active and Passive Euthanasia', *The New England Journal of Medicine* **292**, 78–80.

24. Ramsey, P.: 1978, *Ethics at the Edges of Life*, Yale University Press, New Haven, Connecticut.

25. Shaw, M. W. and Doudrea, A. E. (eds.): 1983, *Defining Human Life: Medical, Legal, and Ethical Implications*, AUPHA Press, Ann Arbor, Michigan.
26. Shelp, E. E.: 1987, 'Choosing Among Evils', in this volume, pp. 211–231.
27. Singer, P.: 1983, 'Sanctity of Life or Quality of Life?', *Pediatrics* **62**, 128–129.
28. Tillich, P.: 1957, *The Protestant Era*, J. L. Adams (trans.), The University of Chicago Press, Chicago, Illinois.
29. Tooley, M.: 1979, 'Decisions to Terminate Life and the Concept of Person', in J. Ladd (ed.), *Ethical Issues Relating to Life and Death*, Oxford University Press, New York, pp. 62–93.
30. Weir, R. F.: 1984, *Selective Nontreatment of Handicapped Newborns*, Oxford University Press, New York.
31. Weiss, R.: 1978, 'The Perils of Personhood', *Ethics* **89**, 66–75.

SECTION V

DECISIONS IN THE PRESENCE OF TRAGEDY

RAYMOND S. DUFF AND ALEXANDER G. M. CAMPBELL*

MORAL COMMUNITIES AND TRAGIC CHOICES

We presented a family-centered policy of deciding the care of severely handicapped infants in 1973 [11]. Since then, much debate, often furious and more legal or political than ethical [29], has occurred about this issue. The policy we proposed in 1973 seemed reasonable then, and it seems even more reasonable and necessary today (although the particulars of some decisions have changed as a result of advances in technology). In order to explain why this is so, we have to say some things about medicine, people, nurture, culture, caring, tragedy, and a strategy of decision-making that is caring and respectful of the people involved. In doing this, we can only point in the direction of some very important, often irrational or unconscious meanings, which are central to what we have seen in real life.[1]

Patient care decisions may be considered in three prognostic groups. Figure 1 provides a rough schematic representation of the way most people apparently think about decision making in the care of the sick. Decisions in Group I concern all treatments known to be more or less effective. Those in Group II concern treatments of doubtful value in the larger picture of caring. Some people seek such treatments, even though the treatment may be harmful; others reject them even though earlier death may be the result (more about this presently). Decisions in Group III concern treatments that are futile. While some people seek such treatment because they want to believe in its effectiveness, most eventually become convinced that in the interest of kindness and common sense it should be rejected. Benefits from treatment fall as prognosis changes from good to poor. Economic costs, suffering, and inconvenience rise as prognosis worsens, slowly at first and then very rapidly as prognosis becomes bleak.

Group I decisions are the most common in day-to-day practice. Future life (prognosis) is expected to be reasonably good if treatment is adequate, patients cooperate, and the fates smile. Group III decisions

R. C. McMillan, H. T. Engelhardt, Jr., and S. F. Spicker (eds.),
Euthanasia and the Newborn, 273–289.
© 1987 by D. Reidel Publishing Company.

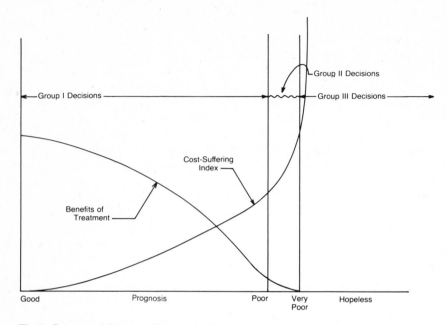

Fig. 1. Conceptual Scheme of Prognosis, Costs, Benefits, and Decision-Making.

concern treatment that is futile. Prognosis for life is hopeless. Death is near. Usually, rescue efforts are stopped to prevent hurting people, and comfort is provided by human caring and appropriate medications. When prognosis is at all promising or better on one hand or hopeless on the other, decision-making is relatively easy and controversy is rare.

Any thorough examination of decision-making in modern medicine draws attention to two conditions: technology has brought increased control over living and dying, thus broadening the range of choices; and people vary widely in their evaluation of these choices. As a result, Group II decisions have become more common and more visible, and we must learn to deal with them because sooner or later all people, more or less under the control of technologists, pass through a phase of very poor prognosis. But these decisions are problematic. Although the threat of death may vary, there is no hope for a healthy life. Sustaining life may be unkind to the patient, and it is usually costly in money and human effort; benefits of treatment are often rated as low or negative; human and economic resources, always limited, spent to sustain these lives, are not available to others who can benefit much from care known to be effective. This last condition, related to resource limitations, is central to the definition of tragic choice [6]. Some benefits for some people can only be had when other people are put at risk, are harmed, or are neglected.[2]. While some decison-makers may secretly or openly wish for death, people facing this state of affairs, particularly in acute care hospitals, have tended to adopt the comforting illusion that their decisions belong solidly in Group I where treatment is considered mandatory ([12], pp. 306–330). Then, most patients and families can maintain hope (but perhaps only its appearance), and health professionals can practice their art and justify their fees. Ambiguity, always painful, is bypassed; but so is responsibility. These conditions were at the root of the hospice movement, which encouraged recognition of approaching terminal illness and development of plans for acting accordingly. Doing otherwise was considered irresponsible. At the other extreme, a few decisionmakers may have supposed the prognosis was hopeless; but that can be a dangerous assumption in some circumstances. Thus, there is a predicament here. On one hand, if treatment is provided in all doubtful situations (and there is almost always doubt because absolute certainty is rarely poosible), we surely will harm many patients but achieve little or no gain. On the other hand, if we do not treat, we may harm persons because patients may be damaged from neglect and yet survive, or they may die when possibly they might have found additional life worthwhile. Freeman offers a convincing analysis of this dilemma [16].

In the remainder of this paper, we offer more details about a family-centered approach to these problems. We begin with some observations about the nature of persons and the social networks in which they live.

Medicine is inherently a moral or moral-technical profession because it seeks to achieve what is right and good for persons. It does this in a process of communications and acts in relationships with patients and persons close to patients. Being active, creative, and changing from birth to death, individuals live, suffer, and die differently. Since the values of persons differ, persons even with the same disease cannot be treated alike without great risk of harm. For the sick to be treated as persons, which has profound implications, patients and often those close to them must be full partners with health professionals in deciding and providing care.

Let us look more carefully at what persons are. Persons are 'I-thous'

[5], themselves influenced by others – a point we will develop presently. That is the crux of social life and the source of autonomy, the power or control persons have over their lives. It is also the source of most meaning, most nurture, and much healing (in the sense of feeling whole) in individual human experience. Social life is centered on each person's family of intimates and their advisors, which together we call 'moral community' or government of the family. Within each moral community, people learn about their family histories, teach religious beliefs and practices, allocate economic and other resources, make reproductive choices, rear children, celebrate life, endure hardship, suffer losses, bury and remember the dead, recover from bereavement and eventually die and thus become part of family history. As Isaiah Berlin noted, spiritual (inner or subjective and thus often irrational or unconscious) not political or public events "are the most real, the most immediate experience of human beings" ([2], p. 15). Autonomy is rooted primarily in moral communities, not in the general government of all. It is not something apart from the social fabric of life. Indeed, if an individual ignores relationships with others in his moral community, he is irresponsible. He will then harm both himself and others close to him. Moreover, he may harm seemingly remote others by mocking the best in the lives of people now dead or by creating adverse conditions for future people. Those who view autonomy as a state in which one does only self-serving things for immediate gains sooner or later must cope with the resulting alienation, a very distressing modern problem [13, 21, 25, 30, 31].

Autonomy is a characteristic of healthy persons. When we speak of particular persons, we ask: "Who am I?" or "Who are you?" We usually do not ask: "Who are we?" Our language tends to emphasize individuals as if there were little or no social reality within or between us. But when we try to answer a basic question like "Who am I?", we do so almost always in terms of social relations in family and work. The boundaries between us usually are so blurred that most individuals cannot logically be considered purely apart from others. Life is made possible and in fact is lived best in a dynamic, nurturing interdependence. When a child is born, major changes take place in the family. When a person dies, parts of others in that person's life die. Survivors are bereft (robbed) of part of themselves and hence must make major adjustments in their lives. If two people separate after long association, both are affected for better or worse by the void that is created. In life generally and in dependency particularly, there is strong support for the 'I-thou' idea presented by Martin Buber who wrote:

The attitude of man is twofold, in accordance with the twofold nature of the primary words which he speaks . . . One primary word is the combination *I-thou* . . . If *thou* is said, the *I* of the combination *I-thou* is said along with it . . . There is no *I* taken in itself, but only the *I* of the primary word *I-thou* ([5], p. 54).

In this view, each person is an individual, an 'I' who is embodied in a living organism. Also, each person is so related biologically and socially to significant others that there is a major other or 'thou' component within himself. (And, of course, he exists in significant others, too.) These others, the thous within each individual, vary with age and personal and social circumstances, but they are almost always there – an exception perhaps being extreme alienation. We live in, through, and with each other much of the time; and even conflict (usually rooted in ambivalence) may be a negative form of affirmation of this reality.

There is another set of terms that may help explain the meaning of I-thou. They are nature, the genetic patterns and tendencies within individuals, and nurture, which is supplied regularly from the physical and social environments. A child may be very active by nature and his parents may enhance or moderate this by nurture, thus creating the whole child as he is: the I (nature)-thou (nurture) combination. Also, since the child influences the parents, their I-thou identities change because the child becomes part of their thous. Since these influences are bilateral and usually profound, they account for the agonies and the ecstasies of family and friendship relationships, and they also explain why most great joys and sorrows are rooted in common intimate ties.

Buber coined 'I-thou' to emphasize the close association between intrapersonal and intimate interpersonal conditions. He coined 'I-it' to refer more or less to person-object relationships. In general, I-thou relationships between persons imply nurture, intimacy, and full reciprocity between persons. Responsibility and power are shared, though not necessarily equally, because people differ in their capacities and interests. Ethics is exoteric. All persons are moral agents. In decision-making, their consciences and passions count, as do their principles. Loyalty towards intimates is vital to social cohesion and to the enhancement of individual autonomy. Without loyalty at the intimate level, there is likely to be diminished loyalty in the larger social order. Of course, there are some exceptions to this.

I-it relationships between persons, on the other hand, imply that *I* (one person) controls *it* (another person or persons) or at least tries to. All or most power is held by *I*. Ethics is esoteric, understood and controlled by a few experts. People have unequal footing in moral discourse. The principles and conscience of *I* prevail over lesser *it* whose principles, reasons, and passions are not quite trusted. I-it relationships have a long history, Plato's presentation being most effective. The central belief is that ordinary people cannot be trusted to govern themselves. Stone claims this is "the oldest and hoariest idea of political philosophy" [37] in which power, not reason, is the primary rule of the game. Loyalty of *I* toward other persons is minimal because *I* behaves in accordance with the interests, principles, and beliefs of *I* – all quite Machiavellian. Note that in the care of the sick, health professionals may (sometimes necessarily) dominate decision-making but fail to ask whether their choices, though cloaked in benevolence, are really best for patients. In an almost unconscious way, I-it relationships subtly can replace I-thou relationships and yet ironically leave the mask of I-thou intact. There is here a curious detached benevolence, which is, however, not always benevolent. We believe Jay Katz has recently analyzed this problem superbly well [23].

The meaning here can be understood also in language used by Fuller, who describes two principles of human association: *shared commitment* and *legalistic associations* [17]. Shared commitment, corresponding closely to our use of I-thou, is concerned with conditions of mind and inner resolution as these bear on friendship, love, and family affairs where through intimacy the boundaries between individuals are blurred. We speak of a man and a woman becoming 'one' in their marriage union. If lucky, they often are one in body (sexual union) and mind (shared values). Generally, we acknowledge the importance of parent-child 'bonding' or attachment [24]. These relationships are extremely important because they provide the only known basis for nurture (vital in childhood and illness), a condition essential for healthier, longer life [3], and for the discovery of meaning in an otherwise alien world. Legalistic associations, corresponding closely to our use of I-it, set boundaries about rights and duties and are more formal, discrete, and individualistic. Legalistic associations commonly guided by law are blunt, quite intolerant of variations, creativity, and hence adaptation. Although benevolence is intended and is usually claimed by those in power, it is in fact coercive because it is removed, detached from the lives of those most intimately involved. Fuller contends, as does Schoeman, that as emphasis in human association shifts toward formal or legalistic modes, shared commitment and thus the source of meaning and nurture in life "tends to sink out of sight" [34]. Then, the most sacred meanings of life may be placed in peril. It may be recalled too that a plethora of laws to insure harmony is as tyrannical as anarchy [33].

Moral communities are as diverse as persons and their families, friends, and advisors. Also, particular decisions imply selective inclusion of persons. The choice to start a pregnancy may be made by two persons between sheets, or somewhere else. But such a choice is rarely made in a vacuum, and it has far-reaching social meaning, which with time or place differs greatly – a contrast being represented by Spain and China. The choice of a person to change jobs and move commonly involves several parties. Choices related to illness or symptoms usually involve the ill person, close family members or friends, and health advisors. Each time a health professional is consulted, he or she becomes a member of a client's moral community and accordingly is obliged as a caring person to share the quest of decision-making.

We summarize our main points. People are social beings (I-thous) by design, not by choice. Appreciation of this fact is essential for an understanding of nurture, autonomy, and the source of most human values. Social conditions particularly at the intimate level will determine the extent and nature of shared commitments and the quality of moral communities. Finally, since the meaning in hard or tragic choices (which Group II decisions tend to be) is centered primarily in shared commitments of persons in moral communities, individual moral communities should assume responsibility for examining issues, making the choices, and living with the consequences.

How should people in moral communities wrestle with dilemmas and tragic choices? We reach the following, perhaps oversimplified, answer. People rightly place themselves at the center of deliberations ([27], p. 169). That is the only way to cope with life responsibly. Subjective feelings of persons in respective moral communities concerning suffering and the meaning of life and death (all personal, philosophical, or religious issues) are important considerations along with objective facts about illness and prognosis with or without treatment. This does not assume, however, that people are the only value or in some situations even the highest value. This thorny issue is central in all Group II decisions because deep in human nature is the individual drive for survival, power, and mastery, a yearning for a safe place in this life or hereafter. This drive creates and sustains an 'anthropocentric' view of man in which man is seen as being above nature and entitled to control nature for his own interests and the glory of God. The idea here seems to be that God will (or a least should) protect all, but man first of all. Such a doctrine is at odds with the 'biocentric' view in which man is seen as part of nature where individual, social, and ecologic interests must be considered together as part of a really little understood whole [15]. In this second view, humility and awe in a deeply religious sense are appropriate though distressing attitudes. They foster learning and bridle pretense and arrogance. God's part is mysterious, and He, She, or It may or may not be able or willing to protect people the way people desire or believe.

Since life is complex and people vary greatly in their abilities, principles, goals, beliefs, needs, and desires, there is much ambiguity. That may be good because it is conducive to zest, freedom of choice, and adaptation [14], but ambiguity is agonizing, and agony and occasional error are the price to be paid for freedom; for freedom is essential for learning about or creating the deeper meanings of life often found in highest concentrations in extreme situations. Listening to suffering or dying persons or those close to them is instructive. People in the hospice movement, for example, can teach us much. Consider this comment by a 56-year old man who recently was found to have a fatal illness: "My highest, middle range, and lowest priorities used to be work, work, and work. I thought that was most rewarding because it gave me power. But it gave me little else. Now my priorities are family, friends, and work." We suggest this man has told us something about how he and perhaps others can best write the final chapter of their lives.

Unless those who wrestle with these decisions are blind, they will be aware that while they try to choose wisely, they may in fact choose foolishly or unjustly. However, usually they cannot know whether their choices are best. They can only try to choose what seems to be the better good or the lesser of evils, a humbling task indeed. Those who see only horror in the transition from flesh to dust (we have in mind here things like bed sores, wasting of flesh, cyanosis, gasping for breath, dehydration, starvation, and so on) and find only good meaning in dust-to-flesh renewal have much difficulty either as members of moral communities or onlookers, of which there are many in the vast, sometimes inhospitable arenas of caring. Failing to get beyond appearances, the real picture may be scrambled in their minds. Good may be labelled evil, and evil good. Such people willingly become moral busybodies, and in this age they get a lot of support and attention for that. But until people understand more clearly what is most likely good or evil in particular situations and are willing to assert this, there is no way to control busybodies or to measure how much good or evil they do. However, if the foregoing analysis is correct, great harm is done when moral communities are disrupted or destroyed; and it seems unlikely that much good comes from it.[3]

To make our position clearer, we draw attention to some problems of using technology in situations with very poor prognoses. Freeman, for example, offers a mixture of technological fixes [16]. On one hand, he advocates full freedom in applying technology in all doubtful situations, and we think he implies that professionals primarily, not patients or families, should decide what is doubtful. On the other hand, he offers a technological fix (euthanasia) as an exit from life if the first fix fails. By proceeding thus, we suspect that responsibility and all the priceless safety and learning associated with it in ambiguous situations may be bypassed because of an implicit pretense that moral ambiguity and agony can and will be addressed in largely technical deliberations or in situations quite remote from moral communities of patients. Both Dostoyevsky's Grand Inquisitor ([8], pp. 292–314) and Shaw's empiric doctors ([32], p. 58) remind us that illusion is alluring to everyone, particularly in times of stress. Perhaps healers most of all need to take these pitfalls into account.

Besides this, killing horrifies people even if it is benevolent in being causally related to saving lives or reducing suffering. People know how difficult the task of controlling human aggression is, vital for survival yet very problematic in human affairs. We believe that no effort should be made to change laws. In view of the difficulties legislators have even with right to die issues, we believe such an effort would be both futile and destructive, and the consequences of such changes (if they could be made) are very unclear. It seems to us that the ambiguities of decision-making in situations of poor prognosis can be managed best in moral communities where deliberations are, appropriately, mostly a private matter, secret and arbitrary in some degree as befits respective unique situations.

Another problem concerns the proposed use of ethics committees. If these are used to educate, set general policies for making tragic choices, and nurture and protect agonizing moral communities, they might serve the public well. However, there are many problems if they, like casuists, set policies too specifically or are used as decision-making bodies as the Department of Health and Human Services fully intends [7]. Committees do not and cannot understand particular tragic situations, because people on committees do not and cannot enter fully into the subjectivity and hence the protective agony of patients and those close to them. Committees are untested in the roles suggested for them; they are subject to the evils of 'groupthink' [22] and they may readily come under institutional pressures such as the financial ones associated with recently imposed DRG (diagnostic related groups) reimbursement policies in the United States.

The approach we propose fixes primary professional responsibility with all its agonies and ecstasies on *the* responsible (singular) physician, though at times others such as nurses or social workers will play particularly central roles. (Duff has stated the reasons for this assertion elsewhere [9].) This plan, through development of trust, permits communications about complex mixtures of parental feelings (love, hate, guilt, commitment, and so on), which relate to puzzling out what decisions are reasonable and practical. Parents will not share their most intimate feelings with the world because they know that many persons would then abuse them unfairly. But, they will reveal secrets gradually to one or a few persons whom they come to trust. In this way, it is possible to discover or create inner strength, which is essential in making and carrying out good decisions. Then, consistent with loyalty to shared commitments and moral communities, moral issues in patient care should be decided together by patients, intimate others (usually family), and advising health professionals generally in that order of decisional power. All this is in harmony with the best traditions of caring as we understand them [26]. Even if there are a few errors, however those are defined, is there a better way? From our combined total of more than 60 years as clinicians and researchers in this field, from our close association with dying relatives or friends, and from our personal experiences with life-threatening illnesses, our answer to this question is a firm no.

There is another regrettably common problem. Health professionals tend to think of patients as 'cases'. Whenever 'thinging' [20] (referring to people as things) like this takes place, patients and families are very upset because they feel violated, reduced from the status of real live people with an unique history and special ordering of values to a thing, like some object that malfunctions and needs fixing in accordance with the rules of those who have fixes for things. 'Thinging' is widespread because it affords health professionals a partial escape from the pain of ambiguity and from the anxieties generated in them when, close up, they witness human suffering or dying they cannot prevent. This escape permits health professionals to get their work done (which is important) mostly on their own terms (which as Katz has shown is extremely problematic [23]). At the same time, patients and families feel dependent, usually too fearful to challenge those helping persons who offend. The approach we propose will avoid most of these problems. We admit, however, that we have a long way to go. But that is no reason to discard good vision. Indeed, it is reason to cherish and nurture vision as we explore ethical unknowns, like (with good results) we have explored biological ones.

If moral communities are to function as we propose, they need those freedoms now too often extinguished by the efforts of moralistic aggressors [28], perhaps a harsh description but one which regrettably we are obliged to use in the interest of accuracy. These aggressors are insensitive even to the well-considered moral views of others. They are captivated by benevolent-appearing ideologies, which give them an escape from the agonies of ambiguity. Then, while they are no longer free men or women, they feel completely free to use or misuse laws and government to impose their morality on everyone [7, 18, 25]. We bring up this current issue here because we want to suggest that those who advocate making euthanasia licit are very likely to give support to both moralistic aggressors and morally banal health professionals. These two groups in quite different ways urgently seek freedom from the pain of ambiguity. They often support one another, and these two modes of relief (rigid moral ideology and quite blind commitment to technology) sometimes are combined in the same persons who then wear a double cloak of benevolence but in fact are non-caring.

The approach of moral communities as we have outlined it may quietly bypass moral aggressors and improve the caring of health professionals generally. Indeed, the latter may be the chief means of achieving the former. Holder has found that courts consistently support moral communities (or families) in ambiguous situations [19] and both state and federal courts in the case of Baby Jane Doe have supported this policy. It seems to us this support is appropriate; and recognition of this and acting on it are overdue.

By using the examples of hospice, self care, and moral community as we have described it, we may arrive at a policy that directs us to address ambiguity responsibly by facing agony where it is most acutely felt in order to secure the protections only it can confer. Out of this crucible, we may find the strength to assert the freedom to make what we feel deeply are prudent, though sometimes tragic, choices. Then, the tyranny of ideologies may be deflated as it is replaced by better, perhaps sacred, things. But it must be remembered that occasionally the sacred is blurred with the obscene and that some error is inevitable. That is part of the tragedy of life, and rejection of that tragedy will only add to the senseless suffering in the world, while acceptance provides the opportunity for hope and even joy through learning and creating.

In brief, practical terms, we suggest that moral communities decide: (1) whether, in doubtful situations, to use technology freely and fully or not at all; (2) how far to go if technology is used; (3) when and how to stop rescue attempts; and (4) how to care for people suffering with extremely poor prognoses. In every step, ambiguities abound. We should honor them, suffer with them, and do our best to act wisely, particularly when we feel compelled to make that irreversible choice of death. Finally, we should review the medical, nursing and other human results of all Group II decisions whether the choice was for continued treatment or death. Only in this way can the science of medicine inform the art of medicine and thus give better guidance to future choices.

In the overall scheme of care, then, health professionals should try to persuade their clients to accept treatment when prognosis with treatment is improved and life seems really promising. That is an easy task. They should try to persuade their clients to forego treatment (but yet continue caring) when treatment is futile and prognosis is hopeless. That is a more difficult task, often requiring passage of time. When prognosis is such that the benefits of treatment are much in doubt and treatment may cause more harm than non-treatment, clients should be invited to wrestle with these ambiguities and decide with professional advisors what choices best fulfill their duties to the sick and their loyalties to principles of justice, utility, and possibly other values. Brandt [4] has stated some general guides that seem reasonable and that people frequently use in any case when facing their own trials with Group II decisions.

There is one other difficulty to be considered. Withholding treatment sometimes will result in protracted, miserable living, which in the minds of many is a far greater evil than death. In dealing with this predicament, we can see no kind or caring way out, except to ask moral communities one by one to do their best to choose wisely and to carry out what they believe they can document as the most caring behavior, which may include choosing death and presiding over dying. If moral communities are to do this, however, they must have reasonable protection from those who would gladly misuse homicide laws to force all others to live and die by their morality.

We said we were strongly opposed to making euthanasia licit, and yet in some sense we advocate it. We hold to this view because as a matter of social policy we believe there is a vast difference between making the choice of death licit by legislation and making the choice of death a matter of caring. The former way might place all caring in peril; the latter should bring major improvements in caring and perhaps substantial reductions in economic costs. What might be done to put reasonable legal protections in place is beyond the scope of this paper. However, we must point out that current law or at least the way it is used or abused prohibits serious discussion of important caring alternatives, often results in people hiding acts that are thought to be caring but have a bad appearance, and finally creates conditions in which repeated, oppressive episodes of public notoriety must be endured along with heavy burdens of grief, sorrow, and economic expense. It seems to us that a caring profession should aim for something better.

Many persons will not be pleased with this approach, and they may offer solutions (particularly, in this era, technological ones) alleged to be superior. To them we say: speak as you wish, but do not coerce, for you cannot really know how devastating detached benevolence can be when it is so blind to conditions of inner lives of persons in moral communities. Three years ago, one of us used 'medical Vietnam' (a metaphor suggested by a chaplain) in referring to ideologically guided technology [10]. Thus far, no one has suggested that such usage was unfitting.

In conferences, classes, and other forums, people can throw light on the dilemmas and tragic choices we have been discussing; and that is very useful. But no one remote from the lives of involved persons can decide what is best in specific situations. Such decisions, if they are to be truly caring in the sense of treating people not as means but as ends, must arise in large part from persons in respective situations. That is a sobering but realistic comment on the limits of caring by remote persons. It follows that we all should take great care to avoid what we suspect is a very common alienating condition described by Pappenheim:

> We do not relate to the other person as a whole or to the event as a whole, but we isolate the one part which is important to us and remain more or less remote observers of the rest. . . . The person who thus splits the real into parts becomes divided in his own self. . . . We seem to be caught in a frightening contradiction. In order to assert ourselves as individuals, we relate only to those phases of reality which seem to promote the attainment of our objectives and we remain divorced from the rest of it. But the further we drive this separation, the deeper grows the rift within ourselves ([30], pp. 12–13).

This pessimistic observation emphasizes that making prudent choices requires not only better vision about the human condition; it also demands courage to deal more satisfactorily with the saddening ideological nonsense of our times.[4] It seems we have lost our way. Since we resist accepting tragedy as part of human experience, we fail too often to deal with tragedy, and thus we cannot discover and adopt the least tragic choice in situations where only tragic choices exist.

Yale University School of Medicine
New Haven, Connecticut, U.S.A.

and

University of Aberdeen
Aberdeen, Scotland.

ACKNOWLEDGEMENT

* The opinions presented in this paper are strictly those of the authors. They do not represent the policies or practices of any institution with which the authors have been or are affiliated. We join in writing this paper because we have found that while political conditions on opposite sides of the Atlantic Ocean are different, the basic problems are the same. Selected philosophical portions of this chapter were first developed in Chapter 9 of a manuscript (Children, Families, and Pediatricians by Duff and others) as yet unpublished. Partial support for preparation of this chapter was provided by the Seymour L. Lustman Fund.

NOTES

[1] The policy we suggest in this chapter for deciding care of severely defective infants was first formulated from earlier research concerning the care of adults with poor prognoses [12]. We believe this policy is applicable to the care of sick or handicapped persons of all ages. It is needed more and more as medical technology is used increasingly to control living and dying. Sooner or later, all people have to pass through a phase of very poor prognosis (see Figure 1). Most of us will pass slowly in a more or less controlled way. We suggest that common sense and ordinary feelings about decency be taken into account in exercising that control.

[2] The argument that society must expand resources or reallocate them to respond to particular felt needs has merit. But societal resources will always be limited, and allocation of these necessarily will be decided in untidy, occasionally capricious political processes. This is so because people believe there are competing, meritorious interests about which they feel strongly. In light of this observation, both the American Academy of Pediatrics [1] and the Department of Health and Human Services [7] misguide us all when they ignore resource limits in setting policy. Beyond this, the Reagan Administration demonstrates a curious hypocrisy in insisting on rescue of practically all handicapped persons while cutting funds to care for them.

[3] The Stinsons offer a dramatic illustration of these problems [36].

[4] Shelp argues that courage particularly in the form of a 'sustained presence' is a neglected virtue in the patient-physician relationship. He notes that both its presence and absence may be ignored [35]. Thus, inappropriate timidity is not identified as something to be discouraged, and appropriate courage is not recognized and rewarded – hardly sound policy.

BIBLIOGRAPHY

1. American Academy of Pediatrics: 1984, 'Joint Policy Statement, Principles of Treatment of Disabled Infants', *Pediatrics* **73**, 559–560.
2. Berlin, I.: 1953, *The Hedgehog and the Fox, An Essay on Tolstoy's View of History*, Simon and Schuster, New York.
3. Berkman, L. F. and Breslow, L.: 1983, *Health and Ways of Living*, Oxford University Press, New York.
4. Brandt, R.: 1987, 'Public Policy and Life and Death Decisions Regarding Defective Newborns', in this volume, pp. 191–208.
5. Buber, M.: 1970, *I and Thou*, W. Kaufman (trans.), Charles Scribner's Sons, New York.
6. Calabresi, G. and Bobbitt, P.: 1978, *Tragic Choices*, Norton and Company, New York.
7. Department of Health and Human Services, Office of the Secretary: 1984, 'Nondiscrimination on the Basis of Handicap; Procedures and Guidelines Relating to Health Care for Handicapped Infants', *Federal Register* **49**, 1622–1654.
8. Dostoyevsky, F.: 1950, *The Brothers Karamazov*, C. Garnett (trans.), Modern Library, New York.
9. Duff, R. S.: 1979, 'Guidelines for Deciding Care of Critically Ill or Dying Patients', *Pediatrics* **64**. 17–23.

10. Duff, R. S.: 1981, 'Counseling Families and Deciding Care of Severely Defective Children: A Way of Coping with "Medical Vietnam"', *Pediatrics* **67**, 315–320.
11. Duff, R. S. and Campbell, A. G. M.: 1973, 'Moral and Ethical Dilemmas in the Special Care Nursery', *New England Journal of Medicine* **289**, 890–894.
12. Duff, R. S. and Hollingshead, A. B.: 1968, *Sickness and Society*, Harper and Row, New York.
13. Durkheim, E.: 1951, *Suicide*, Free Press, New York.
14. Eiseley, L. C.: 1957, *The Immense Journey*, Random House, New York.
15. Elder, F.: 1969, 'Two Doctrines of Nature', in D. Cutler (ed.), *The Religious Situation*, Beacon Press, Boston, Massachusetts, pp. 12–21.
16. Freeman, J.: 1987, 'If Euthanasia were Licit, Could Lives be Saved?', in this volume, pp. 153–168.
17. Fuller, L.: 1969, 'Two Principles of Human Association', in J. R. Pennock and J. W. Chapman (eds.), *Nomon XI: Voluntary Associations*, Atherton Press, New York, pp. 22–34.
18. Geertz, C.: 1964, 'Ideology as a Cultural System', in D. A. Apter (ed.), *Ideology and Discontent*, Free Press, New York, pp. 47–76.
19. Holder, A.: 1983, 'Parents, Courts, and Refusal of Treatment', *Journal of Pediatrics* **103**, 515–521.
20. Howard, J. *et al.*: 1977, 'Humanizing Health Care: The Implications of Technology, Centralization, and Self-care', *Medical Care* **15** suppl., 11–26.
21. Insel, P. M. and Moos, R. H.: 1974, 'The Social Environment', in P. Insel and R. H. Moos (eds.), *Health and the Social Environment*, D. C. Heath and Company, Lexington, Massachusetts, pp. 3–12.
22. Janis, I. L.: 1972, *Victims of Groupthink*, Houghton Mifflin Company, Boston, Massachusetts.
23. Katz, J.: 1984, *The Silent World of Doctor and Patient*, Free Press, New York.
24. Klaus, M. H. and Kennell, J. H.: 1982, *Parent-Infant Bonding*, C. V. Mosby Company, St. Louis, Missouri.
25. MacIntyre, A.: 1981, *After Virtue*, University of Notre Dame Press, Notre Dame, Indiana.
26. Mayeroff, M.: 1971, *On Caring*, Harper and Row, New York.
27. Morison, E.: 1974, *From Know-how to Nowhere, The Development of American Technology*, Basic Books, New York.
28. Morison, R. S.: 1981, 'Bioethics After Two Decades', *Hastings Center Report* **11**, 8–12.
29. Murray, T. H.: 1984, 'On the Care of Imperiled Newborns', *Hastings Center Report* **14**, 24.
30. Pappenheim, F.: 1959, *The Alienation of Modern Man*, Monthly Review Press, New York.
31. Rilke, R. M.: *Fifty Selected Poems*, C. F. MacIntyre (trans.), University of California Press, Berkeley, California.
32. Shaw, B.: 1954, *The Doctor's Dilemma*, Penguin Books, Baltimore, Maryland.
33. Sisk, J. P.: 1977, 'The Tyranny of Harmony', *The American Scholar* **46**, 193–205.
34. Schoeman, F.: 1980, 'Rights of Children, Rights of Parents, and the Moral Basis of the Family', *Ethics* **91**, 6–19.

35. Shelp, E. E.: 1984, 'Courage: A Neglected Virtue in the Patient-Physician Relationship', *Social Science and Medicine* **18**, 351–360.
36. Stinson, R. and Stinson, P.: 1983, *The Long Dying of Baby Andrew*, Little, Brown and Company, Boston, Massachusetts.
37. Stone, I. F.: 1977, 'Plato's Ideal Bedlam, Another Look at Those Philosopher Kings', *Harper's Magazine* **262**, 66–72.

APPENDIX

MARY ANN GARDELL AND H. TRISTRAM ENGELHARDT, JR.

THE BABY DOE CONTROVERSY:
AN OUTLINE OF SOME POINTS IN ITS DEVELOPMENT

The Baby Doe controversy is a complicated one. There are many elements to the drama: judicial, legislative, and regulatory. We have selected some of the high points below in order to give the reader some reference points. The outline is not meant to be exhaustive. In fact, it focuses on only some of the court cases and the regulations and leaves out of consideration the discussion in the medical literature, which has been extensive and continuing.

I. INFANT DOE. On April 9, 1982, a baby boy known to the public as 'Infant Doe' was born in Bloomington, Indiana, with Down's syndrome and tracheoesophageal fistula. The infant's parents, believing that their child's conditions were so severe that survival would not be in his best interest, refused to authorize the surgery required to feed the baby by mouth. Bloomington Hospital sought authorization to perform the surgery. However, the Indiana Courts upheld the parents' treatment refusal decision.[1] Infant Doe died on April 15, 1982. On November 7, 1983, the U.S. Supreme Court[2] refused on grounds of mootness to review the Indiana rulings, thus leaving the lower court's ruling intact.

II. NOTICE TO HEALTH CARE PROVIDERS (May 18, 1982). On the strength of the *Bloomington* case, President Reagan[3] instructed Richard Schweiker, then Secretary of the U.S. Department of Health and Human Services (DHHS), to notify recipient hospitals (approx. 7000) that "[i]t is unlawful under Sec. 504 of the Rehabilitation Act of 1973[4] for a recipient of Federal financial assistance to withhold from a handicapped infant nutritional sustenance or medical or surgical treatment required to correct a life-threatening correction if (1) the withholding is based on the fact that the infant is handicapped, or (2) the handicap does not render the treatment or nutritional sustenance medically contraindicated."[5] Noncompliance with this notice was to be met with the loss of federal funds.

R. C. McMillan, H. T. Engelhardt, Jr., and S. F. Spicker (eds.),
Euthanasia and the Newborn, 293–299.
© *1987 by D. Reidel Publishing Company.*

III. BABY DOE REGULATIONS I (March 7, 1983). In emergency regulations, the DHHS required that, as of March 22, 1983, the substance of the May 1982 notice must be conspicuously displayed on a 17 inches by 14 inches announcement in every delivery ward, maternity ward, pediatric ward, nursery, and neonatal intensive care unit. Included in the notice was a toll-free, 24-hour 'hotline' number that any individual suspecting discriminatory care among handicapped newborns could call. DHHS officials (i.e., the 'Baby Doe Squad') were given the authority to take immediate action to protect infants. This action included on-site investigations of any reported case, including the patient's medical records.[6]

IV. AMERICAN ACADEMY OF PEDIATRICS V. HECKLER (1983). The American Academy of Pediatrics, along with the National Association of Children's Hospitals and Related Institutions and Children's Hospital National Medical Center, brought suit against DHHS and its new Secretary, Margaret Heckler, to enjoin the 'Interim Final Rule' on March 18, 1983, four days before it was to become effective.[7] On April 14, 1983, U.S. District Court Judge Gerhard Gesell found the regulations in violation of the Administrative Procedure Act because they were issued without consideration of, for example, the risks due to the 'Baby Doe Squad's' disruptive actions, the rights and preferences of parents, the ambiguity of 'current medical standards', the scope and applicability of Section 504, and the mandatory procedures for advance notice of and public comment on the rules.

V. BABY DOE REGULATIONS I: REVISED (July 5, 1983). Taking into consideration some of the concerns raised by Judge Gesell, the DHHS revised the March 1983 regulations, publishing the revisions in July 1983.[8] Except for certain procedural changes (e.g., permitting the size of the posted notice to be smaller, 8 ½ inches by 11 inches, shifting investigative responsibilities from the Federal to the State level, and allowing for a 60-day comment period on the revised rules), the 'revised' July regulations were virtually unchanged.

VI. BABY JANE DOE. On October 11, 1983, a baby girl with hydrocephalic spina bifida was born in Port Jefferson, New York, and transferred to the Stonybrook University Hospital. Her parents, wishing that she be treated conservatively, decided against authorizing surgery. The case was brought to the State Court's attention by an out-of-state lawyer, who successfully sought the appointment of a guardian *ad litem* for the infant and an order directing the hospital to perform the surgery. Judge Leonard D. Wexler of the New York State Appellate Court reversed the lower court's decision, holding that the parents' decision was based on responsible medical decisionmaking. In addition, the hospital could not be held responsible for discriminatory care since they were simply carrying out the expressed wishes of the patient's parents. On procedural grounds, the New York Court of Appeals affirmed this decision.[9] The Justice Department then sought through federal court to gain access to the treatment records, but the Second Circuit Court examined the legislative history of the 1974 Rehabilitation Act and decided that it never had been intended to apply to clinical decision-making situations.[10]

VII. BABY DOE REGULATIONS II (January 12, 1984). Following the consideration of some 16,739 responses to the July rules, the DHHS published in January, 1984, its final rules.[11] Three significant revisions are notable: (1) the notice now required that "nourishment and medically beneficial treatment (as determined with respect to reasonable medical judgments) should not be withheld from handicapped infants solely on the basis of the presence of anticipated mental or physical impairments"; (2) the required size of the notice was again decreased (to 5 inches by 7 inches) and the location of the notice was permitted to be "where nurses . . . will see it"; and (3) the rules encouraged hospitals to set up an Infant Care Review Committee charged with the responsibilities of (a) developing policy; (b) reviewing ongoing cases, and (c) reviewing former problematic cases. These regulations were to take general effect on February 13, 1984.

VIII. PUBLIC LAW 98–457: AMENDMENTS TO THE CHILD ABUSE PREVENTION AND TREATMENT ACT (October 9, 1984). In order to regulate clinical decisionmaking in neonatalogy, Congress sought another path of action, namely, to modify the definition of child abuse so that state child abuse agencies could then be held responsible for initiating legal proceedings in cases involving the withholding of care from handicapped infants. Two different bills[12] proposing amendments to federal legislation regarding child abuse[13] were passed. The final version was approved at a joint House-Senate conference on October 9, 1984, and signed by President Reagan on October 11, 1984.[14] According to this legislation, withholding medically indicated treatment is to be understood as "the failure to respond to the infant's life-threatening conditions by providing treatment (including appropriate nutrition, hydration, and medication) when, in the treating physician's or physicians' reasonable medical judgment, (a) the infant is chronically and irreversibly comatose; (b) the provision of such treatment would (i) merely prolong dying, (ii) not be effective in ameliorating or correcting all of the infant's life-threatening conditions; or (iii) otherwise be futile in terms of the survival of the infant; or (c) the provision of such treatment itself under such circumstances would be inhumane." All state child protective agencies were to have by October 9, 1985, mechanisms for investigating and handling reports of child abuse in the hospital setting. In addition, DHHS regulations elaborating this point were to follow (see IX and X).

IX. CHILD ABUSE AND NEGLECT PREVENTION AND TREATMENT PROGRAM: PROPOSED RULES (December 10, 1984). Based on Public Law 98–487, DHHS published in December, 1984, the interim final rules[15] and the guidelines[16] for states' use in developing child abuse programs designed to handle cases of discriminatory care toward handicapped infants.

X. CHILD ABUSE AND NEGLECT PREVENTION AND TREATMENT PROGRAM: FINAL RULES (April 15, 1985). The final regulations remain for the most part unchanged from previous formulations of the rules.[17] Three exceptions are notable. First, unlike the proposed rules, the final ones do not include a series of detailed medical situations and treatment alternatives that were to be used as case study examples to guide clinical practitioners in their practices. Second, those definitions that were the focus of unresolved debate were removed from the text of the final regulations to an attached explanatory appendix. These definitions include, for example, those for the terms "withholding of medically indicated treatment", "life-threatening conditions", "merely prolong dying", and "virtually futile". Third, it was decided that the word 'imminent' be deleted from the final rules because of a failure to agree on its meaning and use.

The final regulations became effective on May 15, 1985. States were to have in effect measures to handle child abuse cases in the health care setting by October 9, 1985.[18]

XI. EXCERPTS FROM THE APRIL 15, 1985, REGULATIONS. Below is offered a selection from the regulations that came into effect as of May 15, 1985. The interpretative sections, as well as other sections, are omitted.

1340.15 Services and treatment for disabled infants.

(a) *Purpose*. The regulations in this section implement certain provisions of the Child Abuse Amendments of 1984, including Section 4(b)(2)(K) of the Child Abuse Prevention and Treatment Act governing the protection and care of disabled infants with life-threatening conditions.

(b) *Definitions*. (1) The term 'medical neglect' means the failure to provide adequate medical care in the context of the definitions of 'child abuse and neglect' in Section 3 of the Act and 1340.2(d) of this part. The term 'medical neglect' includes, but is not limited to, the withholding of medically indicated treatment from a disabled infant with a life-threatening condition.

(2) The term 'withholding of medically indicated treatment' means the failure to respond to the infant's life-threatening conditions by providing treatment (including appropriate nutrition, hydration, and medication), which, in the treating physician's (or physicians') reasonable medical judgment, will be most likely to be effective in ameliorating or correcting all such conditions, except that the term does not include the failure to provide treatment (other than appropriate nutrition, hydration, or medication) to an infant when, in the treating physician's (or physicians') reasonable medical judgment any of the following circumstances apply:

(i) The infant is chronically and irreversibly comatose:

(ii) The provision of such treatment would merely prolong dying, not be effective in ameliorating or correcting all of the infant's life-threatening conditions, or otherwise be futile in terms of the survival of the infant; or

(iii) The provision of such treatment would be virtually futile in terms of the survival of the infant and the treatment itself under such circumstances would be inhumane.

(3) Following are definitions of terms used in paragraph (b)(2) of this section:

(i) The term 'infant' means an infant less than one year of age. The reference to less than one year of age shall not be construed to imply that treatment should be changed or discontinued when an infant reaches one year of age, or to affect or limit any existing protections available under State laws regarding medical neglect of children over one year of age. In addition to their applicability to infants less than one year of age, the standards set forth in paragraph (b)(2) of this section should be consulted thoroughly in the evaluation of any issue of medical neglect involving an infant older than one year of age who has been continuously hospitalized since birth, who was born extremely prematurely, or who has a long-term disability.

(ii) The term 'reasonable medical judgment' means a medical judgment that would be made by a reasonably prudent physician, knowledgeable about the case and the treatment possibilities with respect to the medical conditions involved.[19]

XII. OTIS R. BOWEN, SECRETARY OF HEALTH AND HUMAN SERVICES, PETITIONER V. AMERICAN HOSPITAL ASSOCIATION ET AL. (June 9, 1986). The court, by a vote of 5 to 3, held that the Baby Doe regulations of January 12, 1984, and their ancestors were without legislative authority. Justices Stevens, Marshall, Blackmun, and Powell wrote an opinion for the plurality with Justice Burger concurring in their judgment. Justice Rehnquist took no part in the consideration of the case. In their opinions, Stevens *et al.* held that "A hospital's withholding of treatment when no parental consent has been given cannot violate Sec. 504, for without the consent of the parents or a surrogate decisionmaker the infant is neither 'otherwise qualified' for treatment nor has been denied care 'solely by reason of his handicap.' Indeed, it would almost certainly be a tort as a matter of state law to operate on an infant without parental consent."[20] Though the Court held that "Section 504 does not authorize the Secretary to give unsolicited advice either to parents, to hospitals, or to state officials who are faced with difficult treatment decisions concerning handicapped children",[21] it did not in any way address or invalidate the amendments to the child abuse prevention and treatment act of October 9, 1984, and the rules made on the basis of the act. See VIII, IX, and X. In short, major restrictions still remain in place regarding the freedom of parents to make medical decisions in the best interests of their children.

Baylor College of Medicine
Houston, Texas, U.S.A.

NOTES

[1] The court records in this case are sealed and the decision is unreported.

[2] Doe v. Bloomington Hospital, Indiana Ct. App. (Feb. 3, 1983), *cert. denied*, 104 S.Ct. 394 (1983).

[3] President's Directive of April 30, 1982.

[4] Rehabilitation Act of 1973, Public Law No. 93–112, Title V., Section 504, 87 Stat. (1973), as amended, 29 U.S.C. 794 (1976).

[5] Department of Health and Human Services, Office of Civil Rights: 1982, 'Notice to Health Care Providers', *Federal Register* 47 (May 18), 26027.

[6] Department of Health and Human Services: 1983, 'Nondiscrimination on the Basis of Handicap, Interim Final Rule', *Federal Register* 48 (March 7), 9630–9632.

[7] American Academy of Pediatrics v. Heckler, 561 F. Supp. 395 (D.D.S. 1983).

[8] Department of Health and Human Services: 1983, 'Nondiscrimination on the Basis of Handicaps Relating to Health Care for Handicapped Infants; Proposed Rules', *Federal Register* 48 (July 5), 30846–30852.

[9] Weber v. Stony Brook Hospital, 60 N.Y.2d 208, 456 N.E.2d 1186, 469 N.Y.S.2d 65 (1983).

[10] U.S. v. University Hospital of New York, 575 F. Supp. 607 (E.D.N.Y. 1983), *aff'd*, 729 F.2d 144 (2d Cir. 1984).

[11] Department of Health and Human Services: 1984, 'Nondiscrimination on the Basis of Handicap; Procedures and Guidelines Relating to Health Care for Handicapped Infants', Final Rules', *Federal Register* 49 (January 12), 1622–1654.

[12] H. R. 1904 (S. 1003), 98th Congress (1984).

[13] Child Abuse Prevention and Treatment Act, Pub. L. 93–247, 42 U.S.C. 5111 *et seq.* (1976).

[14] Child Abuse Prevention and Treatment and Adoption Reform Act Amendments of 1984, Pub. L. 98–457, 42 U.S.C. 5101 *et seq.* (1984).

[15] Department of Health and Human Services: 1984, 'Child Abuse and Neglect Prevention and Treatment Program; Proposed Rule', *Federal Register* 49 (December 10), 48160–48173.

[16] Department of Health and Human Services: 1985, 'Interim Model Guidelines for Health Care Providers to Establish Infant Care Review Committees: Notice', *Federal Register* 50 (December 10), 48170.

[17] Department of Health and Human Services: 1985, 'Child Abuse and Neglect Prevention and Treatment Program; Final Rule', *Federal Register* 50 (April 15), 14878–14901.

[18] Stevenson, D. K. *et al.*: 1986, 'The "Baby Doe" Rule', *Journal of the American Medical Association* 225 (April 11), 1909–1912.

[19] See Note 18, pp. 14887–14888.

[20] Otis R. Bowen. Secretary of Health and Human Services, Petitioner v. American Hospital Association *et al.*, Supr. Ct. 84–1529 (June 9, 1986), p. 19.

[21] *Ibid.*, p. 35.

MEDICAL SELF-REGULATION OF BABY DOE CASES IN THE FEDERAL REPUBLIC OF GERMANY

Clinical-moral decision-making regarding the treatment or non-treatment of defective newborns is a challenge in all developed countries having sophisticated medical technology. The structure for decision-making in the Federal Republic of Germany is quite different from the situation in the United States, as highlighted by U.S. federal guidelines for treatment, which place treatment decisions under child protection and child abuse laws, and the regulating role of hospital infant care review committees [3, 8].

In the absence of highly emotional public and legal debates regarding cases like Baby Doe, Baby Jane, and Baby Fae, decision-making has remained within the traditional domain of the physician. There is no special legislation or regulation, nor are there infant care review committees, or specially appointed committees to make, share, or supervise clinical decision-making. The recently published Recommendations of the Deutsche Gesellschaft für Medizinrecht are very close to the actual day-to-day decision-making processes in neonatal intensive care units. These Recommendations offer a promising framework for moral-clinical decision-making through balancing the interests of the newborn, the mother, the family, society, and the medical profession [4].

Among the major moral positions the Recommendations take are the following.

1. *Protection of human life* and its dignity are established as having the highest moral and political value. The life of a child has the same value and is due the same protection as the life of an adult. No reference has been made to the person/non-person debate, which has arisen in the U.S. [5]. It is noted that differentiating between higher and lower values of human life, its physical and intellectual capacities or usefulness, would be contrary not only to natural law but also to German constitutional law, especially Sections 1, 2 and 7, which were responses to the Nazi attempt to judge the worthiness of human life.

R. C. McMillan, H. T. Engelhardt, Jr., and S. F. Spicker (eds.),
Euthanasia and the Newborn, 301–306.
© 1987 *by D. Reidel Publishing Company.*

2. *Decisions to forego treatment* are part of the process of ethical clinical decision-making, which should not restrict itself to considering technical possibilities (Section 4). As Schara has observed: "Intensive care aims at supporting the body so as to reestablish organ functions. If such a restitution of function is not possible, a fact that normally will be established within a short period of treatment, then intensive care not only is no longer mandated, it is no longer permitted" ([7], p. 117). The Roman Catholic theologian Boeckle defines the situation in perinatal intensive care more specifically: "There are no moral arguments for infanticide that could be substantiated by pediatric disease. However, there are cases in which we should postnatally not prolong life artificially by means of surgery or intensive care, and should prenatally in comparable cases after thorough prenatal diagnosis not require the continuation of pregnancy" ([1], p. 24).

3. *Case-by-case decision-making* is required. Only a few of the most severe handicaps are mentioned, for which non-treatment would usually be recommended (Section 5). This is in line with a rule established by the neonatologist von Loewenich: "Decisions to continue treatment or to let die may not be generalized; they have to be made on a case-by-case basis" ([6], p. 203; cf. [2]).

4. *Parental involvement* in decision-making is required. If consent for the indicated treatment is unattainable or if there is a conflict between the parents, the court for guardianship [Vormundschaftsgericht], a specialized court consisting of federally appointed lawyers, will have to share decision-making.

The contrast between German self-regulation and U.S. governmental regulation invites the analysis and assessment of the values underlying these different approaches to neonatal treatment decisions.

Kennedy Institute of Ethics
Georgetown University
Washington, D.C., U.S.A.

and

Institut für Philosophie
Ruhr-Universität
Bochum, F.R.G.

ADDENDUM

LIMITS ON THE DUTY TO PROVIDE MEDICAL CARE FOR SERIOUSLY DEFECTIVE NEWBORNS [4]

Recommendations of the German Society for Medical Law, developed at the First Conference of Experts, held at Einbeck, Germany, June 27–29, 1986.

I

1. Human life is a value of the highest order within our legal and moral framework.

Its protection is a public duty (Article 2, Section 2, Basic Law of the Federal Republic), its maintenance is a primary medical task.

2. To rank the importance of protecting life according to social value, usefulness, bodily condition, or mental capacity violates the moral law and the Constitution.

II

Death is defined, according to both medical and judicial opinion, as the irreversible cessation of brain function (brain death).

The duty to treat ends with the determination of the death of the newborn.

III

The intentional shortening of a newborn's life by means of active intervention violates the commitments of the medical and judicial professions.

IV

1. The physician is required to do that which is best and most effective in maintaining life and mitigating or eliminating existing deficiencies.

2. The physician's duty to treat is not determined solely by what treatment is medically possible.

It is also to be determined by taking into consideration human-ethical criteria of judgment and the physician's mandate to heal.

3. Therefore, there are cases in which the physician must not employ all means of medical treatment, especially the establishment and maintenance of vital functions and/or massive surgical intervention.

V

These conditions apply whenever, from the standpoint of actual medical experience,

1. life cannot be maintained for any length of time, but rather certain death will be postponed, e.g., in the case of severe dysrhaphia-syndrome [incomplete closure of the primary neural tube] or inoperable heart defects;

2. in spite of treatment it is determined that the newborn will never have the possibility of communicating with his environment, e.g., severe microcephaly, very severe brain damage;

3. the newborn's vital functions can be maintained for any length of time only by means of intensive medical intervention, e.g., breathing difficulties without possibility of correction, loss of kidney function without possibility of correction.

VI

1. Treatment falls within the realm of the physician's judgment whenever the treatment of a newborn would only afford a life with the most severe, non-remediable deficiencies, e.g., the most severe brain damage or Potter-syndrome [bilateral renal agenesis], with which the duty to treat does not already cease under V.

When determining whether to initiate or discontinue treatment, the physician should be guided by the duty to treat as it pertains to adults with similar probable outcomes.

2. The same holds true with multiple defects, which in their aggregate are just as severe as those individual defects in 1.

A conclusive enumeration of all conceivable case descriptions and their legal evaluation is not possible.

3. The need for the consent of the parents/guardian remains unaffected by these considerations.

VII

The fact that the newborn would have life with disabilities, e.g., caudal dysplasia, mongoloidism, which do not conform to the levels of impairment listed above, does not justify omitting or terminating life-sustaining treatment.

VIII

1. Even if a duty to employ life-sustaining treatment does not exist, the physician must maintain basic care of the newborn.
2. Interventions to mitigate the defects must be carried out, if they are in due proportion to the expected decrease in suffering.

IX

1. The parents/guardian are to be informed about the newborn's affliction and the possibilities for treatment.
They should be included in the decision process from the beginning through the provision of counseling and information.
2. The rights and duties of the parents/guardian to approve of the medical intervention depend on judicial determination.
This means: If the parents/guardian refuse to agree to medically advised treatment, or if they cannot agree, then the court dealing with guardianship [Vormundschaftsgericht] must make the decision. If this is not possible, the physician may carry out urgently indicated medical treatment (emergency measures).

X

The above-mentioned findings, the measures adopted, as well as the bases for refusal of life-sustaining treatment, should be documented in an explicit and conclusive form.

E. DEUTSCH, A. DOENICKE, H. EWERBECK, A. G. BAUMANN, J. GRUENDEL, H.-D. HIERSCHE, G. HIRSCH, A. HOLSCHNEIDER, B. JAEHNKE, E. G. LOCH, V. VON LOEWENICH, U. SCHLAUDRAFF, E. SEIDLER, W. SPANN, H. STEINBERGER, K. ULSENHEIMER, W. WEISSAUER, I. ZANDER.
Translated by S. G. M. ENGELHARDT.

BIBLIOGRAPHY

1. Boeckle, F.: 1982, 'Grundlagen ärztlicher Ethik', in *Ethische Probleme in der Medizin*, ed. H. Olbing and H. Mueller, Urban & Schwarzenbach, München, pp. 19–28.
2. Brodehl, J.: 1982, 'Grenzen der konservativen Therapie bei Kindern mit infauster Prognose', in *Ethische Probleme in der Paediatrie*, ed. H. Olbing and H. Mueller, Urban & Schwarzenbach, München, pp. 210–224.
3. Department of Health and Human Services: 1985, 'Child Abuse and Neglect Prevention; Model Guidelines . . . to Establish Infant Care', *Federal Register* 50, 72 (April 15), 14878–14901.
4. Deutsche Gesellschaft für Medizinrecht: 1986, 'Grenzen der ärztlichen Behandlungspflicht bei schwerstgeschädigten Neugeborenen', *Medizinrecht* 4, 281–282.
5. Engelhardt, H. T., Jr.: 1986, *The Foundations of Bioethics*, Oxford University Press, New York.
6. von Loewenich, V.: 1982, 'Grenzen der neonatalen Intensivbehandlung', in *Ethische Probleme der Paediatrie*, ed. H. Olbing and H. Mueller, Urban & Schwarzenbach, München, pp. 194–204.
7. Schara, J.: 1975, 'Die Grenze der Behandlungspflicht in der Intensivmedizin', *Münchner Medizinische Wochenschrift* 36, 117.
8. Weir, R. F.: 1984, *Selective Non-Treatment of Handicapped Newborns*, Oxford University Press, New York.

INDEX

NOTES ON CONTRIBUTORS

Darrel W. Amundsen, Ph.D., is Professor of Classics, Department of Foreign Languages and Literatures, Western Washington University, Bellingham, Washington.

Richard B. Brandt, Ph.D., is Professor of Philosophy, Department of Philosophy, The University of Michigan, Ann Arbor, Michigan.

Alexander G. M. Campbell, M. B., F.R.C.P. (Edin.), is Professor of Child Health, University of Aberdeen, Aberdeen, Scotland.

Raymond S. Duff, M.D., is Professor of Pediatrics, Yale University School of Medicine, New Haven, Connecticut.

H. Tristram Engelhardt, Jr., Ph.D., M.D., is Professor, Departments of Medicine and Community Medicine, and Member, Center for Ethics, Medicine, and Public Issues, Baylor College of Medicine, Adjunct Research Fellow, Institute of Religion, and Professor of Philosophy (Part-Time), Rice University, Houston, Texas.

Gary B. Ferngren, Ph.D., is Associate Professor of History, Department of History, Oregon State University, Corvallis, Oregon.

John M. Freeman, M.D., is Professor, Neurology and Pediatrics, Johns Hopkins University School of M[...] Baltimore, Maryland.

Mary Ann Gardel[...] [...]losophy, Baylor College [...]

Nancy M. P. King[...] [...]e Medicine, The Unive[...]

Marvin Kohl, Ph[...] [...]y, State University of N[...]

Richard C. McMi[...] [...], Mercer University Scho[...]

Hans–Martin Sass[...] [...]Institute of Ethics, Geor[...] [...] Philosophie, Ruhr–Un[...]

Margery W. Sha[...] [...]ofessor of Medical Genet[...] [...]as.

Earl E. Shelp, Ph[...] [...]Religion, and Assistant [...] [...]Medicine, Baylor College[...]

John C. Sinclair[...] [...]Hamilton, Ontario, Cana[...]

Stuart F. Spicke[...] [...]Medicine, Department o[...] [...]University of Connecticu[...]

Kenneth L. Vaux, Dr. Theol., is Associate Professor of Ethics, [...] of Internal Medicine, School of Medicine, University of Illinois, Chicago, Illinois.

313